Hereditary Retinal and Choroidal Diseases

Volume I. Evaluation

Hereditary Retinal and Choroidal Diseases

Volume I.   Evaluation

Alex E. Krill, M.D.*

Professor of Ophthalmology
Pritzker School of Medicine
University of Chicago
Chicago, Illinois
*Deceased

HARPER & ROW, PUBLISHERS

HAGERSTOWN

Cambridge		London
New York		Mexico City
Philadelphia		Sao Paolo
San Francisco		Sydney

1817

Hereditary Retinal and Choroidal Diseases: Volume I. Evaluation. Copyright © 1972 by Harper & Row, Publishers, Inc.

First edition

Standard Book Number: 06–141490–5

Library of Congress Catalog Card Number: 72–82–836

*Dedicated to
Suzanne and Eileen*

Contents

Preface

Our knowledge of hereditary diseases of the eyegrounds has increased leaps and bounds within the past decade. In large part this is due to the clinical utilization within this period of several relatively new testing techniques, such as dark adaptation, more sophisticated color vision testing, electroretinography, electrooculography, and fluorescein angiography. It thus behooves the clinician to know something about these methods: what they mean, what they tell us, and particularly, where they can help.

Indeed, a certain amount of knowledge of these techniques is essential in understanding some of the key information on hereditary diseases. Some examples are: A characteristic dark-adaptation profile is seen in early retinitis pigmentosa. Specific color vision findings help identify cone degenerations, total congenital color blindness, and dominant optic atrophy. An abnormal electrooculogram identifies the carrier of vitelliruptive (vitelliform) macular degeneration and perhaps of butterfly-shaped pigment macular dystrophy as well. In X-linked (juvenile) retinoschisis there is usually an abnormality only of the ERG b-wave, whereas in autosomal recessive (Goldmann-Favre) retinoschisis the entire ERG is markedly abnormal. Drusen are easily distinguished from the typical lesions of fundus flavimaculatus on fluorescein angiography.

Therefore, I have devoted a good portion of this first volume to these techniques. The remaining portion deals with the general area of genetics. Volume 2 covers specific hereditary retinal and choroidal diseases.

Since I felt retinal function evaluation, fluorescein angiography, and genetics to be important enough in their own right to warrant a separate volume, my coverage in these areas goes beyond possible relationships to hereditary retinal and choroidal diseases. I have tried to provide a brief basic background on all of the retinal function tests discussed in this volume. Furthermore, the clinical usefulness of these tests is considered in all areas, not just those related to the hereditary diseases discussed in the second volume. Desmond Archer has taken the same approach in his chapter on fluorescein angiography.

Although visual evoked responses are presently of little value in the diagnosis of hereditary retinal and choroidal diseases, we have included a short chapter on this technique, since it may prove to be useful in the future. A short section on electronystagmography is included in the chapter on electrooculography. It explains how this technique can also be used to measure eye movements.

It goes without saying that some knowledge of genetics is necessary for a thorough understanding of any hereditary disease. In view of the many recent advances throughout all areas of genetics, I have provided a review which covers a broad spectrum of subjects, including most of the subdivisions of genetics which relate in some way to clinical medicine.

Acknowledgments

I have had the good fortune to work with some very knowledge-able people who are experts in areas covered in this work. Their influences have made these two volumes possible. Bertha Klien and Harold Falls stimulated my interest in the fundus. Bertha Klien and I have had many long discussions on retinal disease, usually to my benefit. Mathew Alpern helped me acquire some knowledge of retinal physiology. Most important of all, he made me develop a more critical attitude towards clinical retinal function testing. For the last five years I have had the pleasure of working on several projects with Joel and Vivianne Porkorny, both Doctors of Psychology. They have helped me particularly in the area of color vision.

I have worked with three superb retinal fellows since 1965. In their process of learning, Muhammad Chishti, Desmond Archer, and August Deutman have taught me much and I express my gratitude. Desmond Archer has contributed a chapter to each volume and August Deutman has contributed two chapters in the second volume.

I must pay tribute to the intellectually stimulating environment at the University of Chicago which allowed me to carry out such a project. For this I give credit to my fellow staff members, particularly to Frank W. Newell, Chairman of the Department, who has helped in countless ways during my years at the University.

Several people, not acknowledged in the text, assisted in various ways in the preparation of the first volume. Dr. Janet Rowley and Judith Mikuta furnished several of the photographs used in Chapter 1, particularly those of the abnormal karyotypes. Yvonne Mangnall provided the electron micrographs used in Chapter 2. Marlene Fishman, Miriam Creeden, and my wife, Suzanne, assisted in proofreading. Peach Coke and Donna Lenhoff typed the manuscript.

Hereditary Retinal and Choroidal Diseases

Volume I. Evaluation

1

Principles of Genetics

In the past 20 years great strides have been made in genetics. In this chapter the basic material necessary for an understanding of the subject will be covered, with the emphasis on some of the more important concepts that have evolved, particularly in relation to human genetics. The diverse material in this area is organized under major subdivisions, and appropriate references are given. In addition, a list of general textbooks [1-7] is included at the beginning of the reference section.

MOLECULAR GENETICS

In the nucleus of each cell is a substance called chromatin. As reproductive activity begins and a cell starts to divide, the chromatin takes the form of threadlike bodies called chromosomes. The chromosomes carry the hereditary pattern in the form of genes. Genes vary in size, according to the species of organism, from about 0.00001 to 0.0001 mm. The number also varies, but there are several thousand genes in every cell.

DNA

Classically, the gene is the basic unit of inheritance. Biochemically the basic genetic material is deoxyribonucleic acid (DNA) found primarily in the cell nucleus in the chromosomes.* DNA carries the blueprint for the organism and is the storehouse of genetic information. In a given species the amount of DNA in all somatic cells is the same, and the germ cells (sperm or ova), which contain half the number of chromosomes, contain half the amount of DNA. This substance is a chain of deoxyribose (a five-carbon sugar) molecules, linked by phosphate, each carrying a single nitrogenous base (Fig. 1-1). The nitrogenous base is a purine (adenine or guanine) or one of the pyrimidines (thymine or cytosine). A sugar-phosphate unit, together with a nitrogenous base, is called a nucleotide.

There are four kinds of nucleotides, since there are four kinds of bases. It has been estimated that in a single human cell there are 5 billion nucleotide pairs, or enough information to make 1.7 billion letters or 340 million words averaging 5 letters. This would provide 1,000 volumes of 500 words per page, 600 pages per volume, or 9 times the entire content of the *Encyclopaedia Britannica*—yet the DNA of the ova resulting in the entire earth's population would fit into a $\frac{1}{8}$-inch cube.

GENETIC CODE

Electron microscopic and x-ray diffraction patterns have revealed that the complete genetic unit consists of two DNA chains, wound into entwined, counterrotating helices, held together by hydrogen bonds between the nitrogenous bases (Fig. 1-1). Each base is so shaped that it can form a hydrogen bond with only one of the other three types of bases: adenine always pairs with thymine, guanine with cytosine.

This structure can also be likened to a spiral staircase in which the sides of the staircase consist of alternating phosphate and deoxyribose, and the steps are the paired nitrogenous bases.

According to this model, the code that passes on genetic information (the gene) consists of two symbols, adenine-thymine (AT) and guanine-cytosine (GC), repeated with varying frequencies along the DNA molecule in a sort of biological Morse code.

Cellular reactions are controlled by enzymes. Enzymes are made of proteins based on various combinations of 20 different amino acids.

---

* It has been recently discovered that DNA occurs in the mitochondria of the cytoplasm as well.[8] This DNA may also have a genetic role.

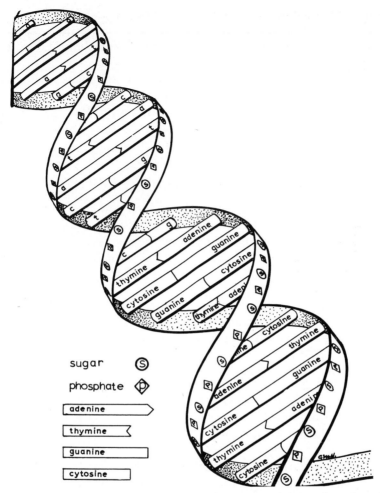

sugar   Ⓢ

phosphate   Ⓟ

| adenine |⇒

| thymine |◁

| guanine |

| cytosine |

FIG. 1-1. *Diagrammatic representation of a DNA molecule. The sides of the molecule are twisted to form two long chains consisting of alternating phosphate and deoxyribose molecules, in the shape of a spiral staircase. Each "stair" of the spiral staircase consists of paired nitrogenous bases, which always occur in specific combinations; adenine pairs only with thymine and guanine with cytosine.*

The sequence of the 4 bases in DNA spells out instructions for particular amino acids. This sequence is the key to the genetic code. Since there are 20 different amino acids and only 4 different kinds of nucleotides in DNA, the nucleotides must work in groups of 3, called codons, to represent a given amino acid.

The genetic code has been compared to a four-letter "alphabet" (the four bases) from which three-letter "words" (sequences of three bases) are spelled out. Each three-base sequence (triplet) codes for one amino acid. A series of triplets specifies the order in which amino acids are arranged in a polypeptide chain.

A modern concept of the gene is that it is a sequence of triplets that contains the code for one polypeptide. The polypeptide may be a complete protein (e.g., pancreatic ribonuclease) and, in this case, the gene codes for a protein. However, usually several polypeptides must come together to form a protein (e.g., hemoglobin).

RNA

Protein synthesis actually occurs in the cytoplasm. Being limited mostly to the nucleus, DNA cannot carry out a cell's reproductive function by itself. It is assisted by other nucleic acids, called ribonucleic acids. Ribonucleic acid (RNA) can pass from the nucleus, where the "plan" is picked up, out into the cytoplasm, where the protein is actually put together.

RNA differs from DNA in that it is single-stranded rather than double-stranded, contains the sugar ribose instead of the sugar deoxyribose, and contains uracil instead of thymine as one of the four nitrogenous bases (the other three are the same). Three kinds of RNA take part in protein synthesis: messenger RNA, transfer RNA, and ribosomal RNA. Messenger RNA transmits the genetic information from the DNA molecule to the cytoplasm; transfer RNA brings amino acids into the site of protein synthesis, the ribosome, and ribosomal RNA functions in connection with the ribosome in some manner that is not fully understood as yet.

The interested reader is referred to the recommended textbooks [1-7] and particularly several references [8-11] for more details.

CYTOGENETICS

This area has progressed considerably during the past 15 years.[1-7, 13, 19, 27] The advances are a reflection of prior technical developments in the evaluation of chromosomal morphology. These technical advances include primarily the following:

1. The improvement of cell culture techniques. Culturing of cells dates back to the turn of the century; however, it did not become a fairly simple laboratory technique until the discovery of antibiotics, which eliminated the requirement for extremely rigorous asepsis.

2. The discovery that colchicine arrests cells in mitosis during meta-

phase, at the time when they are ready for separation and are most easily visible.

3. The discovery that hypotonic saline causes cells to swell and spread, making examination of cellular contents much simpler.
4. The discovery that phytohemagglutinin, which had been employed for years to separate white from red cells in blood samples, stimulates mitosis in peripheral blood leukocytes, making possible chromosome preparations from peripheral blood. Previously, tissue biopsies were required for this purpose.

The first breakthrough was the discovery in 1956 that the human cell has 46 instead of 48 chromosomes.[28] Since then, several discoveries have been made, but particularly important to clinical genetics are the characteristic conditions caused by specific chromosomal abnormalities, which will be discussed in a later section, *Chromosomal Aberrations*.

TECHNIQUE FOR CHROMOSOMAL STUDY

A small sample of heparinized blood is obtained. (A skin biopsy may also be taken if mosaicism, to be discussed later, is considered a possibility.) Phytohemagglutinin is added to clump the red cells and stimulate division of the leukocytes. The red cells are removed and the white cells placed in a culture medium. Further developments now make it unnecessary to separate the leukocytes, and only a few drops of whole blood are required.

In two or three days the leukocytes begin dividing. When division is profuse, colchicine is added to arrest the process. A hypotonic saline solution is added to swell the cells and separate the chromosomes, which are then further separated by air-drying the cells as they are mounted on a slide. After staining, the separated chromosomes can be easily examined and photographed.

CHROMOSOMAL ANATOMY

The next step is classification of the chromosomes. A photograph at an enlargement of 3,000 or 4,000 is cut apart so that each of the 46 chromosomes can be paired with its identical member (homologue). In the enlarged photograph each chromosome appears to be split lengthwise into two segments called chromatids and joined at a sharply constricted region called the centromere (kinetochore) (Fig. 1-2). The chromosomes are paired and classified into groups according to their length

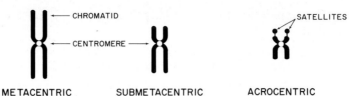

METACENTRIC   SUBMETACENTRIC   ACROCENTRIC

FIG. 1-2. *Diagrammatic representation of three types of human chromosomes seen during the metaphase stage of mitosis. Note that each chromosome is split lengthwise, except at a sharply constricted region called the centromere, into two segments designated as chromatids. The chromosomes with a centromere midway between the ends are called metacentric. Those with the centromere a little off center are called submetacentric. And those with this structure near one of the ends of the chromosome are called acrocentric; note the small heterochromatic bodies connected with the ends of the chromosomes by a thin filamentous stalk (arrow). These latter bodies are called satellites. (From Thompson, J. S., and Thompson, M. W.* Genetics in Medicine. *Philadelphia, W. B. Saunders Co., 1966.)*

and the location of the centromere, which may be found midway between the ends of the chromosome (metacentric), a little off center (submetacentric), or near one of the ends (acrocentric). In addition, the presence of satellites (small heterochromatic bodies connected with chromosomes by a thin filamentous stalk) and secondary constrictions are sometimes used for classification.

Denver Classification

A microphotograph of the chromosomes cut out and arranged according to the various structural features used for classification is called a karyotype (Fig. 1-3). The Denver classification, in almost universal use until recently,* was adopted in 1960 at a meeting in Denver. It is impossible to distinguish each of the 23 pairs, but they can easily be categorized into seven groups identified by the letters A through G in order of decreasing length and position of chromatid (Fig. 1-3). Only chromosome pairs Nos. 1, 2, 3, 16, 17, and 18 are distinguished by routine methods.

Audioradiography and Fluorescein and Giemsa Staining

Audioradiographic characteristics after labeling with ^{3}H-thymidine may also aid in identifying certain chromosome pairs.[18] These

---

* A newer classification, called the Chicago classification, is rapidly gaining in popularity.

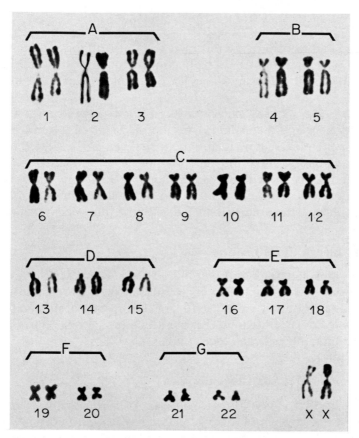

FIG. 1-3. A microphotograph of the chromosomes cut out and arranged primarily according to length of each chromosome and position of centromere. This is called a karyotype. The arrangement into seven groups identified by the letters **A** through **G** is according to the "Denver classification." Note the two similar chromosomes at the end of the bottom row which are called X chromosomes and which identify this subject as a female. The X chromosomes are sometimes placed in the **C** group before pair No. 6, which they resemble in structure.

include Nos. 4, 5, 13, 14, 15, occasionally Nos. 21 and 22, and all X chromosomes in excess of one. Recently fluorescent materials, quinacrine mustard or quinacrine dihydrochloride have been used to bind chromosomal DNA and presumably give each type of chromosome a characteristic fluorescent band-like pattern that can be identified by photoelectric sensors.[17, 25] This technique, which requires less than an hour for analysis of chromosomes in interphase cells and about 72 hours for dividing cells, has been useful in identifying the Y chromosome and chromosome pairs, Nos. 6 through 12 and 21 and 22.[24a, 25] In contrast, autoradiography may take weeks. Furthermore, autoradiography may not always be a reliable method of identifying chromosomes because of asynchronous DNA replication, which creates different or similar patterns at different stages in different or identical chromosomes.[14, 26]

The fluorescein staining technique has a few disadvantages: the stain is not permanent and a special microscope is required to examine the fluorescent material. A new technique utilizing a Giemsa stain offsets these disadvantages, since the stained material is permanent and can be examined with an ordinary microscope.[16a] Furthermore, a similar banding pattern is produced which allows identification of the same additional chromosome pairs detected with the fluorescein technique.

The Chicago Classification

Two other meetings, in London in 1963 and in Chicago in 1966, were held on the nomenclature of chromosomes. This resulted in the Chicago classification, a more useful, flexible system of nomenclature than the Denver classification. This classification will be referred to in the section on chromosomal aberrations.

Autosomal and Sex Chromosomes

As indicated, every human cell has 46 chromosomes with the exception of the sperm and the ova, which have 23 chromosomes each. Forty-four of the 46 chromosomes are called autosomes and can be grouped into 22 pairs of identical partners (Fig. 1-3). Each pair, though, is different in genetic content and frequently in appearance from other pairs. All pairs, except one, are the same in males and females. The pair of chromosomes that is not identical in the two sexes was named the sex chromosomes by Wilson[29] in 1909. This unique pair consists of two similar chromosomes in women called X chromosomes (Fig. 1-3) and two dissimilar chromosomes in males (Fig. 1-4). One male sex chromosome resembles the two female X chromosomes and is therefore also called an X chromosome; the second is unique and is called the Y chromosome. The Y chromosome, in some unknown manner,[21] is very strongly male-determining; the development of testes and some secondary sex characteristics are dependent on the Y chromosome.[20, 23]

Female Sex Chromosomes

The two X chromosomes of a female, although similar in length and position of centromere, show a number of differences. During the

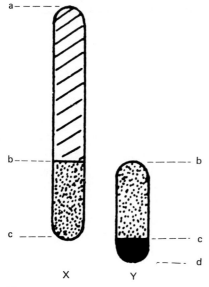

FIG. 1-4. *Diagrammatic representation of the X and Y chromosomes. The Y chromosome is considerably shorter than the X chromosome. Segment* **ab** *of the X chromosome carries all of the known X-linked genes. Segments* **bc** *on the X and Y chromosomes are similar in morphological appearance and are said to be homologous. On the other hand, segments* **ab** *of the X chromosome and* **cd** *of the Y chromosome are entirely different in size and morphological appearance. It is only in segment* **bc** *that interchange of material between the two chromosomes can occur.*

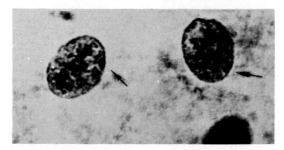

FIG. 1-5. *The arrows point to the Barr body, a small very intensely staining structure at the periphery of the nucleus as shown above and present in close to 40 percent of the cells from a buccal mucosa smear of a female.*

prophase of cellular division, one of the two X chromosomes is more heavily condensed, takes a darker stain, and is said to be heterochromatic.[23, 24] This heterochromatic chromosome has a later DNA replication pattern.[22] This same chromosome is frequently seen in the resting phase (interphase) of somatic cells as a small, very intensely staining body, most commonly situated at the periphery of the nucleus, just inside the nuclear membrane and called the Barr sex-chromatin body or the Barr body (Fig. 1-5). This peculiarly staining body, first identified by Barr and Bertram [12] in cat nerve cells, has been identified in most mammalian somatic cells. In humans it is usually searched for in buccal mucosa smears and normally is seen in close to 40 percent of such cells from a female. The appearance is similar in most cells except in polymorphonuclear leukocytes, where it appears as a darkly staining lobule attached to the nucleus by a stalk, and is called a drumstick [16] (Fig. 1-6). The distinctive morphology of the Barr body in these cells is a reflection of the peculiar shape of the nuclei of the polymorphonuclear leukocytes.

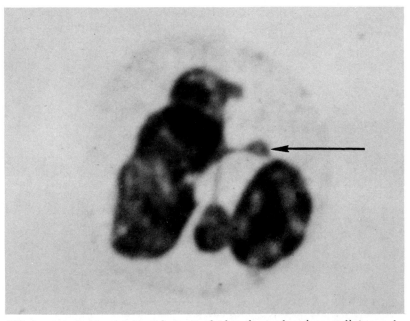

FIG. 1-6. *A darkly staining lobule attached to the nucleus by a stalk in a polymorphonuclear leukocyte is called a drumstick (arrow). The structure is seen in females and represents the appearance of the Barr body in a polymorphonuclear leukocyte.*

Male Sex Chromosomes

The two male sex chromosomes differ considerably in length, with the Y chromosome being much shorter (Fig. 1-4). These chromosomes have homologous segments which are similar in morphological appearance and nonhomologous segments which are dissimilar. The nonhomologous segment of the X chromosome is considerably larger. It is only in the homologous sections of the X and Y chromosomes that interchange and crossing-over of genetic material can occur. The Y chromosome can now usually also be identified with a buccal smear using the fluorescein dye assay test alluded to previously.[17, 25]

It should be emphasized that variability in human chromosomal morphology is common. From family to family there is a prominent variability in length of the human Y chromosome; [15] Japanese and Jews are said to have very long Y chromosomes. In some families the long arm of the No. 16 pair is elongated, and in others one arm of the No. 1 pair is attenuated. Variability in the mass of the short arms or satellites of acrocentric chromosomes is commonly encountered. Several other variations have been reported. More investigations on normal variability, including age and other factors, are needed.

Diploid and Haploid Numbers

In each somatic cell of a human there are 23 pairs of chromosomes, one member of each pair from each parent, so that the number of chromosomes is said to be a diploid or doubled number. A cell that is not actively dividing is said to be in interphase. The chromosomes are not individually distinguishable at this time. There are two types of divisions a cell may undergo. One type of cell division, mitosis, retains the same chromosomal number as the parent cell. The other type of cell division, meiosis, occurs in the sex cells (ovum and sperm) and results in a halving of the total number of chromosomes. The number of chromosomes in the sex cells is said to be a haploid number.

MITOSIS

Mitosis is the type of cell division by which the body grows and replaces discarded cells. The cytoplasm divides by simply cleaving in half, but the nucleus undergoes a complicated series of activities which result in transmission to the daughter cells of precisely the same chromosomal complement as that of the parent cell. Four stages of mitosis are distinguished: prophase, metaphase, anaphase, and telophase.

During prophase the chromosomes first become visible. The chromosomes have doubled and consist of two chromatids held together at a nonstaining spot, the centromere (Fig. 1-7A). During this phase two structures appear, each of which contains a centriole with an aster and a group of filaments called the spindle. By the end of this phase the nuclear membrane and nucleoli have disappeared.

Metaphase begins when the chromosomes line up at the equatorial plane of the cell, essentially at the equator of the developing spindle. The chromosomes are connected at their centromeres with the spindle (Fig. 1-7B). Longitudinal splitting through the centromere occurs, dividing the chromatids.

During anaphase the divided chromatids move apart and travel toward the poles of the cell as if drawn by the spindle (Fig. 1-7C).

When the chromosomes arrive at the poles of the cell, telophase begins (Fig. 1-7D). The division of the cytoplasm (cytokinesis) now also occurs. Eventually, a complete membrane is formed across the cell, and the nucleoli and nuclear membranes reappear. Two new cells are thus formed. The chromosomes unwind, become less densely stained, and eventually can no longer be identified.

MEIOSIS

Meiosis is the special type of cell division occurring in sex cells, or gametes. In meiosis, the homologous pairs of chromosomes of the dividing gamete sort themselves out, and each chromosome of a pair lies close to its partner. This process is called synapsis. The cell then divides into two parts, with each chromosome of a pair going to a separate part. Each new cell, therefore, receives half the number of chromosomes of the parent cell, the haploid number. If it were not for this reduction division, the chromosomes in each cell would double in number with each successive generation. Actually, there are two stages to meiosis, resulting in four new haploid cells from each parent cell. Meiosis will be discussed in greater detail under the heading *Other Properties of Genes*.

The union of male and female gametes at fertilization is called sexual recombination. The union results in a fertilized egg, called a zygote, which has the combined number of chromosomes of both gametes. The zygote, therefore, has the same diploid number as a somatic cell. The zygote develops into a new organism, producing somatic cells by normal mitotic cell division.

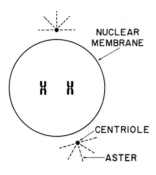

NUCLEAR
MEMBRANE

CENTRIOLE

ASTER

A. PROPHASE

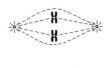

B. METAPHASE

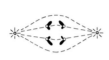

C. ANAPHASE

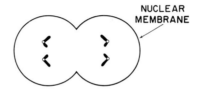

NUCLEAR
MEMBRANE

D. TELOPHASE

FIG. 1-7. *The four stages of mitosis, the somatic cell division, which results in the formation of two cells, each with the same chromosome complement as the parent cell. During prophase (Fig. 1-7A) the chromosomes have doubled and are seen to consist of two chromatids held together at a nonstaining spot, the centromere. During this phase, two structures appear, each of which contains a centriole with an aster and a group of filaments called the spindle. By the end of this phase, the nuclear membrane and the nucleoli have disappeared.*

During metaphase (Fig. 1-7B) the chromosomes line up at the equatorial plane of the cell, which is at the equator of the developing spindle. The chromosomes are connected at their centromeres with the spindle. Longitudinal splitting occurs during this phase through the centromere dividing the chromatids.

During anaphase (Fig. 1-7C) the divided chromatids move apart and travel toward the two poles of the cell along the spindle.

The telophase (Fig. 1-7D) begins when the chromatids arrive at the poles of the cell. Division of the cytoplasm (cytokinesis) now occurs, and a complete membrane is formed across each cell with eventual reappearance of the nucleoli and nuclear membranes forming two completely new cells.

INHERITANCE

A "familial" condition is one that occurs in more than one member of a family, but this does not mean it is inherited. "Genetic" conditions are presumably inherited, and the concept of the gene in relation to inheritance will be developed in this section. "Genetic," used in this sense, and "inborn" are synonymous. A congenital condition is manifest at birth but is not necessarily inherited. An embryopathy is an abnormality developed during embryogenesis and induced by in-utero environmental agents, either physical, chemical, or toxic.

Some diseases are inherited in a number of different ways (e.g., retinitis pigmentosa). In general, such diseases are most severe in the autosomal recessive form and least severe in the autosomal dominant form, and intermediate in the X-linked recessive form.

ALLELES

Genes occupying the same position on each chromosome of an identical pair are called alleles. An individual carrying alleles for the same trait (for example, two genes for blue eyes) is said to be a homozygote for that trait (Table 1-1). Anyone carrying alleles for different traits (for example, one gene for blue eyes and one gene for brown eyes) is said to be a heterozygote for either trait. Usually, there are only a single pair of alleles possible at two loci on homologous chromosomes. When there are more than two alternative alleles possible at any one locus, the alleles are called multiple alleles. A common example of multiple allelism is provided by the series of alleles that determine the ABO blood groups. The alleles are designated as O, A^1, A^2, and B. At the locus for one type of color blindness the possible alleles are genes for protanomaly, extreme protanomaly (according to some workers), protanopia, and normal color vision.

A hemizygote is a male carrying a gene on the X chromosome. Since he only has one X chromosome, he has no opposing normal gene.

Genotype, Phenotype, Phenocopy

Genotype refers to the genetic makeup of an individual (for example, the alleles present at a locus). Phenotype refers to the actual physical, physiological, and biochemical characteristics of the individual which are determined by his or her genotype. Obviously, the phenotype can be modified by the environment of the individual. On the other hand, a clinical picture in an individual produced entirely

TABLE 1-1

Designation	Number of Alleles for Trait	Number of Opposing or Normal Alleles
Heterozygote	1	1
Homozygote	2	0
Hemizygote	1	0

by an environmental factor, but nevertheless closely resembling, or even identical with, a phenotype (which is determined primarily by the individual's genotype) is known as a phenocopy.

Dominant and Recessive

An allele that is always expressed in the phenotype, whether homozygous or heterozygous, is dominant; an allele that is expressed only when homozygous is recessive. It is the trait (phenotypic expression of a gene) rather than the gene itself that is dominant or recessive, but the terms "dominant gene" and "recessive gene" are in common use. In general, dominant traits are determined by basic structural defects (e.g., cell membrane), whereas recessive traits are determined by enzymatic defects.

In general, then, the patterns followed by simple inherited genetic traits within families are determined by whether the trait is dominant or recessive, by whether the gene is autosomal (on an autosome) or sex-linked (on a sex chromosome), and by the chance distribution of the gene from parents to children through the gametes. These patterns can be altered or obscured by various factors, such as heterogeneity, pleiotropy, reduced penetrance, variable expressivity, variability of onset age, sex limitation (either complete or partial), interaction of two or more gene pairs, and environmental effects.

PEDIGREE ANALYSIS

Family data can be summarized in a pedigree chart, which is merely a shorthand method of classifying the data for ready reference. The affected individual who first brings a family to the attention of the physician is the propositus (proband or index case) and is indicated

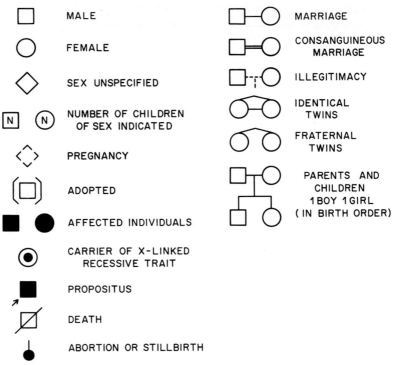

FIG. 1-8. *Commonly used symbols for pedigree analysis.*

by an arrow; most of the other commonly used symbols are shown in Figure 1-8.

In general, if there is only one affected individual in a family, and if there is no history of consanguinity among the parents, then the physician must be very cautious in the information he gives to a family.

AUTOSOMAL DOMINANT INHERITANCE

Autosomal dominant inheritance is associated with a number of specific terms, which are described below:

Regular dominance—Gene always manifest in single dose

Irregular dominance—Gene not always manifest in single dose

Expressivity—The extent to which a gene shows effect

Penetrance—Frequency of expression of a genotype

Skipped generation—Individual with normal phenotype in spite of abnormal genotype

Pleitropic gene—Gene with multiple effects

Formes frustes—Attenuated form of a disease or syndrome

Autosomal dominant diseases which always show full expression with only one defective gene show regular dominance, and those with variable expression show irregular dominance. An abnormal gene that does not always produce the full expression of the disease is said to manifest variable expressivity. A gene that is pleiotropic (responsible for numerous clinical abnormalities) is frequently characterized by variable expressivity. A dominant disease determined by such a gene may be present in an abortive form or *formes frustes*. Occasionally, a gene that ordinarily produces an autosomal dominant disease will have no effect at all in some individuals. The gene is said to show lack of penetrance in such individuals, who represent a skipped generation. The penetrance of an abnormal gene in a given pedigree can be calculated and expressed as a percentage. In families where the gene has 100 percent penetrance (regular dominance) 50 percent of the offspring of affected members, on the average, will show the same disease. There is no predilection for either sex. A conclusive demonstration of autosomal dominant inheritance requires that the disease occur in three successive generations in both sexes. The precise criteria for autosomal dominant inheritance, assuming 100 percent penetrance of the gene and full or close to full expression, are summarized as follows:

1. The trait appears in every generation.
2. The trait is transmitted by an affected person to 50 percent of offspring (on the average).
3. Unaffected persons do not transmit trait to their children.
4. There is an equal sex incidence.

The risk of siblings of an affected individual having the same disease are shown in Table 1-2.

TABLE 1-2
Risk of Recurrence in Siblings

Example	Risk (%)
Both parents with same recessive disease	100
Autosomal dominance, regular	50
Autosomal dominance, irregular	25 (variable)
Autosomal recessive	25
Congenital malformation of unknown cause	5 or less

AUTOSOMAL RECESSIVE INHERITANCE

An autosomal recessive disease does not show full expression unless two defective genes are present. A carrier of one defective gene, the heterozygote, may show minimal evidence of the gene, particularly at the biochemical level. Genes for autosomal recessive, as well as autosomal dominant, diseases may be pleiotropic. Variability in the phenotype of the homozygote is not unusual in such conditions (for example, Wilson's disease). The incidence of autosomal recessive diseases is higher among the offspring of related (consanguineous) parents, since they have a greater frequency of similar genes than two unrelated parents. On the average, one out of four offspring of two parents with the same gene for an autosomal recessive disease will be affected (homozygote), two will be carriers (heterozygotes), and one will be normal. All offspring of an affected individual will be carriers. If an affected individual marries a carrier, then 50 percent of the offspring will be affected and 50 percent will be carriers. There is no predilection for either sex. The specific criteria for autosomal recessive inheritance are summarized as follows:

1. The trait appears only in siblings, not in their parents, offspring, or other relatives.
2. Parents of affected child may be related.
3. There is an equal sex incidence.
4. One fourth of siblings of propositus, on the average, are affected.

The chances of siblings having the same disease are shown in Table 1-2.

A carrier of a recessive gene can have affected children only if his or her spouse is also a carrier. By definition, a recessive gene produces no clinically significant disease, but nevertheless its presence may be detected by appropriate means of study, particularly at the biochemical level (for example, carriers of Tay-Sachs disease, cystic fibrosis, galactosemia, and phenylketonuria [7, 33, 36]). Occasionally, a heterozygote for an autosomal recessive disease may show minimal clinical findings. For example, the heterozygote for cystinuria may develop renal calculi, and the heterozygote for sickle-cell hemoglobin may develop a retinopathy. Carrier identification is useful in genetic counseling, since the relatives of an affected individual might want to know if they are carriers, and if so, what the status of their prospective males is.[35, 36, 38]

Certain rare traits may show up in fairly high frequency in isolated populations where intermarriage is common.[31, 34] Furthermore, "new" diseases may come to light in such populations (for example, in the

Amish [34]). Certain recessive conditions may occur fairly frequently because of the high frequency of the gene in the population. Such conditions may at times even mimic dominant traits (pseudodominance).

SEX-LINKED INHERITANCE

A trait determined by genes carried on any of the sex chromosomes is called sex-linked. Traits determined by genes carried on the homologous segment of the male X chromosome are called partially sex-linked. However, no trait or disease has been convincingly traced to a gene supposedly present on this portion of the X chromosome. Traits determined by genes carried on the Y chromosome are called holandric, but only one trait, hairy ears, is thought to reflect a gene on the Y chromosome. [12] All other sex-linked traits or diseases are believed to be due to genes on the nonhomologous segment of the X chromosome. Therefore, since almost all sex-linked traits or diseases are thought to be a result of genes carried on the nonhomologous segment of the X chromosome, sex-linked traits or diseases are commonly referred to as X-chromosomal-linked or X-linked.

A male has only one representative of any X-linked gene, and so is said to be hemizygous for the gene, rather than homozygous or heterozygous. Since there is no normal gene to oppose a defective X-linked gene in the male, its resulting trait or disease, whether dominant or recessive, will always be manifest. On the other hand, a female may be heterozygous for a gene (present on one of the two X chromosomes) or homozygous (the gene is present on both X chromosomes). Since most sex-linked traits or diseases are said to be recessive, two defective genes are usually necessary in the female before the typical condition occurs. If only one defective gene is necessary, then the condition is dominant. Obviously, the terms "dominant" and "recessive" are meaningless in the male.

The distinctive feature of X-linked inheritance, both dominant and recessive, is the absence of father-to-son transmission, since the male X chromosome passes only to daughters. All daughters of an affected male will inherit the defective gene. One half of the sons of females carrying the defective gene and one fourth of the sons of all daughters of carrier females will be affected. If the trait is recessive, no daughters of affected males should be affected, although all will be carriers. If the trait is dominant, all daughters of affected males will be affected and 50 percent of the daughters of an affected female will be affected. The proportion of affected sons of carriers and of carriers' daughters will be the same as with an X-linked recessive condition. Occasionally, an X-linked dominant trait is lethal in the male, so that the affected trait is seen only in females. An excess of affected females in a pedigree should suggest the possibility of X-linked dominant inheritance. The criteria for X-linked recessive inheritance and those for X-linked dominance are as follows:

Criteria for Sex-Linked Recessive Inheritance
1. The incidence of trait is much higher in males.
2. Trait is passed from affected male through all his daughters to half their sons.
3. Trait is never transmitted from father to son.
4. Affected males in a family are brothers or related to one another through carrier females.

Criteria for Sex-Linked Dominant Inheritance
1. Affected males transmit trait to all daughters but none of sons.
2. Affected females transmit trait to half their children of either sex as in autosomal dominant inheritance.
3. Incidence of trait is usually higher in females.

An X-linked trait or disease is manifest in the female when (1) the condition is dominant; (2) the condition is recessive but the female is carrying two defective genes; (3) the condition is recessive and she is carrying only one defective gene, but she has, similar to the male, only one X chromosome (Turner's syndrome); (4) the female is a "manifest" heterozygote. There are many examples of females with two X chromosomes who are carrying only one defective gene for a "recessive" condition, but nevertheless show either partial manifestation or, very rarely, full manifestation of the condition. It is here that the classical notions of "recessive" and "dominant" have required modification in relation to X-linked inheritance. This will be discussed later in more detail in a special section, *The Sex Chromosomes*.

CODOMINANCE AND INTERFERENCE

If both alleles of a pair are fully expressed in the heterozygote, without either allele modifying the other, the genes are said to be codominant. Interference refers to the phenomenon of each allele contributing an effect on the phenotype, but there is modification of each allele by the other.

INTERMEDIATE DOMINANCE

This refers to a condition (for example, thalassemia) where there are always clinical manifestations in the heterozygote state, but these manifestations are more severe in the homozygote state.

SEX-LIMITED AND SEX-INFLUENCED TRAITS

There are many traits, not carried on the sex chromosome, in which the disease is more common or almost solely in one sex. This is not surprising, because the milieu in which any gene acts depends partly upon the sexual constitution. Theoretically, a trait that appears in only one sex is said to be sex-limited; however, there is no proven example of an entirely sex-limited abnormality in man. Sex-linked recessive traits are easily distinguished from sex-limited traits by the *absence* of male-to-male transmission. However, if males do not reproduce, this distinction may be impossible. Testicular feminization, where males do not reproduce, presents such a problem, but the weight of the evidence seems to favor sex limitation rather than sex linkage.

MULTIFACTORIAL (POLYGENIC) INHERITANCE

So far, we have considered only traits in which there is a clear-cut difference between normal and affected individuals. However, there are many other human traits, such as stature, pigmentation of the skin, and intelligence, in which no such distinct difference exists, but in which there is variation over a wide range.[30, 37] Certain diseases, such as diabetes, have this type of variation, with no sharp distinction between normal and abnormal phenotypes, or perhaps with a threshold level beyond which the measurements may be regarded as abnormal. The inheritance in these conditions is termed multifactorial or polygenic. Probably the best example of polygenic inheritance in man is the fingerprint ridge counts.

Traits produced by multiple genes are usually influenced considerably by the environment and are distributed in the population in accordance with the normal curve of probability. Therefore, proof of this type of inheritance is difficult. It is usually entirely indirect and based upon statistical tools that are used to measure phenotypic similarity among relatives and to compare phenotypic variation among relatives with that of the general population. If the trait is determined purely by heredity, the genes concerned are strictly additive in their effects. The theoretical correlations between relatives for the trait should be proportional to the number of genes both have inherited from a common ancestor. However, since multifactorial characteristics may be affected by unpredictable or undetected environmental factors and by segregation (see the next section, *Other Properties of Genes*) at a large number of gene loci, clear-cut phenotypic classes are frequently not evident. Some of the other factors that aid in this difficult diagnosis are outlined elsewhere.[5]

Counseling may be difficult in this type of inheritance. If one offspring has the defect and the parents are normal, the chance of a subsequent child inheriting a similar set of genes and having the same type of malformation is of low magnitude, approximately 5 percent or less for common single defects. The risk figure may be slightly greater if the defect in the affected child is severe and slightly less if the anomaly is mild. The risk of an affected individual having an affected offspring is also about 5 percent, similar to the sibling recurrence risk.

OTHER PROPERTIES OF GENES

MEIOSIS

Some of the properties to be considered here necessitate a more detailed study of meiosis, the type of cell division occurring only in sex cells and during which the chromosome number is halved. There are two meiotic divisions in reality, but it is only during the first meiotic division that the events occur which are unique and of importance for understanding many of the basic genetic properties. The second meiotic division, which resembles an ordinary mitotic division, will not be discussed here. The following features of this first meiotic division are important (Fig. 1-9):

1. Homologous chromosomes pair and lie parallel to each other in point-for-point association (Fig. 1-9A). This pairing does not occur in mitosis.
2. Each chromosome then splits longitudinally, except at its centromere (Fig. 1-9B). Thus, the two homologous chromosomes have formed four chromatids.
3. Actual points of contact, called chiasmata, form between the strands of each chromosome pair (Fig. 1-9C). It is at these sites that genetic interchange, called crossing-over or recombination, can occur; and in this way, new combinations of genes can arise. Remember that

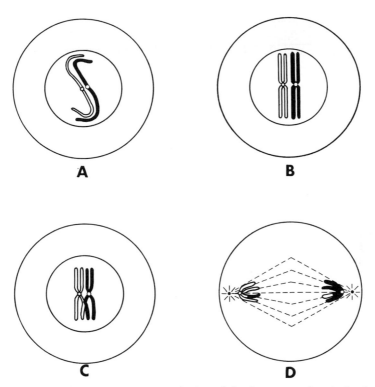

FIG. 1-9. Diagrammatic representation of the first stage of meiosis, the special type of cell division occurring in the gonads resulting in cells (gametes) that contain half the chromosome complement as the parent cells. During this division, homologous chromosomes pair and lie parallel to each other in point-for-point association (Fig. 1-9A). Each chromosome then splits longitudinally, except at its centromere (Fig. 1-9B), forming four chromatids. Actual points of contact, called chiasmata, form between the strands of each chromosome pair (Fig. 1-9C) where crossing-over (genetic interchange) can occur, giving rise to new combinations of genes. The two homologous chromosomes (each consisting of two chromatids) separate, each going to a different pole of the cell (Fig. 1-9D), and each forming a different germ cell or gamete with half the original number of chromosomes and reconstituted chromosomal structure. (From Thompson, J. S., and Thompson, M. W. Genetics in Medicine. Philadelphia, W. B. Saunders Co., 1966.)

the two members of the pair of homologous chromosomes were from the parents of the individual, one being maternal and the other paternal in origin.

4. These genetic exchanges can occur several times along the length of the paired chromosomes.

5. After these interchanges the two homologous members (each consisting of two chromatids) separate, each going to a different pole of

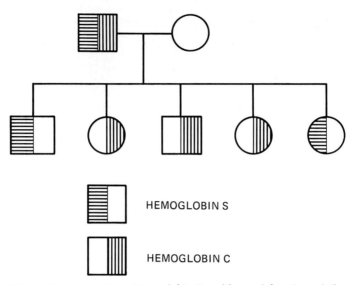

FIG. 1-10. *Segregation. Hemoglobin S and hemoglobin C result from genes that occupy the same genetic loci, and they are therefore called allelic genes. These two genes cannot occur together in an offspring and are said to segregate. A child inherits one or the other type of hemoglobin, as shown above.*

the cell (Fig. 1-9 *D*), and each ultimately forming a different germ cell, or gamete. These chromosomes, received originally as purely maternal and paternal in origin, have each now become mixtures of paternal and maternal chromosomes.

SEGREGATION

Two genes which are alleles — that is, occupy the same genetic locus on two homologous chromosomes — separate with the separation of the two homologous chromosomes during meiosis, and each goes to a different gamete (Fig. 1-10). These two genes are said to segregate, a property of only allelic genes, and they *cannot* occur together in the same offspring. For example, if one parent has hemoglobin S and hemoglobin C, both of which occupy the same genetic locus on homologous chromosomes, none of his or her children inherit both or neither hemoglobin (Fig. 1-10); all inherit one or the other. By definition, these are segregating traits and their genes have to be allelic.

INDEPENDENT ASSORTMENT

On the other hand, genes on homologous chromosomes that are not at identical loci (nonalleles) may or may not separate during meiosis when each "revised" chromosome separates and goes to the opposite pole of the cell. Remember that interchange of chromosomal material occurs during meiosis, so that two genes originally on different chromosomes may end up together on either one of the two chromosomes or remain separated. Thus, with two nonallelic traits there are four possibilities in the offspring (Fig. 1-11). A child may inherit either trait (the genes remained on different chromosomes), both traits, or neither (the genes are now on one chromosome, and the child has inherited either the chromosome that contains neither gene or contains both genes). This scheme of inheritance of nonallelic traits is based on the

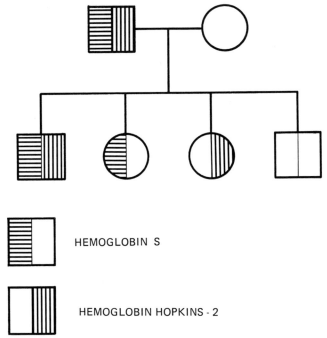

HEMOGLOBIN S

HEMOGLOBIN HOPKINS - 2

FIG. 1-11. *Independent assortment. The two hemoglobins shown reflect genes at different loci. During meiosis, when each revised chromosome separates, there may be interchange of chromosomal material, so that these two genes may end up together on either one of the two homologous chromosomes or be separated (depending on their original positions and the sites of genetic interchange). Thus, with two nonallelic traits, there are four possibilities. A child may inherit either trait, both traits, or neither, depending on whether the genes were originally on the same chromosome or homologous chromosomes and on what occurred during meiosis. The scheme of inheritance of nonallelic traits is based on the principle of independent assortment, which reflects the behavior of the chromosomes at the first meiotic division.*

principle of independent assortment which, obviously, reflects the behavior of the chromosomes at the first meiotic division.

LINKAGE

Nonallelic genes with loci on the same or homologous chromosomes tend to be transmitted together from generation to generation and are said to be linked. Such genes are linked in coupling if they are on the same chromosome, but in repulsion if they are on homologous chromosomes (Fig. 1-12).

The closer together the two genetic loci are, the less likely they are to be affected by crossovers. The concept of linkage is involved in mapping out the positions of genes on chromosomes; such mapping studies have been done principally for the X chromosome.

To understand how linkage is determined, it is necessary to first consider what happens to two dominant traits in an individual that are dependent on two nonallelic genes. There are four possible classes of offspring (Fig. 1-12):

Class 1. Those carrying both genes
Class 2. Those carrying neither gene
Class 3. Those carrying the dominant gene from locus A
Class 4. Those carrying the dominant gene from locus B

With nonallelic genes on nonhomologous chromosomes (or very far apart on the same or homologous chromosomes), the four classes of

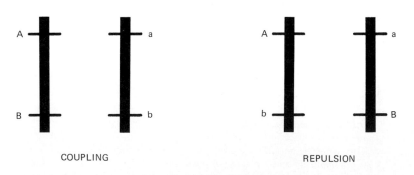

COUPLING　　　　　　　　　　　　　　　REPULSION

A,B = ABNORMAL GENES

FIG. 1-12. Genes that tend to be transmitted together from generation to generation are said to be linked. If two such genes (**A** and **B**) are on the same chromosome, they are said to be linked in coupling, but if they are on homologous chromosomes, they are said to be linked in repulsion.

progeny will occur with equal frequencies (each 25 percent), given a sufficient number of progeny. This represents independent assortment. With linked nonallelic genes there will be significantly more offspring from classes 1 and 2 than from 3 and 4 if the two genes are on the same chromosome, but vice versa if the two genes are on homologous chromosomes. The closer genetic loci are, the less frequently crossover (also called recombination) will occur. The fewer the crossovers, the greater the difference in frequency between classes 1 and 2 compared with classes 3 and 4. With no crossovers, either classes 1 and 2 or classes 3 and 4 (depending on whether the two genes are on the same or homologous chromosomes) will occur in 100 percent of the offspring.

The actual measurement of linkage is provided by the proportion of crossover or recombinant individuals among offspring of informative matings.* In the case of X-linked traits, the phenotype of the sons and the father of double heterozygous females may provide enough information to calculate linkage. In actual practice, data are pooled from many families, and the most recent methods utilize programs on the electronic computer to derive the best estimates of the probability of linkage and the distance between the loci.[38b, 39, 39a, 40] Certain red-cell antigens and enzymes and serum protein serve as marker genes for some of the autosomal chromosomes.[39, 39a] For the X chromosome there are several known genes, in terms of probable position on this chromosome, which are used as markers, such as those that determine partial color blindness, hemophilia, and glucose-6-phosphate dehydrogenase deficiency. In fact, tentative maps of the X chromosome have been published.[38b, 41]

MUTATION

Any change in the structure of a gene is called a mutation, and the changed gene is called a mutant. The mutant is an allele of the old form of the gene. Mutation is sometimes used to describe a change in the number or arrangement of chromosomes, which, of course, will usually result in a permanent hereditable change in the genetic material. However, it is more likely to be used in reference to a single gene (sometimes called a point mutation). In molecular genetic terminology, a mutation results from the miscopying or mispairing of two of the usually complementary base pairs on a DNA molecule, so that a change in base order in a daughter strand results. This change of one base for

* This would be the mating of a person who is doubly heterozygous (one gene at each of two different loci) for two specific dominant traits mated to a person who is homozygous for the recessive gene at each locus. The phenotype of the offspring reveal the genotype of the heterozygous parent.

another at some point in the sequence of the several hundred or thousand bases contained in the DNA of a particular gene may occur more or less at random anywhere along the sequence.

Mutations may occur spontaneously in nature from causes not fully understood. They may also be produced by a variety of agents called mutagens, such as radiation, certain chemicals,[38a] and perhaps viruses.

Some mutations in the gametes are lethal, causing the destruction of the offspring. Others are less harmful or are even beneficial to the new organism and are passed on to the next generation. In time, variations produced by mutation, as well as by chromosomal rearrangement, lead to new species, preserve the fit and eliminate the unfit, and thus carry on the process of evolution.

Mutagens may produce mutations in somatic as well as in germ cells, but these, of course, are not transmitted to future generations. Somatic mutations in humans are difficult to identify and evaluate, but it has been theorized that somatic mutations may account for the inception of some cancers.

THE SEX CHROMOSOMES

According to classical genetic theory, females carrying a gene for a recessive trait or disease on only one X chromosome (heterozygous for the gene) should show no manifestations of the defect. The usual explanation is that the defective gene of one X chromosome is recessive to the normal allele at the same locus on the other X chromosome. However, there are many examples of structural and functional abnormalities in females supposedly heterozygous for recessive traits. For example, such abnormalities, usually mild, but occasionally moderate or severe, have been reported in carriers of choroideremia, X-linked retinitis pigmentosa, ocular albinism, X-linked sutural cataracts, and protan and deutan color defects.[54]

The status of the carrier has been explained by some workers as follows: An X-chromosomal-linked disease is called "recessive" when the female is normal, "intermediate" when the female has mild to moderate abnormalities, and "dominant" when the female has defects almost as severe as those in the involved male. The most obvious problem with this explanation is the intrafamilial variability among carriers. This variability among heterozygotes has been explained by hypothesizing dominant sex-linked inheritance with variable penetrance.

Some of the other semantic explanations noted in the past to explain both the presence of defects and the variability among heterozygotes are (1) varying physiological constitution [67]; (2) differences in exposure to intrauterine or postnatal stress; and (3) effects of another gene,[54, 70] such as "mutual penetrance," "sensitization" or an "expression increasing effect." Sensitization is a particular effect of another pathological gene (for example, a gene for macular degeneration or for esotropia).

LYON INACTIVATION HYPOTHESIS

An entirely new theory for X-linked inheritance was advanced by Lyon [57] in 1961. She proposed that early in embryonic life in each cell of the female, one X chromosome becomes inactive with the other remaining active; the descendants of these cells then have the same active X chromosome as their parent cells. Since the selection is random and either X chromosome may become inactive, the tissues of a female are a mosaic of cell patches, some with maternally derived, others with paternally derived, active X chromosomes. The size of the patches depends on the embryonic stage at which inactivation occurred and hence on the number of cells in the developing tissue at that time. Patch size also depends on the number of all divisions between the time of inactivation and that of observation (Fig. 1-13).

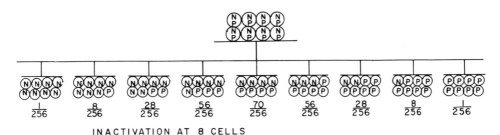

INACTIVATION AT 8 CELLS

N = Female X Chromosome
P = Male X Chromosome

FIG. 1-13. *Theoretic model, based on the binomial theorem, for inactivation at an eight-cell stage of embryogenesis. There is a 1/256 chance of a completely normal female resulting with each cell containing only the female X chromosome and a similar chance of a completely abnormal female resulting with each cell containing the abnormal male X chromosome. Most commonly, as shown, the female should have almost an equal mixture of cells containing the male X chromosome and cells containing the female X chromosome.*

Some possible clinical implications of this hypothesis are as follows:

1. The abnormalities of carriers from different families and even within the same family should vary greatly in degree because of random inactivation.
2. A large sample should have as many severely as mildly affected carriers.
3. In the case of X-linked retinal disease, both normal and abnormal areas would be predictable if a known retinal defect could be mapped in carriers. Or if a test measured a smaller or larger area than the size of a normal or abnormal patch, great variability would be anticipated in the data obtained from area to area (the amount of overlapping would vary from area to area). If inactivation occurs early during embryogenesis, at approximately the same time as the formation of the Barr body, the patches should be fairly large and presumably easily detected.

Supporting Data at a Cellular Level

Impressive data supporting this hypothesis concern genetic effects at a cellular level. There are several diseases in which tissue cultures of skin fibroblasts or lymphocytes from female heterozygotes have been shown to be mixtures of normal cells and cells that are identical with those in the affected male hemizygote. Such diseases include glucose-6-phosphate dehydrogenase (G6PD) deficiency,[49] sex-linked agammaglobulinemia,[51] the Hunter syndrome or mucopolysaccharidosis II,[47] X-linked uric aciduria [48] (Lesch-Nyhan syndrome), and hypoxanthine-guanine-phosphoribosyl transferase.[59, 60] Cell cultures of leiomyomas (which presumably arise from a single cell) from Negro women heterozygous for G6PD deficiency contain only one type of electrophoretic band (either normal or abnormal), suggesting that only one X chromosome was active in the parent cell.[56] Two red blood cell populations (enzyme-deficient and normal cells) have been demonstrated in carriers of G6PD deficiency [44–46] and in 1967 also in carriers of the Xgᵃ blood group.[61]

The occurrence of "dosage compensation" suggests inactivity of one X chromosome.* This term was introduced by Muller [64] in 1932 to

---

* Substances controlled by genes on autosomal chromosomes occur in twice the amount when a controlling gene is present on both members of a pair, than when a controlling gene is present on only one chromosome. However, the same amount of substance occurs with either one or two governing genes on X chromosomes.

describe the fact that in *Drosophila* the effect of genes borne on the X chromosome is about the same in males, where they occur in single dose, as in females, where they are present in double dose. This relationship also holds true for the quantity of certain products in humans controlled by genes on the X chromosome, such as glucose-6-phosphate dehydrogenase,[51] clotting factors, and antihemophilic globulin.

Microscopic and metabolic differences between the two X chromosomes previously referred to (one is hyperpyknotic with a Barr body and is definitely late in replication) have been thought to support the inactivation hypothesis.

Objections to These Data. Although these data, particularly the tissue culture and tumor studies, are impressive, some workers feel that they do not constitute prima facie evidence for the inactivation hypothesis. Apparently two distinct cell populations may also occur in tissue cultures of skin fibroblasts from heterozygotes of an autosomal recessive disease, the classic Hurler's syndrome (mucopolysaccharidosis I).[48] Since autosomal inactivation is highly unlikely,[44, 69] another basis for the two cell populations in such tissue culture must be assumed, at least for heterozygotes with Hurler's syndrome and possibly also for heterozygotes of sex-linked disorders. Multiple myelomas (presumably arising from one plasma cell) in heterozygotes for gamma globulins regulated by autosomal loci produce gamma globulins of only one type,[50] suggesting that there is only one active autosomal chromosome of the pair concerned with the production of gamma globulins. Since it is unlikely that inactivation causes only one active autosomal chromosome, it may be that the finding of only one active X chromosome in cells of a leiomyoma can be explained in another manner.

Unanswered Questions. If inactivation does occur, it is uncertain how much of the X chromosome is affected. A study, by autoradiographic techniques, of ribonucleic acid synthesis during prophase in chromosomes of human lymphocytes revealed synthesis in both X chromosomes, which indicates that inactivation, if it exists, is not complete.[42]

Data from the study of leiomyomas and normal myometrium samples from women heterozygous for G6PD deficiency suggest that individual patches are indeed very small and probably very numerous.[56] Such minute patches could result from inactivation occurring either late in development—hence in a large number of cells—or early in development, if accompanied by extremely thorough mixing of descendent cells so that they are finely and evenly spread. There are no data to help resolve this question.

Supporting Data at a Multicellular Level

Genetic effects at the multicellular level have been cited to support inactivation. Some of the points made are (1) the frequent presence of abnormalities in heterozygotes; (2) the greater variability among carriers of sex-linked diseases; (3) patches of normal and abnormal muscle found in individuals heterozygous for the Duchenne type of muscular dystrophy;[66] (4) carriers of anhidrotic ectodermal dysplasia who have patches of normal skin alternating with severely affected skin;[52] and (5) an extra or absent autosomal chromosome of the size of the X chromosome causing embryonic death early in gestation, whereas extra or absent X chromosomes are well tolerated.[43]

Objections to These Data. Objections can be raised to each of these arguments. Manifestations in the carrier more often than not are mild; only rarely are they severe. If random inactivation were the case, there should be just as many severely affected as mildly affected "normal" females. Furthermore, female monozygotic twins should show greater interpair variability than male monozygotic twins in regard to X-linked traits; however, this has not been proved to be true.[62] The two eyes of carriers are usually the same. If random inactivation were the case, differences should be frequent.

It is questionable whether heterozygote carriers of sex-linked diseases really show greater variability than individuals with some autosomal diseases. Some autosomal diseases, reflecting pleiotropic manifestations of a mutant gene (e.g., the dominant phacomatoses or Wilson's disease, which is recessive), tend to show great variability, even within the same family. Even certain X-linked diseases (for example, choroideremia) show great variation among affected males in the same family.

Since two populations of muscle fibers have been found in affected males with early Duchenne type of muscular dystrophy,[66] such findings in heterozygotes cannot be called upon to support the inactivation hypothesis. The significance of patches in carriers of anhidrotic ectodermal dysplasia is questionable.[50]

Although an extra or missing X chromosome is compatible with life, it appears that such individuals are never normal,[43] implying some function of the second X chromosome.

Ocular Studies

Tests for mosaicism have been done using perimetric threshold determinations in carriers of choroideremia,[53] X-linked retinitis pigmentosa,[53] protan defects,[55] and X-linked congenital night blindness.[54] Although threshold elevations, usually mild in degree, were noted in many carriers, in none was threshold variability from area to area greater than in normal control groups.

Possible Mechanisms

With certain ad hoc assumptions or speculations, the inactivation hypothesis could still explain genetic effects at the multicellular level in carriers of the X-linked ocular diseases mentioned. A preponderance of patches with normal X chromosomes might occur (regardless of the situation at the time of inactivation) because a normal gene may give one X chromosome a selective advantage over the other [44] when random inactivation occurs. If inactivation occurred early during embryogenesis, even a relatively small selective advantage of the normal cell type would result in a negligible incidence of the abnormal cell type. In essence, then, inactivation may not be random.

Furthermore, cells may mingle or migrate during embryogeny, and if so, patches may be extremely small, forming only when cells settle. If mingling of cells continues indefinitely, the effect will be an overall, uniform intermediate effect.[59, 60]

Many aspects of visual function may depend on an all-or-none phenomenon (that is, an enzyme, pigment, etc., must be deficient to a certain degree before a clinically observable or measurable defect can be noted). Thus, if the functions tested do not have a directly proportional relationship to a possible enzymatic defect, then no abnormal results to any degree would be found.

Finally, the possibility must be considered that inactivation is incomplete, so that it occurs without affecting the loci for the ocular diseases evaluated, or the whole X chromosome, for that matter. However, if the hyperpyknotic chromosome is actually an inactivated one (as many postulate), the human retinal cones are definitely affected. Each retinal cone cell of the female contains a sex-chromatin body not present in comparable material from the male.[68]

It is obvious that there is no completely satisfactory explanation for the status of carriers of X-linked diseases.

INBORN ERRORS OF METABOLISM

An inborn error of metabolism is a genetically determined biochemical disorder in which a specific enzymatic defect produces a metabolic block which may have pathological consequences. This term was first introduced into medicine by Garrod [74] in his now classical Croonian lectures given to the Royal College of Physicians in 1908. Garrod's concept of the pathogenesis of these disorders was largely based on his studies of alkaptonuria, a rare condition characterized by the continuous and lifelong excretion of homogentisic acid in the urine in large amounts. Essentially, he made two points: (1) He believed that the basic disorder was due to the patient's lack of ability to perform one specific metabolic step. And (2) he noted a characteristic familial distribution. Two or more of a set of brothers and sisters might show the abnormality, but it was rarely seen in the parents, children, or other relatives of affected patients. Furthermore, there was clearly an increased incidence of cousin marriage among the parents of alkaptonurics. This was indeed the first example of so-called autosomal recessive inheritance to be recognized as such in man.

Thus, Garrod interpreted alkaptonuria as being caused by the congenital deficiency of a specific enzyme due to the presence of an abnormal mendelian factor, or gene. He predated by many years the now well-established generalization that genes exert their effects in the organism by directing the synthesis of enzymes and other proteins. This was followed in time by the "one gene–one enzyme" theory of Beadle and Tatum, derived from their work with the mold *Neurospora* and the fruit fly *Drosophila*. This has been rephrased in the light of more recent knowledge of protein synthesis as "one gene–one polypeptide chain." This is the accepted definition of the function of any structural gene (see the section *Molecular Genetics*).

Garrod also predicted that in due course other inherited diseases would be found to have a similar underlying basis, and he also suggested that other kinds of abnormalities, such as drug idiosyncrasies, might occur as a result of analogous enzyme defects. His predictions have been amply fulfilled. At the present time, there are at least 125 conditions that might properly fit Garrod's concept of "inborn errors of metabolism." [77, 79, 80]

ORIGIN OF THE ERROR

The most likely explanation for the origin of inborn errors is a simple point mutation (spontaneously or due to an environmental factor). A classical example is that of sickle-cell anemia. This results from a mutant form of the gene which defines the sequence of amino acids in the beta-polypeptide chain of adult hemoglobin. In sickle-cell hemoglobin the sixth position in the beta-polypeptide chain, which in normal hemoglobin is occupied by glutamic acid, is replaced by valine. It has been calculated that this difference is probably caused by an abnormality in the DNA of the gene confined to the region of a specific base where adenine is substituted for thymine.

The substitution of a glutamic acid by a valine residue in this position, though apparently a very slight alteration in the overall structure of the protein, produces a very dramatic change in one of its properties. It causes a profound reduction of solubility when the hemoglobin is deoxygenated,[8] so that red cells tend to become deformed into a characteristic sickle-cell shape when the partial pressure of oxygen is low. The change in shape of the red cells, by leading to increased blood viscosity and red-cell fragility and by impeding circulation in the smaller vessels, is probably the main immediate cause of the chronic hemolytic anemia, the multiple scattered infarcts, and other characteristic features of sickle-cell anemia such as the retinopathy.

Thus, gene mutations involve the random exchange of one base for another at some point in the sequence of the several hundred or thousand bases contained in the DNA of the particular gene. So it follows that many different alternative genes or alleles may in principle be generated by different mutations in a given gene. For example, from a gene with 900 bases coding for a polypeptide chain 300 amino acids long, as many as 2,700 different alleles might arise from different mutations, causing the replacement of a single base, since each of the 900 bases may be altered to one of three others by different mutational events. In theory, each of the large number of different mutant alleles may be expected to have its own specific effects on the synthesis and structure of the corresponding enzyme.

Mutation Effects

It should be emphasized, though, that not all mutations are harmful. In some cases, because the base change simply alters a triplet coding for one particular amino acid to another triplet coding for the same amino acid, no alteration in the structure of the protein will occur at all. As indicated previously, a mutation may even be beneficial for the individual (and for the species). However, most mutations are harmful to some degree.

Metabolism is performed as a stepwise series of reactions, each of which is catalyzed by a specific enzyme. The pathway may be blocked by nonfunction of a required enzyme at any step. Or a deficiency of enzyme may greatly retard metabolism. A partial or complete block may lead to deficiency or lack of a product normally produced by the

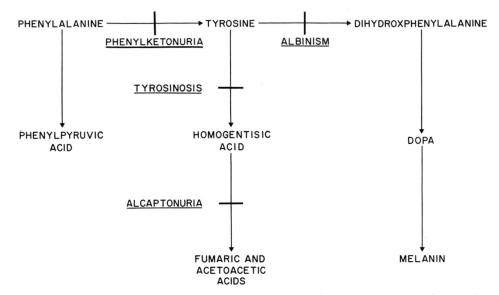

FIG. 1-14. *Some steps in the metabolism of phenylalanine and the possible diseases that may result from blocks at different stages in metabolism of this single product. Phenylketonuria results from a block in the conversion of phenylalanine to tyrosine; tyrosinosis is the consequence of a block in the degradation of tyrosine to homogentisic acid; alkaptonuria is caused by lack of the enzyme that converts homogentisic acid to fumaric and acetoacetic acid; albinism results from blockage of stages in the conversion of tyrosine to melanin and is not yet fully understood. (From Thompson, J. S., and Thompson, M. W. Genetics in Medicine. Philadelphia, W. B. Saunders Co., 1966.)*

retarded or missing reaction, or a more distal one; the accumulation of precursors proximal to the reaction; failure of coupled reactions to be completed; or opening of accessory pathways. Any of these reactions can lead to unfavorable phenotypic consequences.

A good example to illustrate the multiple possible diseases that may result from blocks at different stages in the metabolism of a single product is shown for phenylalanine (Fig. 1-14). Note that phenylketonuria, tyrosinosis, alkaptonuria, and albinism are all possible resulting diseases, depending on the site of an abnormality.

The foregoing conditions are examples of disorders of amino acid metabolism. However, any type of metabolism can be affected. Disorders of lipid metabolism (e.g., amaurotic familial idiocy), copper metabolism (e.g., Wilson's disease), carbohydrate metabolism (e.g., galactosemia), and defects in active transport mechanisms (e.g., cystinuria) are well known. Lists of specific conditions that have been identified are described in recent reviews of this area.[73, 75, 76, 79–81]

CLINICAL FEATURES

A wide variety of clinical features characterize the inborn errors of metabolism, but there are two points of particular note: (1) There is a high incidence of mental retardation associated with these disorders. For example, over 50 percent of the inborn errors of amino acid metabolism are associated with a moderate to severe degree of mental retardation. However, there is no special characteristic or feature of mental retardation that would point to an inborn error of metabolism. (2) A good many of the hereditary inborn errors of metabolism, caused by defects in single enzyme systems, have been found to exhibit varying clinical forms, presumably the result of different mutations that have produced qualitative or quantitative changes in the enzymes involved. Thus, the recent literature contains increasingly frequent references to genetic heterogeneity, giving evidence of a new awareness of the extent of human genetic variation and of the recognition that a given character can turn out to be due to one of many alleles or to genes at different loci.[72]

It is not surprising that a wide variety of ocular abnormalities have been described in the inborn errors of metabolism. For example, the cornea shows the macromolecular polysaccharides of Hurler's disease, the cystine crystals in cystinosis, the copper deposits of Wilson's disease, and unknown deposits in Fabry's disease. The sclera shows characteristic pigmentation in alkaptonuria. The iris shows the lack of pigmentation in various types of albinism. The lens is cataractous in galactosemia and dislocated in homocystinuria. The vitreous is opacified in familial amyloidosis. The retina shows different and characteristic deposits in the diseases of Tay-Sachs and Niemann-Pick and in metachromatic leukodystrophy and Farber's lipogranulomatosis. The retinal veins show pronounced tortuosity with Fabry's disease and perhaps optic neuropathy with glucose-6-phosphate dehydrogenase deficiency.

INHERITANCE OF INBORN ERRORS

Nearly all the inborn errors are inherited as autosomal recessive, a few as sex-linked traits. Some conditions classified as inborn errors show a less clear-cut pattern of transmission (for example, diabetes mellitus, gout) and may represent examples of polygenic or multifactorial inheritance.

As is characteristic of autosomal recessive disease, the parents and offspring of an affected individual and, on the average, two thirds of the unaffected siblings are heterozygotes (see *Autosomal Recessive Inheritance*). Many heterozygotes, who appear to be normal when usual clinical examinations are performed, can be identified by biochemical means. In fact, in over 50 metabolic diseases (autosomal and X-linked recessive) there is clear identification of the carrier either by the demonstration of abnormal enzyme levels or by abnormal response to loading tests, which stress the enzyme system.[79] Such identification is important for those individuals who want to avoid having children with the disease. A carrier theoretically would obviously not choose another carrier for a mate.

THERAPY

Several types of treatment have been developed, some of which prevent the disease effects and others that minimize defects. These include the following:

1. Replacement of the deficient factor. This is becoming a fairly common possibility and can be quite useful in the case of extracellular deficiencies. Appropriate plasma proteins may be used in corrections of certain defects, such as agammaglobulinemia and afibrinogenemia. Ideally, replacement of the "missing" or "defective" enzyme is desirable, but this is not possible to date.

   In some conditions with deficient enzymatic activity, administration of large amounts of the vitamin cofactor, e.g., vitamin B_6 or vitamin B_{12}, allows the crippled enzyme to function adequately.[79b] One form of homocystinuria displays this phenomenon.

2. Elimination diets. These are particularly useful in cases of intracellular defects, and have been widely used to control phenylketonuria, galactosemia, and certain types of hyperlipemia.[71] Such therapy eliminates toxic metabolites; however, for greatest effect, treatment must begin very early in life. With the increasing usage of screening methods for many hereditary metabolic defects in the newborn,[78] the effectiveness of dietary restriction at the proper age in certain conditions has become obvious.

3. Dietary supplementation. In orotoaciduria, uridylic and cytidylic acids are not synthetized, but can easily be added to the diet.

4. Avoidance of drugs. As noted, some genetic diseases—for example, G6PD deficiency—can be triggered by certain drugs, which can be prevented by simple avoidance.

5. Provision of an alternate pathway. In congenital methemoglobi-

nemia, the administration of methylene blue results in the conversion of methemoglobin to hemoglobin by the hexose monophosphate shunt.

6. Elimination from the body. In hemochromatosis, if iron is removed from the body (by venesection in males; females lose enough iron in menstruation), iron accumulation is prevented, along with the symptoms of the disease.

7. Surgical therapy. Removal of the spleen, for instance, can correct anemia in cases of hereditary spherocytosis even if not done before the appearance of the anemia.

8. Competitive inhibition. The overproduction of some product because of a blockage in the metabolic chain may be stopped by inhibition of the reaction leading to the detrimental product—as in oxalosis, the conversion of glyoxalate to oxalate may be inhibited by sodium hydroxymethane sulfonate.

9. Abortion. It now has become possible to identify certain metabolic diseases (for example, Fabry's disease) in the fetus from enzyme assays on aminotic fluid obtained through a new technique called aminocentesis.[47, 74a, 79a] Obviously, certain individuals may consider abortion under these circumstances.

PHARMACOGENETICS

Pharmacogenetics deals with drug responses and their genetic modification. The variability of response of human beings to many drugs is usually continuous and gives a unimodal normal distribution curve for the drug action measured. These unimodal distribution curves are consistent with multifactorial inheritance and are difficult to analyze for the genetic influences involved.

Pupillary response to atropine-like drugs is probably in this category. Many factors are important, such as age, sex, initial iris diameter, color of iris and race.[82a, 83a] Race is one of the most important factors, as it is well known that Negroes are often less responsive than Caucasians to similar doses of atropine.

On the other hand, some drugs produce responses in a few individuals that clearly stand out from the rest of the population.[83, 84] When the data from a large number of persons with such a drug are plotted, a discontinuous variation is noted with bimodal or even trimodal curves. This multimodal distribution curve of drug response is usually the result of an alteration in drug metabolism in these individuals which "stand out." Each mode probably represents a distinct phenotype from which a single genotype may be inferred.

The altered drug response may be the only clinical manifestation of a particular genotype; some conditions in this category are listed in Table 1-3. In fact, the use of the drug may have resulted in the discovery of the genetic system defect. Two examples in Table 1-3 that have received much publicity in the glaucoma literature are the presence or absence of taste for phenylthiourea (there is a higher incidence of nontasters among glaucoma patients than among the normal population) and the occurrence of a pressure elevation of a certain degree in an eye after using topical corticosteroids for a period of time in that eye [82] (much more likely to occur in those carrying one or two genes for glaucoma than in those not carrying this gene). Another example in Table 1-3 of great importance to the ophthalmologist is a deficiency of an enzyme in the plasma called pseudocholinesterase. Extremely prolonged apnea, lasting hours, may result from modest therapeutic dosages of relaxant agents such as succinylcholine (suxamethonium) in individuals with low levels of this enzyme.[82b] This deficiency is inherited in an autosomal recessive manner.

It is also possible that an altered drug response may be associated with other characteristic clinical abnormalities. Both the unusual drug response and the disease may be secondary to a specific abnormal genotype or, in some cases, a chromosomal abnormality. Some heredi-

TABLE 1-3
Abnormalities Revealed Only by the Use of Drugs

Abnormality	Drug
Tasters-nontasters	Thiouracil derivatives, thiopeutone
Glucose-6-phosphate dehydrogenase deficiency	Sulfa drugs, chloroquine, etc.
Slow acetylation	Isoniazid, certain sulfa drugs (e.g., sulfamethazine)
Plasma pseudocholinesterase deficiency	Succinylcholine
Coumarin resistance	Warfarin
Hemoglobin Zurich	Sulfonamides
Acatalasia	Hydrogen peroxide
Slow-rapid parahydroxylation	Diphenylhydantoin
Elevated ocular tension	Topical glucocorticosteroids

tary diseases with altered drug responses are shown in Table 1-4. Note that patients with Down's syndrome (mongolism) are abnormally sensitive to atropine.

TABLE 1-4
Hereditary Diseases with Altered Drug Response

Disease	Drug	Effect
Crigler-Najjar syndrome	Menthol Salicylates Tetrahydrocortisone	Impaired conjugation
Hereditary-methemoglobinemia (diaphorase I deficiency)	Nitrite	Failure of methemoglobin reduction
Von Gierke's disease	Epinephrine Glucagon	No effect on blood sugar
Pentosuria	Aminopyrine Glucuronolactone	Increased urinary xylulose
Hemoglobin H disease	Sulfonamides	Hemolytic anemia
Down's syndrome	Atropine	Sensitive

CHROMOSOMAL ABERRATIONS

Lejeune and associates [97] opened a new era in medical genetics in 1959 when they demonstrated that mongols have 47 instead of the normal 46 chromosomes. However, it should be emphasized that 27 years before, in 1932, Waardenburg,[108] in a treatise on ophthalmology published in a Dutch journal, correctly surmised that mongolism is caused by an extra chromosome. Chromosome aberrations are now known to occur in an estimated 0.3 to 0.5 percent of live births and to be a significant cause of mental and physical defects. In this section, we will discuss some of the more prominent chromosomal abnormalities, particularly in relation to the eye, but first we will consider the vocabulary of chromosomal abnormalities and the possible causes of such abnormalities.[93, 95, 102, 104, 106, 107, 112]

KARYOTYPE

As pointed out in the section *Cytogenetics*, chromosomes are studied during the metaphase of mitosis under the microscope. The karyotype is used for the definitive evaluation and consists of a microphotograph of the chromosomes cut out and arranged according to the various structural features used for classification, described in the cytogenetics section. There is now a tendency for the popular Denver classification to be replaced by the Chicago classification,[87] actually a modified version of the first classification with many more details. The Chicago classification will be briefly described after defining most of the terms used to describe abnormalities.

As has been pointed out, a chromosomal study is a procedure that may take many days. Obviously, one should have some very definite indications in mind before ordering such a procedure.

The present-day indications for chromosomal studies include mongolism, chronic myelogenous leukemia and perhaps some other types of malignancies, certain sexual abnormalities (e.g., ambiguous external genitalia or bilateral cryptorchidism in a male), perhaps certain neuropsychiatric disorders (particularly with aggressive behavior [103]), frequent spontaneous abortions,[95a] and multiple congenital anomalies. There is a greater likelihood of finding a chromosomal abnormality when most of the following congenital abnormalities are noted in a child: (1) a low birth weight; (2) mental retardation; (3) failure to thrive; (4) congenital heart disease; (5) an abnormality of the eyes, teeth, or kidneys; (6) abnormal dermatoglyphics; (7) persistent embryonic or fetal hemoglobin; (8) skeletal malformations; and (9) abnormal enzyme levels. Since most patients with chromosomal abnormalities exhibit mental deficiency, some geneticists feel that many mental defectives, particularly of unknown cause, should be screened for chromosomal abnormalities. It is now possible to obtain amniotic fluid from a pregnant mother and evaluate a chromosome karyotype in the fetus.[99a]

ABERRATIONS OF CHROMOSOME NUMBER

In describing an abnormal number of chromosomes, the terms "euploidy" and "aneuploidy" are used. Euploid refers to a situation where the total number of chromosomes is an exact multiple of the haploid number (23, the number in the sex cells). Triploid describes a chromosome number of 69 (where each cell contains three representatives of each type of chromosome), and tetraploid a chromosome number of 92 (where each cell contains four representatives of each type of chromosome).

A chromosome number is aneuploid if it is not an exact multiple of the haploid number, and the majority of chromosomal numeral aberrations compatible with life are of this type. A chromosomal numerical abnormality of 47 is by far the most common, but 48 and 45 are occasionally described.

If a particular chromosome is extra, the individual has a trisomy. For example, in mongolism there is an extra chromosome No. 21, and this is called trisomy 21 (Fig. 1-15). If a chromosome is missing, the individual has a monosomy of that chromosome. The only instance of monosomy for a whole chromosome is Turner's syndrome in which only one X chromosome is present in a female (Fig. 1-16). Partial monosomies are described under abnormalities of chromosomal structure. Mosaicism is a term used to describe the presence in somatic tissues of two or more cell types, differing either in chromosome number or in chromosome morphology. Generalized mosaicism involving either the sex chromosomes or some autosomes have been described, but sex chromosome mosaicism occurs more frequently.[90,92] Some mosaics have monosomy in a certain proportion of their cells, and this seems to be a viable arrangement if cells with a normal karyotype are also present.

How Polyploidy Arises

Polyploidies (triploidy, etc.) presumably arise by division of the chromosomes with increase in their number without division of the cytoplasm to increase the number of cells that should accommodate them.

How Aneuploidy Arises

The chief cause of aneuploidy is the failure of a pair of chromosomes to separate during the first meiotic division (called nondisjunction), so that two daughter cells result where one contains both members of a particular pair of chromosomes and one contains neither (Fig. 1-17). If the cell with an extra chromosome unites with a normal cell, the new individual will have 47 chromosomes with 3 of that particular set of chromosomes rather than the usual 2 and will be said to be trisomic for that chromosome. If the cell that is missing a chromosome unites with a normal one, the new individual will have only 45 chromosomes. Nondisjunction can also occur during the second meiotic division or during mitosis, at which time homologous chromatids fail to separate (Fig. 1-17). If nondisjunction occurs during the first meiotic division, a cell with 3 chromosomes will contain both the paternal and the maternal representatives of that chromosome; whereas if it occurs during the second meiotic division, a cell with 3 chromosomes will

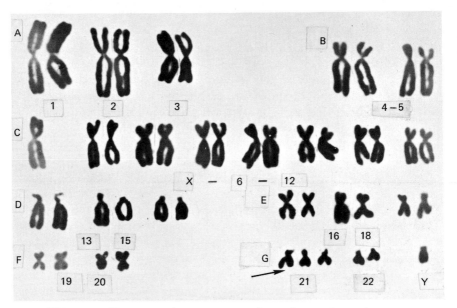

FIG. 1-15. Karyotype of most common form of mongolism, showing an extra chromosome No. 21 (arrow).

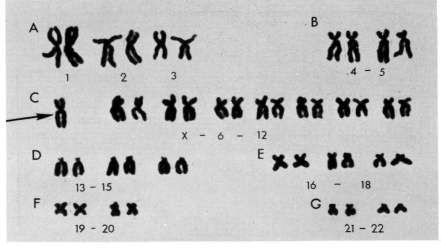

FIG. 1-16. Karyotype for Turner's syndrome in which only one X chromosome (arrow) is present in an affected female.

44

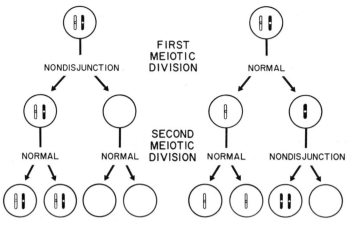

FIG. 1-17. *Examples of nondisjunction at first and second meiotic divisions shown in diagrammatic fashion. Nondisjunction at the first meiotic division produces gametes containing both members of the pair of homologous chromosomes or neither member. Nondisjunction at the second meiotic division produces gametes containing (or lacking) two identical chromosomes, both derived from the same member of the homologous pair. (From Thompson, J. S., and Thompson, M. W. Genetics in Medicine. Philadelphia, W. B. Saunders Co., 1966.)*

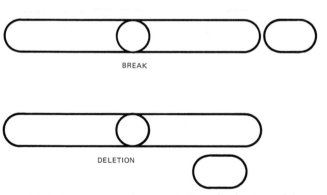

FIG. 1-18. *Diagrammatic representation of a fracture of the end of the chromosome, called a break, shown at the top of the photograph. In the bottom portion of the photograph, a loss of the broken portion has occurred, and this is known as a deletion of this portion of the chromosome.*

contain a double complement of either the paternal or maternal chromosome. Nondisjunction occurring at mitosis after formation of the zygote at the time of an early cleavage division will result in trisomic and monosomic cell lines and, thus, a mosaic (if the mosaic cell line survives).

ABERRATIONS OF CHROMOSOMAL STRUCTURE

In order to be recognized under the microscope, chromosomal structural abnormalities usually must involve at least one tenth of the chromosome. The common types of structural aberrations are breaks, deletions, translocations, duplications, inversions, and isochromes.

Break

This is a fracture in a segment of a chromosome with retention of the fractured segment (Fig. 1-18). Spontaneous healing usually occurs. A certain number of breaks are found under physiological conditions, but under certain stresses, such as exposure to x-ray, various drugs, and viral infections, the number of breaks increase, probably owing to a delay in the spontaneous healing process.

Deletion

In deletions, part of a chromosome breaks off and is lost (Fig. 1-18). Such abnormalities, particularly if they involve sizable amounts of the genetic material, could be expected to be lethal in many cases, but large deletions are in fact not commonly found. If the deleted portion does not involve the centromere, the abnormal chromosome will replicate and divide in the normal way at succeeding cell divisions. A ring chromosome (Fig. 1-19) is a type of deletion chromosome in which both ends have been lost and the two broken ends have united to form a ring-shaped figure.

Translocation

This is the transfer of material from one chromosome to a non-homologous chromosome (Fig. 1-20). A fragment that breaks off a chromosome without a centromere cannot survive unless it becomes attached to another chromosome, which, by also having suffered breakage, has a raw end. Translocation may take place by reciprocal exchange between two nonhomologous chromosomes. If one of the parts exchanged contains the centromere, one of the two resulting chromosomes will be dicentric (with two centromeres) and the other will be acentric (with no centromere).

A translocation will not lead to an abnormal phenotype if there is minimal loss of genetic material. For example, a composite chromosome formed from a No. 15 and No. 21 may contain all of the genetic

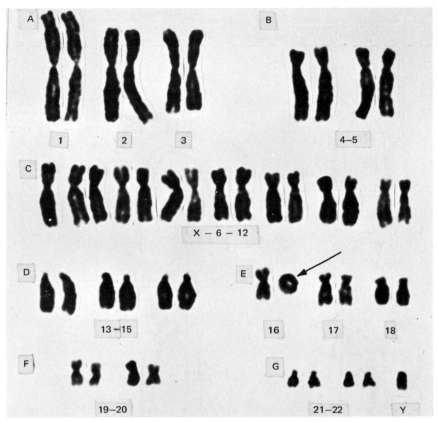

FIG. 1-19. A ring chromosome (arrow), a type of deletion chromosome in which both ends have been lost and the two broken ends have reunited to form a ring-shaped figure.

FIG. 1-20. A translocation mongol, in which there is transfer of material from one of the D-group chromosomes to an extra chromosome No. 21 (arrow).

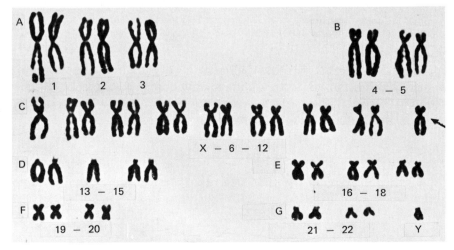

ISOCHROMOSOME
FORMATION

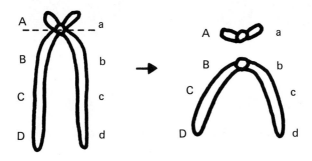

INVERSION

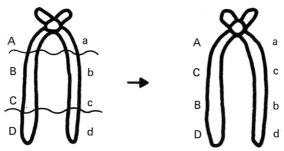

FIG. 1-21. *The top half shows how an isochrome is formed. Cell division occurs perpendicular to the long axis of the chromosome, instead of parallel to it. Therefore the chromosome, instead of dividing into two identical halves, divides into a long and short chromosome, both with metacentric centromeres.*

The bottom half shows an example of inversion in which there is fragmentation of a chromosome followed by 180-degree rotation of one fragment and reunion of the fragment, so that one section of the reformed chromosome is now inverted.

material (Fig. 1-20) on the unsatellited arms of each in the one chromosome. This individual, with a normal phenotype, is said to be a translocation carrier. The carrier can produce offspring lacking genetic material and thus having an abnormal phenotype.

Duplication

A duplication is the presence of an extra piece of chromosome which may be a duplication within a chromosome or attached to a nonhomologous chromosome (see *Translocation*). Duplications are more common and much less harmful than deletions. Small duplications ("repeats") may be an evolutionary mechanism for the acquisition of new genes.

Inversion

This involves fragmentation of a chromosome followed by a 180-degree rotation of one fragment and reunion of the fragments (Fig. 1-21, *bottom*). One section of the reformed chromosome is now inverted and this may (1) interfere with pairing between homologous chromosomes and thus cause suppression of crossing-over and (2) cause nondisjunction of the imperfectly paired homologous chromosomes.

Isochromes

These occur when the centromere of a chromosome divides perpendicularly instead of parallel to the long axis of a chromosome (Fig. 1-21, *top*). The two halves are known as isochromes. This has been described for the X chromosome (Fig. 1-22) and for chromosome No. 21.

THE CHICAGO CLASSIFICATION OF 1966

This system (Table 1-5) retains some of the features of the Denver classification originated in 1960 and the London classification originated in 1963, and is being used more and more in the genetic literature throughout the world.[87]

Autosomes are numbered 1 through 22 and the groups are A to G, as before. As previously mentioned, the short arm of a chromosome is called p, the long arm q. Shortening or absence of an arm of a chromosome is indicated by a minus sign, lengthening or an extra entire chromosome by a plus sign. For example, the abbreviation 47,XY,21+ describes the standard trisomy 21 of mongolism in a male. The abbreviation 46,XX,5p— describes the complement of a girl with the cri du chat syndrome, with the short arm of a No. 5 shortened by deletion of a segment. Structural alterations are designated by several lower-case symbols. For example, a translocation between the long arms of a D-group chromosome and the long arms of a G-group chromosome in an otherwise normal individual is indicated as 45XX,D—,G—,t (DqGq)+. Note that the first item to be recorded is the total number of chromo-

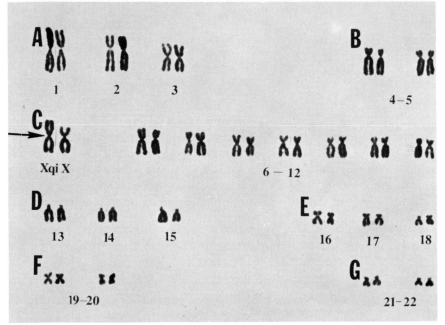

FIG. 1-22. *An example of an isochrome of the X chromosome (arrow), in which one of the X chromosomes contains two long segments instead of a short and long segment as in the normal X chromosome. The symbol Xqi is from the Chicago classification; q indicates a long arm of the X chromosome and i indicates an isochromosome (see Table 1-5).*

somes, including the sex chromosomes, followed by the sex chromosome constitution. The autosomes are specified only when there is an abnormality present, such as in the preceding example. Table 1-5 lists the nomenclature symbols. For more detailed information, the report of the Chicago Conference, available free of charge from the National Foundation, should be consulted.[87]

ETIOLOGY OF CHROMOSOMAL ABERRATIONS

The precise causes and mechanisms of chromosomal aberrations remain unknown; and at present, progress is still hindered by our ignorance of mammalian chromosomal fine structure. Nevertheless, certain facts concerning the etiology of chromosomal aberrations have received attention within the past few years.

TABLE 1-5
Nomenclature Symbols for Chicago Classification

A–G	the chromosome groups
1–22	the autosome numbers (Denver System)
X,Y	the sex chromosomes
diagonal (/)	separates cell lines in describing mosaicism
plus sign (+)	when placed immediately after the autosome number or group letter designation indicates that the particular chromosome is extra or missing
minus sign (−)	when placed immediately after the arm or structural designation indicates that the particular arm or structure is larger or smaller than normal
question mark (?)	indicates questionable identification of chromosome or chromosome structure
asterisk (*)	designates a chromosome or chromosome structure explained in text or footnote
ace	acentric
cen	centromere
dic	dicentric
end	endoreduplication
h	secondary constriction or negatively staining region
i	isochromosome
inv	inversion
inv (p+q−) or inv (p−q+)	pericentric inversion
mar	marker chromosome
mat	maternal origin
p	short arm of chromosome
pat	paternal origin
q	long arm of chromosome
r	ring chromosome
s	satellite
t	translocation
tri	tricentric
repeated symbols	duplication of chromosome structure

Aging

Late maternal age is a major factor in the production of mongolism and is also correlated with the occurrence of 13–15 and 16–18 trisomies and the sex chromosomal trisomies XXX and XXY. The way in which maternal age causes nondisjunction is unknown. Its importance is emphasized by the fact that of all babies born to mothers past 40 years of age, 1 in 40 has Down's syndrome.

Autoimmune Disease

The role, if any, of autoimmunity in the causation of chromosomal aberrations is obscure, but a number of investigators have demonstrated evidence for an association between maternal autoantibodies and chromosomal aberrations.[91] In particular, antithyroid antibodies are relatively frequent in young mothers of children with Down's syndrome, and Hashimoto's thyroiditis has been observed in some patients with Turner's syndrome.

Genetic Determinants

In a small number of families with Down's syndrome, the abnormality may be caused by a gene that enhances nondisjunction.[86, 101] Also a translocation carrier parent has a one-third chance of having a mongolian child. There are genes that may predispose to chromosomal rearrangements. In cultured cells derived from individuals with Bloom's syndrome or Fanconi's anemia (both conditions inherited in an autosomal manner) there is a high incidence of chromosomal rearrangements and breaks, and there is evidence that this tendency exists in vivo as well as in vitro.[93]

Radiation, Viruses, and Chemicals

Radiation, viruses, and certain chemicals are capable of causing human chromosomal breaks and rearrangements in higher incidence than they normally occur; and their significance for man's health is unknown. It is possible that some of these agents could be detrimental to a human germ-cell line.

Adequate data for the assessment of the role of maternal or paternal radiation as a possible cause of nondisjunction are not yet at hand, according to most workers, although there are some claims to the contrary.

SPECIFIC CHROMOSOMAL ABNORMALITIES

Many, if not most, of the common severe chromosomal aberrations are characterized by ocular abnormalities, and these will be outlined in this section. Ocular abnormalities where a chromosomal abnormality was reported only once or twice (for example, Marfan's syndrome), but not subsequently reproduced, will not be cited. One of the possible causes of such "single case chromosomal abnormalities" is that some laboratories call a variation of normal what other laboratories call abnormal. It is obviously important to establish the range of normal variation in each laboratory. In describing the chromosomal abnormalities associated with ocular changes, only the principal features will be summarized. The reader is referred to critical references for each condition under the heading *Chromosomal Aberrations*.

DELETION SYNDROMES

Cri du Chat

The best-known deletion syndrome is the so-called cat-cry or cri du chat syndrome, first described by Lejeune and co-workers [98] in 1963. Young infants affected with this syndrome have a typical cry, comparable to the mewing of a cat, which is caused by a hypoplasia of the larynx and which is present only in the first few months of life. Most cases show deletion of the short arm of the No. 5 chromosome [88, 98] (Fig. 1-23). The most common systemic and ocular findings are summarized as follows:

Systemic Findings in the Cat-Cry Syndrome
Low birth weight
Slow growth
Catlike cry
Severe mental deficiency
Microcephaly
Hypotonia
Round face
Low set and/or poorly formed ears
Simian crease in palm
Micrognathia
Congenital heart disease

Ocular Findings in the Cat-Cry Syndrome
Antimongoloid slant
Hypertelorism

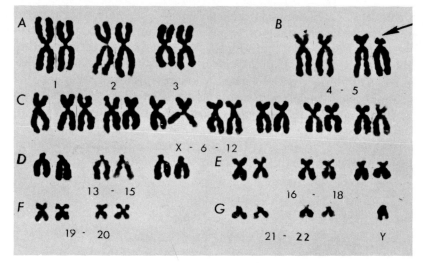

FIG. 1-23. *Karyotype from a patient with the cri du chat syndrome in which there is partial deletion of the short arm of a chromosome of the 4–5 group (arrow).*

Epicanthal folds

Exotropia

Myopia

Iris coloboma

Optic atrophy

Wolf's Syndrome

In 1965, Wolf[111] described a syndrome due to a deletion of the short arm of the No. 4 chromosome which is quite similar to the cri du chat syndrome, except for the absence of the cat cry and the presence of seizures and cleft lip and palate. The ocular abnormalities are the same in the two syndromes, except that exophthalmos and a defect of the medial half of the eyebrows have been reported in Wolf's syndrome.[96, 100, 111]

Partial Deletion Long-Arm No. 13

Allerdice and co-workers[85] recently described a syndrome characterized by deletion of parts of the long arm of a No. 13 chromosome in which ocular findings were common. The most common systemic and ocular findings are as follows:

Systemic Findings in the Long-Arm 13 Deletion Syndrome
Mental retardation
Microcephaly
Trigonocephaly
Micrognathia
Large malformed ears
Facial asymmetry
Congenital heart disease
Anal atresia
Cryptorchidism
Hypospadias and epispadias

Ocular Findings in the Long-Arm 13 Deletion Syndrome
Hypertelorism
Microphthalmia
Epicanthal folds
Ptosis
Uveal coloboma
Congenital cataract

Retinoblastomas have been noted in 2 of the 23 cases reported.[85]

Partial Deletion Short- or Long-Arm No. 18

Ocular findings are also common in the partial deletion syndromes of the No. 18 chromosome.[98a] Partial deletion of either the short or long arm may occur, and each produces characteristic systemic and ocular abnormalities as follows:

Systemic Findings in Partial Deletion Syndromes of Chromosome No. 18
Short-Arm Deletion Syndrome (18p−)
  Mental retardation
  Short stature
  Micrognathia, moon face, depressed angle of mouth
  Floppy, sometimes low-set ears
  Flat bridge of nose
  Caries
  May be webbed neck

Long-Arm Deletion Syndrome (18q−)

Mental retardation

Short stature

Microcephaly and/or oxycaphocephaly, midface retraction

Prominent antihelix, atretic or hypoplastic ear canals

Cardiac defect

Widely separated and/or hypoplastic nipples

Long tapering fingers, anomalies of feet and/or toes, dimples at elbows, shoulders, knees, and knuckles

Cryptorchidism, hypoplastic penis, hypospadias

Ocular Findings in Partial Deletion Syndromes of Chromosome No. 18

Short-Arm Deletion Syndrome (18p−)

Ptosis *

Hypertelorism *

Epicanthal folds *

Strabismus *

Eccentric pupil

Cataract

Corneal opacity

Long-Arm Deletion Syndrome (18q−)

Optic disc abnormalities *

Atrophy

Tilting

Staphyloma

Other varied eyeground abnormalities *

Tapetoretinal dystrophy

Macular scarring

Macular "defects" (not described in detail)

Nystagmus *

Epicanthal folds *

Strabismus *

Narrow palpebral fissure

Oval-shaped pupils

Microcornea

* Most common findings.

AUTOSOMAL CHROMOSOMAL ANEUPLOIDIES

Down's Syndrome (Mongolism Trisomy 21)

This condition was first described by Down[89] in 1866, but its cause remained a deep mystery until 1959 when Lejeune and colleagues[97] showed that these children had 47 chromosomes, the extra one being a No. 21 chromosome. Over 90 percent of the patients with this condition have this characteristic trisomy (Fig. 1-15), but a small percentage have a translocation of the long arm of chromosome No. 21 (Fig. 1-19) onto either a chromosome of the D group (13–15) or another chromosome of the G group (21–22).[86, 101, 107] Translocation mongolism may be inherited from a carrier parent, usually the mother. Down's syndrome is the most common chromosomal abnormality and the most common multiple malformation syndrome in man, with an incidence of 1 in 660 births.[109] The most common systemic and ocular findings are summarized as follows:

Systemic Findings in Down's Syndrome

Hypotonia

Mental deficiency

Tendency toward open mouth with thick protruding tongue

Small stature with awkward gait

Brachycephaly

Thin cranium with late closure of fontanels

Hypoplasia to aplasia of frontal sinuses

Small nose with low nasal bridge

Ears are small; small or absent earlobes

Dental hypoplasia

Short and thick neck

Square hand with short and stubby fingers

Feet are short and broad with poorly developed arch; wide gap between first and second toes

Diastasis recti

Pelvic hypoplasia

Characteristic dermatoglyphics (simian crease, etc.)

Congenital heart disease

Dry hyperkeratotic skin

Hair is fine, soft, and often sparse

Abnormal male and female genitalia

Infertility

Poor response to stress

Ocular Findings in Down's Syndrome

Epicanthal folds

Mongoloid slant

Almond-shaped palpebral fissure

Iris hypoplasia

Brushfield spots

Myopia

Keratoconus

Esotropia

Cataract

Blepharitis

Ectropion

Trisomy-18 Syndrome (E Syndrome, Edward's Syndrome)

This condition, with an extra No. 18 chromosome (Fig. 1-24), is the second most common multiple malformation syndrome in man, having an incidence of 3 per 10,000 newborn babies. The most frequent systemic and ocular findings [94, 94a, 106] are as follows:

Systemic Findings in Trisomy-18 Syndrome

Feeble fetal activity, weak cry

Growth deficiency

Hypoplasia of skeletal muscle, subcutaneous and adipose tissue

Mental deficiency, delay of psychomotor development

Prominent occiput, narrow bifrontal diameter

Diminished response to sound

Small oral opening with narrow palatal arch

Micrognathia

Low-set and malformed ears

Receding chin

Hypertonicity with limbs in flection

Clenched hand, with tendency for overlapping of index finger over third, fifth finger over fourth

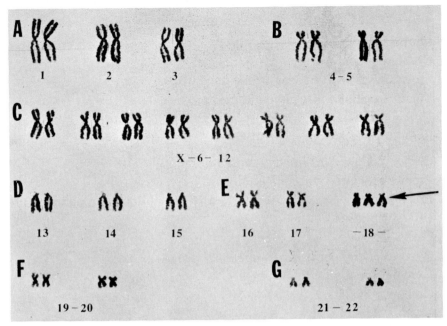

FIG. 1-24. *Karyotype of the trisomy-18 syndrome in which there is an extra No. 18 (arrow) chromosome.*

FIG. 1-25. *Karyotype of the trisomy-13 syndrome in which there is an extra No. 13 (arrow) chromosome.*

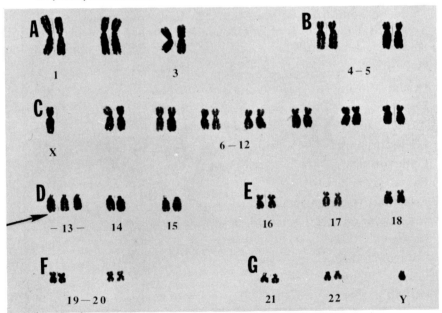

Cardiac abnormality
Cryptorchidism (male)
Small pelvis with limited hip abduction
Inguinal or umbilical hernia and/or diastasis recti
Hypoplasia of nails, especially on fifth finger and toes
Early death

Ocular Findings in Trisomy-18 Syndrome
Prominent epicanthal folds
Blepharophimosis with unusually small or oblique palpebral fissures
Unusually thick lower lid
Ptosis
Hypertelorism; occasional hypotelorism
Hypoplastic supraorbital ridges
Corneal opacities
Microphthalmia
Congenital glaucoma
Uveal colobomas

Trisomy-13 Syndrome (D Trisomy Syndrome, Patau's Syndrome)

This condition, with an extra No. 13 chromosome (Fig. 1-25), has a very high incidence of ocular malformations, many of them quite severe; these are outlined, along with the important systemic findings, as follows:

Ocular Findings in Trisomy-13 Syndrome
Hypotelorism; sometimes hypertelorism
Anophthalmia
Microphthalmia
Optic atrophy
Retinal dysplasia
Persistence of primary vitreous
Intraocular connective tissue, including cartilage
Cataracts
Corneal clouding
Uveal coloboma
Absent eyebrows

Shallow supraorbital ridges

Cyclopia

Systemic Findings in Trisomy-13 Syndrome

Microcephaly

Holoprosencephaly type defect with varying degrees of incomplete development of forebrain olfactory and optic nerves

Severe mental retardation

Wide sagittal suture and fontanels

Apneic spells in early infancy

Minor motor seizures

Apparent deafness

Cleft lip and/or palate

Diffuse capillary hemangiomas, especially on forehead

Rudimentary digits on hands and feet

Congenital heart deformity

Loose skin, particularly on posterior neck

Polydactyly of hands and sometimes feet

Simian crease

Hyperconvex narrow fingernails

Posterior prominence of heel

Thin posterior ribs, with or without missing rib

Increased frequency of nuclear projections in neutrophils

Unusual persistence of embryonic and/or fetal-type hemoglobin

Inguinal or umbilical hernia

Cryptorchidism and abnormal scrotum in male

Bicornuate uterus in female

Failure to thrive and early death, usually within first six months of life

Ring Chromosome-13 Syndrome

This anomaly is not a true aneuploidy, but because some of the same ocular findings as in the trisomy-13 syndrome are seen (to a much milder degree), it was included in this section. These ocular findings include microphthalmos, iris and choroidal colobomas, intraretinal cartilage (near optic nerve), and hypertelorism.[104a]

Cat-Eye Syndrome

This condition is caused by an extra chromosome about half the size of a G-group chromosome.[110, 112] However, clinically it is quite different from Down's syndrome, which usually has a complete extra G-group chromosome. Although this condition is relatively rare, it has specific eye symptoms. The major systemic and ocular findings follow:

Systemic Abnormalities in Cat-Eye Syndrome
Mild to moderate developmental deficiency
Mental deficiency
Auricular fistula
Anal atresia with rectovestibular fistula
Ear tags

Ocular Findings in Cat-Eye Syndrome
Uveal coloboma
Optic atrophy
Derangement of the posterior pole of the retina without evidence of a
   macula
Downward slant to palpebral fissure

The name "cat-eye" is derived from the characteristic iris coloboma, which is always present.

SEX-CHROMOSOMAL ANEUPLOIDIES

Sex-chromosomal aneuploidies have less severe clinical manifestations than autosomal aneuploidies. There are no characteristic eye manifestations in the sex-chromosomal abnormalities except in Turner's syndrome.[106a] This is a condition in females characterized most frequently by a complete absence of one X chromosome in all cells (Fig. 1-16). Some patients may be mosaics with one X chromosome absent in only some of the cells; or the abnormality may be an X-isochromosome, X-short-arm deletion, or X-ring chromosome. The incidence of color blindness should be the same in females with Turner's syndrome as in normal males. The ocular findings are summarized as follows:

Ocular Findings in Turner's Syndrome
Prominent epicanthal folds
Ptosis

Strabismus

Nystagmus

Blue sclera

Pigmented areas on the eyelids

Accentuated antimongoloid inclination of the palpebral fissures

Incidence of color blindness same as in males

Cornea with small horizontal axis

Eccentric pupil

Anterior axial embryonic cataract

DERMATOGLYPHICS

Dermatoglyphics are the patterns of the ridged skin of the palms, fingers, soles, and toes.[113-117] The word means "skin carvings" and was coined by H. Cummins, an anatomist, who published a still-definitive text in the field with C. Midlo [114] in 1943. It is the skin of the palm of the hand that is of particular interest to geneticists. Made up of tiny ridges, averaging 0.48 mm broad in young men and 0.43 mm in young women, this skin provides increased frictional resistance for grasping and also helps stimulate nerve endings. Besides the ridges, which are rich in sweat glands, there are also tiny islands, short ridges, forked structures, and tiny dots. Between these various prominences lie sulci.

Running roughly parallel to each other, the ridges curve and turn about central points called triradii to form distinct patterns, the best known of which are the fingerprints, the patterns found on the skin overlying the volar pads on the tips of the fingers. The various general patterns that the fingerprints may assume are shown in Figure 1-26. Patterns are rare on the middle and proximal sections of the digits, but they are frequently found in certain locations on the palms (designated as I, II, III, IV, thenar, and hypothenar in Fig. 1-26). Wherever they form patterns, the ridges turn about a triradius, the center of three delta-shaped regions (Fig. 1-26). The five principal palmar triradii (labeled a, b, c, d, and t in Fig. 1-26) are usually found at the base of each digit, except the thumb, and near the border of the hand with the wrist. The traits are heritable; and in fact, the fingerprint ridge count is a classical example of polygenic inheritance.

The dermal ridges are formed early in life before the end of the fourth month of embryogenesis. Therefore, disturbances during the first four months of development may produce abnormal dermato-

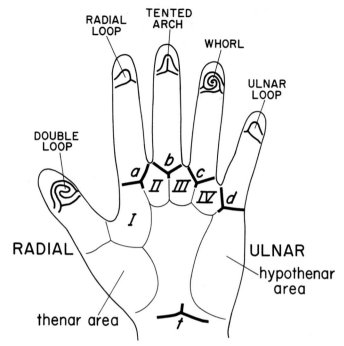

FIG. 1-26. *Normal dermatoglyphics showing some of the features evaluated in prints of the palms and fingers. Various fingerprint patterns are illustrated. Areas on palms that may show patterns are labeled as I, II, III, IV, thenar, and hypothenar. The five principal palmar triradii are labeled* **a, b, c, d,** *and* **t.**

glyphics, regardless of the cause. In fact, abnormalities have been detected in a wide range of disorders, such as chromosomal aberrations, rubella embryopathy, thalidomide embryopathy, and congenital heart disease. In general, these are nonspecific abnormalities, but a characteristic combination of pattern types may be found in mongolism and, to a lesser extent, in some other chromosomal aberrations such as Turner's syndrome and Klinefelter's syndrome.

Dermatoglyphics is now considered to be useful as a screening method for picking out patients who are likely to have chromosomal aberrations, particularly Down's syndrome. Dermatoglyphics have, for these reasons, been referred to as "the poor man's karyotype," and indeed the findings may be sufficiently diagnostic in Down's syndrome, so that the much more expensive and time-consuming chromosomal analysis may not be necessary.

TECHNIQUE

For most medical purposes, scanning the hands and feet with a simple magnifying lens such as is found on an otoscope is adequate. This can be accomplished in seconds and often gives the clinician familiar with this area all the information he needs to screen a given patient for dermatoglyphic features associated with various clinical disorders. If a permanent record of the ridge patterns is desired or certain ridge features have to be counted, a print of the dermatoglyphics may be made by using an inked stamp pad and smooth bond paper. With practice, the optimal amount of ink and pressure required to produce good contrasts and to avoid smudges is determined. The inked finger, palm, or sole is pressed against the paper, placed on a firm surface. Some prefer to use a malleable surface such as sponge rubber to get at hard-to-reach areas of the palm. An inkless method involves powdered talc or graphite which is dusted on fingers, and the patterns are "lifted" with transparent tape. Even photographic techniques have been used.

REFERENCES

General Textbooks for All Subjects

1. Bergsma, D. *Human Genetics.* New York, The National Foundation–March of Dimes, 1968.
2. Emery, A. E. H. *Modern Trends in Human Genetics.* London, Butterworth & Co., 1968.
3. Fraser, Roberts, J. *An Introduction to Medical Genetics,* 5th ed. New York, Oxford University Press, 1970.
4. Hsia, D. Y-Y. *Human Developmental Genetics.* Chicago, Year Book Medical Publishers, 1968.
5. Porter, I. H. *Heredity and Disease.* New York, McGraw-Hill, 1968.
6. Strickberg, M. *Genetics.* New York, Macmillan, 1968.
7. Thompson, J. S., and Thompson, M. W. *Genetics in Medicine.* Philadelphia, W. B. Saunders, 1966.

Molecular Genetics

8. Borst, P., and Kroon, A. M. Mitochondrial DNA: physiochemical properties, replication, and genetic function. *Int. Rev. Cytol. 26:*108, 1969.
8a. Caspari, E. W., and Ravin, A. W. (eds.). *Genetic Organization.* New York, Academic Press, 1969, Vol. 1, Chapters 2–4.
9. Nirenberg, M. Genetic memory. *J.A.M.A. 206:*1973, 1968.

10. Stent, G. S. *Molecular Genetics.* San Francisco, Freeman, 1971.

11. Woese, C. R. *The Genetic Code.* New York, Harper & Row, 1967.

Cytogenetics

12. Barr, M. L., and Bertram, L. F. A morphological distinction between neurons of the male and female and the behavior of the nucleolar satellite during accelerated nucleoprotein synthesis. *Nature 163:*676, 1949.

13. Bartolas, M., and Baramki, T. A. *Medical Cytogenetics.* Baltimore, Williams & Wilkins, 1967.

14. Bloom, G. E., and Gerald, P. S. Localization of genes and chromosome 13: analysis of two kindreds. *Amer. J. Hum. Genet. 20:*495, 1968.

15. Cohen, M. M., Shaw, M. W., and MacCouer, J. W. Racial difference in the length of the human Y-chromosome. *Cytogenetics 5:*34, 1966.

16. Davidson, W. M., and Smith, P. R. A morphological sex difference in polymorphonuclear neutrophil leucocytes. *Brit. Med. J. 2:*6, 1964.

16a. Drets, M. E., and Shaw, M. W. Specific banding patterns of human chromosomes. *Proc. Natl. Acad. Sci. 68:*2073, 1971.

17. George, K. P. Cytochemical differentiation along human chromosomes. *Nature 226:* 80, 1970.

18. German, J. "Audioradiographic Studies of Human Chromosomes. I. A Review," in J. F. Crow and J. V. Neil (eds.). *Proceedings of the 3rd International Congress of Human Genetics.* Baltimore, Johns Hopkins Press, 1967.

19. German, J. Studying human chromosomes today. *Amer. Sci. 58:*181, 1970.

20. McKusick, V. A. *On the X-Chromosome of Man.* Baltimore, Waverly Press, 1964.

21. Mittwoch, U. Do genes determine sex? *Nature 221:*446, 1969.

22. Morishima, A., Grunbeck, M. M., and Taylor, J. Asynchronous duplication of human chromosomes and the origin of the sex chromatin. *Proc. Nat. Acad. Sci. 48:* 756, 1962.

23. Ohno, S. *Sex Chromosomes and Sex-linked Genes.* New York, Springer-Verlag, 1967.

24. Ohno, S., and Makino, S. The single X nature of the sex chromatin in man. *Lancet 1:*78, 1961.

24a. O'Riordan, M. L., Robinson, J. A., Buckton, K. E., and Evans, H. J. Fluorescence distinguishes between chromosomes of Down's syndrome and chronic myeloid leukemia. *Nature 230:*167, 1971.

25. Pearson, P. L., Bobrow, M., and Vosa, C. G. Technique for identifying Y chromosomes in human interphase nuclei. *Nature 226:*78, 1970.

26. Steele, N. W. Autoradiography may be unreliable for identifying human chromosomes. *Nature 221:*1114, 1969.

27. Swanson, C. B., Merz, T., and Young, W. J. *Cytogenetics.* Englewood Cliffs, N.J., Prentice-Hall, 1967.

28. Tjio, J. H., and Levan, A. The chromosome number of man. *Hereditas 42:*1, 1956.

28a. Uchida, I. A., and Lin, C. C. Fluorescent staining of human chromosomes. Identification of some common aberrations. *Canad. Med. Assoc. J. 4:*479, 1971.

29. Wilson, E. B. Recent researches on the determination and heredity of sex. *Science* 29:53, 1909.

Inheritance

30. Carter, C. O. Genetics of common disorders. *Brit. Med. Bull.* 25:52, 1969.
31. Eriksson, A. W., and Forsius, J. Studies of human population genetics and anthropology in isolates on the Aland Islands. *J. Genet. Hum.* 13:60, 1964.
32. Falls, H. F. Significance of genetics in the daily practice of the ophthalmologist, in *Symposium of Surgical and Medical Management of Congenital Anomalies of the Eye*, Trans. of the New Orleans Academy of Ophthal. St. Louis, C. V. Mosby, 1968.
33. Hsia, D. Y-Y. Recent advances in the detection of heterozygous carriers, in *Human Genetics*, ed. by Bergsma, D. New York, The National Foundation–March of Dimes, 1968, pp. 75–87.
34. McKusick, V. A., Hostetler, J. A., and Egeland, J. A. Genetic studies of the Amish. *Johns Hopkins Med. J.* 115:203, 1964.
35. Murphy, E. A. The rationale of genetic counseling. *J. Pediat.* 72:121, 1968.
36. Reisman, L. E., and Matheny, A. P., Jr. *Genetics and Counseling and Medical Practice*. St. Louis, C. V. Mosby, 1969.
37. Smith, D. W., and Aase, J. M. Polygenic inheritance of certain common malformations. *J. Pediat.* 76:653, 1970.
38. Thompson, M. W. Genetic counseling in clinical pediatrics—what to do with enquiries about hereditable disorders. *Clin. Pediat.* 6:199, 1967.

Other Properties of Genes

38a. Curran, W. J. Mutagenicity of chemicals and drugs. *Science* 171:51, 1971.
38b. Edwards, J. The analysis of X-linkage. *Ann. Hum. Genet.* 34:229, 1971.
39. McKusidc, V. A. The mapping of human chromosomes. *Sci. Am.* 224:104, 1971.
39a. Renwick, J. H. Progress in mapping human autosomes. *Brit. Med. Bull.* 25:65, 1969.
40. Renwick, J. H., and Bolling, D. A program complex for encoding, analyzing, and storing human linkage data, in *Proc. 3rd Int. Cong. Hum. Genet.*, ed. by Crow, J. F., and Neel, J. V. Baltimore, The Johns Hopkins Press, 1966.
41. Sanger, R. Genes on the X-chromosome. *Canad. J. Genet. Cytol.* 7:179, 1965.

The Sex Chromosomes

42. Back, F., and Dormer, P. X-chromosome activity in lymphocytes. *Lancet* 1:385, 1967.
43. Barr, M. L. B. The sex chromosomes in evolution and medicine. *Canad. Med. Ass. J.* 95:1137, 1966.
44. Beutler, E. Gene inactivation: the distribution of gene products among populations of cells in heterozygous humans. *Cold Spring Harbor Sympos. Quant. Biol.* 29:261, 1964.
45. Beutler, E., and Baluda, M. C. The separation of glucose-6-phosphate-dehydro-

genase-deficient erythrocytes from the blood of heterozygotes for glucose-6-phosphate-dehydrogenase deficiency. *Lancet 1*:189, 1964.

46. Beutler, E., Yeh, M., and Fairbanks, V. F. The normal human female as a mosaic of X-chromosome activity: studies using the gene for G-6-P-D deficiency as a marker. *Proc. Nat. Acad. Sci. 48*:9, 1962.

47. Boyle, J. A., Raivio, K. O., Astrin, K. H., Schulman, J. O., Graf, M. L., Seegmiller, J. E., and Jacobsen, C. B. Lesch-Nyhan syndrome. Preventive control by prenatal diagnosis. *Science 169*:688, 1970.

48. Danes, B. S., and Bearn, G. A. Hurler's syndrome: genetic study of clones in cell culture with particular reference to the Lyon hypothesis. *J. Exp. Med. 126*:509, 1967.

49. Davidson, R. G., Nitowsky, H. M., and Childs, B. Demonstration of two populations of cells in the human female heterozygous for glucose-6-phosphate dehydrogenase variants. *Proc. Nat. Acad. Sci. 50*:481, 1963.

50. Gruneberg, H. Sex-linked genes in man and the Lyon hypothesis. *Ann. Hum. Genet. 30*:239, 1967.

51. Hirschorn, K., and Firschein, I. L. Genetic activity of the X-chromosome in man. *Trans. N.Y. Acad. Sci. 26*:545, 1964.

52. Kerr, C. B., Wells, R. S., and Cooper, K. E. Gene effect in carriers of anhidrotic ectodermal dysplasia. *J. Med. Genet. 3*:169, 1966.

53. Krill, A. E. Observations of X-chromosomal linked chorioretinal degenerations. *Amer. J. Ophthal. 64*:1029, 1967.

54. Krill, A. E. X-chromosomal-linked diseases affecting the eye. Status of the heterozygote female. *Trans. Amer. Ophthal. Soc. 67*:535, 1969.

55. Krill, A. E., and Beutler, E. Red-light thresholds in heterozygote carriers of protanopia: genetic implications. *Science 149*:186, 1965.

56. Linder, D., and Gartler, S. M. Glucose-6-phosphate dehydrogenase mosaicism: utilization as a cell marker in the study of leiomyomas. *Science 150*:67, 1965.

57. Lyon, M. F. Gene action in the X-chromosome of the mouse (*Mus musculus L.*). *Nature 190*:372, 1961.

58. Lyon, M. F. Sex-chromatin and gene action in the mammalian X-chromosome. *Amer. J. Hum. Genet. 14*:135, 1962.

59. Lyon, M. F. The activity of the sex chromosomes in mammals. *Sci. Progr. 58*:117, 1970.

60. Lyon, M. F. Genetic activity of sex chromosomes in somatic cells of mammals. *Phil. Trans. Roy. Soc. London 259*:41, 1970.

61. MacDiarmid, W. D., Lee, G. R., Cartwright, G. E., and Wintrobe, M. M. X-inactivation in an unusual X-linked anemia and the Xg[a] blood group. *Clin. Res. 15*:132, 1967.

62. McKusick, V. *On the X-Chromosome of Man.* Baltimore, Waverly Press, 1964.

63. Mittwock, V. *Sex Chromosomes.* New York, Academic Press, 1967.

64. Muller, H. J. Further studies on the nature and causes of gene mutation. *Proc. 6th Int. Cong. of Genet.* Ithaca, New York, Vol. 1. Menasha, Wisconsin, Brooklyn Botanical Gardens, 1932.

65. Ohno, S., and Cattanach, B. M. Cytological study of an X-autosome translocation in the *Mus musculus. Cytogenetics 1*:129, 1962.

66. Pearson, C. M., Fowler, W. M., and Wright, W. X-chromosome mosaicism in females with muscular dystrophy. *Proc. Nat. Acad. Sci. 50:*24, 1963.

67. Pickford, R. W. Variability and consistency in the manifestation of red-green color vision defects. *Vision Res. 7:*65, 1967.

68. Teplitz, R. L. Sex chromatin of cone cells of human retina. *Science 150:*1827, 1965.

69. Teplitz, R. L., and Beutler, E. Mosaicism, chimerism and sex-chromosome inactivation. *Blood 27:*2, 1966.

70. Walls, G. L. Peculiar color blindness in peculiar people. *Arch. Ophthal. 62:*13, 1959.

Inborn Errors of Metabolism

71. Brissand, H. E. Diet therapy of disorders of amino acid metabolism. *Sem. Hop. Paris 47:*462, 1971.

72. Childs, B., Vazken, M., and Kaloustian, D. Genetic heterogeneity. *New Eng. J. Med. 279:*1205, 1267, 1968.

73. Effron, M. L. Medical progress. Aminoaciduria. *New Eng. J. Med. 272:*1058, 1107, 1965.

74. Garrod, A. E. Inborn errors of metabolism, reprinted with supplement. New York, Oxford University Press, 1963.

74a. Gertner, M. Use of aminocentesis for prenatal genetic counseling. *Bull. N.Y. Acad. Med. 46:*916, 1970.

75. Ghadini, H. Diagnosis of inborn errors of amino acid metabolism. *Amer. J. Dis. Child. 114:*433, 1967.

76. Harris, H. Molecular basis of hereditary disease. *Brit. Med. J. 2:*135, 1968.

77. Hsia, D. Y-Y. Inborn Errors of Metabolism, 2nd ed. Chicago, Year Book Medical Publishers, 1966.

78. Hsia, D. Y-Y. Screening of hereditary metabolic defects among new-born infants. *Canad. Med. Ass. J. 95:*247, 1966.

79. Hsia, D. Y-Y. Recent advances in the detection of heterozygous carriers, in *Human Genetics*, ed. by Bergsma, D. New York, The National Foundation–March of Dimes, 1968, pp. 75–87.

79a. Milunsky, A. Prenatal genetic diagnosis. *New Eng. J. Med. 283:*1441, 1498, 1970.

79b. Rosenberg, L. E. Inherited aminoacidopathies demonstrating vitamin deficiency. *New Eng. J. Med. 281:*145, 1969.

80. Scriver, C. R. Inborn errors of amino acid metabolism, in new aspects of human genetics. *Brit. Med. Bull. 25:*35, 1969.

81. Stanburg, J. B., Wyngaarden, J. B., and Frederickson, P. S. *The Metabolic Basis of Inherited Disease*, 2nd ed. New York, McGraw-Hill, 1966.

Pharmacogenetics

82. Becker, B., and Hahn, K. A. Topical corticosteroids and heredity in primary open-angle glaucoma. *Amer. J. Ophthal. 57:*543, 1964.

82a. Bertler, A., and Smith, S. E. Genetic influences in drug responses of the eye and the heart. *Clinical Science 40:*403, 1971.

82b. Kalow, W. Pharmacogenetics and anesthesia. *Anesthesiology* 25:3, 377, 1964.

83. LaDu, B. N., and Kalow, W. Pharmacogenetics. *Ann. N.Y. Acad. Sci.* 151:691, 1968.

83a. Marmion, V. J. Pharmacogenetics in Ophthalmology. *Proc. Roy. Soc. Med.* 64:628, 1971.

84. Porter, I. H. The genetics of drug susceptibility. *Dis. Nerv. Sys.* 7:25, 1966.

Chromosomal Aberrations

85. Allerdice, P. W., Davis, J. G., Miller, O. J., Klinger, H. P., Warburton, D., Miller, D. A., Allen, F. H., Abrams, C. A. L., and McGilvray, E. The 13q— deletion syndrome. *Amer. J. Hum. Genet.* 21:499, 1969.

86. Benda, C. E. *Down's Syndrome. Mongolism and Its Management.* New York and London, Grune & Stratton, 1969.

87. Bergsma, D., Hamerton, J. L., and Klinger, H. R. (eds.). *Chicago Conference: Standardization in Human Cytogenetics.* New York, The National Foundation—March of Dimes, 1966.

88. Breg, W. R. Cri du chat syndrome in adolescents and adults: clinical findings in 13 older patients with partial deletion of the short arm of chromosome No. 5 (5p). *J. Pediat.* 77:782, 1970.

89. Down, J. L. H. Observations on an ethnic classification of idiots. *Clinical Lecture Reports. London Hospital* 3:259, 1866.

90. Engel, E. Mosaicism. *New Eng. J. Med.* 272:34, 1965.

91. Fialkow, P. J. Autoimmunity: a predisposing factor to chromosomal aberrations. *Lancet* 1:474, 1964.

92. Ford, C. E. Mosaics and chimaeras. *Brit. Med. Bull.* 25:104, 1969.

93. German, J. Studying human chromosomes today. *Amer. Sci.* 58:181, 1970.

94. Ginsberg, J., Perrin, E. V., and Sueoka, W. T. Ocular manifestations of trisomy 18. Report of two cases with clinical, cytogenetic and pathologic findings. *Amer. J. Ophthal.* 81:18, 1970.

94a. Ginsberg, J., Bove, K., Nelson, R., and Englender, G. S. Ocular pathology of trisomy 18. *Ann. Ophthal.* 3:273, 1971.

95. Jacobs, P. A. Structural abnormalities of the sex chromosomes. *Brit. Med. Bull.* 25: 94, 1969.

95a. Larson, S. L., and Titus, J. L. Chromosomes and abortions. *Mayo Clin. Proc.* 45:60, 1970.

96. Leao, J. C., Bargman, G. J., New, R. L., Kajii, T., and Gardner, L. I. New syndrome associated with partial deletion of short arms of chromosome No. 4. *J.A.M.A.* 202: 434, 1967.

97. Lejeune, J., Turpin, R., and Ganthier, M. Le Mongolisme, premier exemple d'aberration autosomique humaine. *Ann. Genet.* 1:41, 1959.

98. Lejeune, J., Lafourcade, J., Berger, R., Vialatte, J., Boeswillwald, M., Seringe, P., and Turpin, R. Trois cas de deletion partielle des bras courts d'un chromosome 5. *C.R. Acad. Sci.* 257:3098, 1963.

98a. Levenson, J. E., Crandall, B. F., and Sparkes, R. S. Partial deletion syndromes of chromosome 18. *Ann. Ophthal.* 3:756, 1971.

99. Lindsten, J. *The Nature and Origin of X-Chromosome Aberrations in Turner's Syndrome.* A cytogenetical and clinical study of 57 patients. Stockholm, Almqvist & Wiksell, 1963.

99a. Macintyre, M. N. Prenatal chromosome analysis—a life saving procedure. *South Med. J. 64* (supp. 1):85, 1971.

100. Miller, O. J. Partial deletion of short arm of chromosome No. 4 (4p—); clinical studies in five unrelated patients. *J. Pediat. 77:*792, 1970.

101. Penrose, L. S., and Smith, G. F. *Down's Anomaly.* Boston, Little, Brown & Co., 1966.

102. Polani, P. E. Autosomal imbalance and its syndromes, excluding Down's. *Brit. Med. Bull. 25:*81, 1969.

103. Price, W. H., and Whatmore, P. B. Criminal behavior and XYY males. *Nature 213:* 815, 1967.

104. Rowley, J. D. Cytogenetics in clinical medicine. *J.A.M.A. 207:*914, 1969.

104a. Saraux, H., Rethore, M. O., Aussaunaire, M., Dhermy, P., Joly, C., Leloch, J., Praud, E., and Lejeune, J. Ocular anomalies of the phenotype DR (ring-chromosome D). *Ann. Oculist 203:*737, 1970.

105. Schmid, W. Pericentric inversion (report of two malformation cases suggestive of parental inversion heterozygosity). *J. Genet. Hum. 16:*89, 1967.

106. Taylor, A. I. Patau's, Edward's, and cri-du-chat syndrome: a tabulated summary of current findings. *Develop. Med. Child. Neurol. 9:*78, 1967.

106a. Thomas, C., Cordier, J., and Reny, A. Ocular manifestations of Turner's syndrome. *Arch. Ophtal. (Paris) 29:*565, 1969.

107. Valentine, G. H. *The Chromosome Disorders, An Introduction for Clinicians,* 2nd ed. Philadelphia, Lippincott, 1970.

108. Waardenburg, P. J., cited in German, J. Studying human chromosomes today. *Amer. Sci. 58:*182, 1970.

109. Walzer, S., Breau, G., and Gerald, P. S. A chromosome survey of 2,400 normal newborn infants. *J. Pediat. 74:*438, 1969.

110. Weber, F. M., Dooley, R. R., and Sparkes, R. S. Anal atresia, eye anomalies, and an additional small abnormal acrocentric chromosome (47XX mar +): report of a case. *J. Pediat. 76:*594, 1970.

111. Wolf, U., Porsch, R., Baitsch, H., and Reinwein, H. Deletion of short arms of a B-chromosome without "cri-du-chat" syndrome. *Lancet 1:*769, 1965.

112. Zellweger, H. Cytogenetic aspects of ophthalmology. *Survey Ophthal. 15:*77, 1970.

Dermatoglyphics

113. Alter, M. A. Dermatoglyphic analysis as a diagnostic tool. *Medicine 46:*35, 1966.

114. Cummins, H., and Midlo, C. *Finger Prints, Palms and Soles: An Introduction to Dermatoglyphics.* New York, Dover Publications, 1961.

115. Holt, S. B. *The Genetics of Dermal Ridges.* Springfield, Ill., Charles C Thomas, 1968.

116. Mulvihill, J., and Smith, P. W. Genesis of dermal ridge patterning. *J. Pediat. 75:* 579, 1969.

117. Thompson, J. S., and Thompson, M. W. *Genetics in Medicine.* Philadelphia, W. B. Saunders, 1966, Chapter 14.

2

Fluorescein Angiography

Desmond B. Archer

Most methods employed for clinical examination of the ocular fundus, including the ophthalmoscope, the fundus camera, and slit-lamp microscope, permit resolution of fundus details to approximately 25 microns, just short of that required to visualize the smallest retinal arterioles and capillaries. In 1960 Novotny and Alvis [46] combined the optical advantages of the modern fundus camera with the angiographic properties of sodium fluorescein to add a new dimension to the study of the fundus of the eye. This technique permits resolution in the region of five microns and vividly outlines even the smallest retinal capillaries. Further, by providing easy detection of dye leakage from impaired retinal arterioles and capillaries, this procedure offers a sensitive means for assessing the integrity of the blood-retina barrier in vivo. Considerable data have been obtained regarding the dynamics of the retinal and choroidal blood flow in both physiological and pathological states. Also, in conjunction with ancillary techniques, such as ophthalmodynamometry, it is now possible to determine the levels of intraocular pressure at which perfusion of the various retinal and choroidal vessels occurs in health and disease.

This chapter discusses the distribution and fate of fluorescein within the normal and pathological ocular fundus and emphasizes the principal applications of this technique in clinical ophthalmology.

PROPERTIES OF FLUORESCEIN

STRUCTURE

Fluorescein is a weak dibasic acid of the xanthine group. It is poorly soluble and generally used as the sodium salt, which dissolves in an equal weight of water. Sodium fluorescein is a crystalline substance that becomes yellow-red in aqueous solution. The dye has remarkable fluorescent properties, the conversion of absorbed light to fluorescent light being almost 100 percent. The maximum light absorption and excitation of fluorescein is found between 485 and 500 nanometers (nm) in aqueous solution. The emission curve for fluorescein has a maximum between 525 and 530 nm (Fig. 2-1). It has a low molecular weight (376.27), which facilitates its rapid diffusion throughout the body fluids. The fluorescence of the dye is unquenched by oxygen and seems little affected by tissues.

FATE OF SODIUM FLUORESCEIN IN VIVO

Molecular Binding

When injected into the bloodstream, 40 to 80 percent of the dye becomes bound to the plasma proteins, particularly albumin. These bindings are, however, weak and labile and may be influenced by temperature and certain chemical factors such as pH of the blood. The fluorescein albumin conjugate demonstrates only about 50 percent of the fluorescence of the dye in aqueous solution because of reduced absorption of light at the peak excitation wavelength of 490 to 495 nm. Fluorescein also becomes annexed to the surface of the red blood cells, but to a much lesser degree. A substantial portion of the exciting and emitted wavelengths of fluorescein is absorbed by the hemoglobin molecule, resulting in some diminution of fluorescence in whole blood. This is evidenced clinically in the vivid angiograms customary in patients with anemia.

Distribution Throughout the Body

Following intravenous injection of fluorescein, dye becomes rapidly distributed throughout the intravascular and extravascular compartments of the body. Staining of the skin and mucous membranes occurs within a matter of minutes, reaches a peak at about 10 minutes, and then fades over the next 4 hours or so. Fluorescein does not form a firm bond with any vital tissue.

Elimination

The disappearance of fluorescein from the intravascular compartment occurs very rapidly, and it is largely lost for angiographic purposes after its first circulatory passage. Fluorescein is largely eliminated by the liver and kidneys within 24 hours; however, with sensitive techniques, traces may be found up to 10 days after injection. Impaired renal function leads to considerable retention of the dye, although, in our experience, no ill effects have been noted following angiography in such patients.

Coloring of Body Fluids and Skin

The skin will have a jaundiced appearance for 2 to 3 hours after the injection of fluorescein, and the urine will appear yellow for 24 to

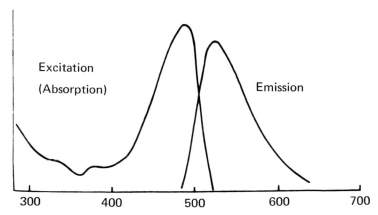

FIG. 2-1. *Absorption and emission spectra of fluorescein. (From Maurice, D. Invest. Ophthal. 6:464, 1967.)*

48 hours afterward. It is of obvious importance to inform both the patient and his physician of these changes. In general, fluorescein ininterferes little with routine hematological investigations, although considerable caution should be exercised when tests employing fluorescent techniques are used. Occasional false-positive results have been recorded using biochemical assays of urinary catecholamines for pheochromocytomas following angiography.[50] In such instances a delay of 36 to 48 hours after angiography should occur prior to using these techniques. The appearance of fluorescein in the urine may lead to a positive sugar reaction (Benedict's test) for several days after injection.

Distribution Throughout the Eye

Our knowledge in this field has been considerably enhanced by fluorescence microscopic studies of the localization of fluorescein within the eye [21,56] and angiographic-histologic correlations of dye-protein complexes such as Lissamine Rhodamine B (RB 200) which has the same angiographic appearance and distribution throughout the eye as sodium fluorescein.[41]

In general the distribution of fluorescein in the extravascular ocular tissues is determined by the permeability of the retinal and choroidal vasculature and the pigment epithelial layer. The localization of dye within the eye is related to the affinity of the various ocular tissues for fluorescein. The normal permeability of the various ocular vessels and tissues is summarized in Table 2-1.

1. *Retinal Vessels.* These vessels are lined by a layer of tightly packed endothelial cells, joined together by junctional complexes unique to the retinal and cerebral systems (Fig. 2-2A). These junctional complexes (of the zonula occludens variety [54]) represent an area of fusion of the cell membranes and completely seal the intercellular space (Fig. 2-2A *inset, arrow*). These junctions can withstand considerable physiological stress, including hypotonic and hypertonic environments as well as the local application of histamine, without measurable changes in permeability occurring.[7] The endothelial cells along with their junctional complexes constitute the blood-retinal barrier.[54] Normally this layer is remarkably impermeable even to small molecules such as sodium fluorescein. Some fluorescein molecules or fluorescein albumin-bound molecules may adhere loosely to the endothelial cells of the retinal vessels, particularly to the larger vascular radicals on the venous side of the circulation. This phenomenon is

TABLE 2-1
Permeability of Ocular Structures to Fluorescein

Tissue	Permeable	Site of Barrier to Fluorescein
Retinal arterioles and capillaries	No	Endothelial cells and their junctional complexes
Large choroidal vessels	No	Probably endothelial cells and their junctional complexes
Choriocapillaris	Yes	—
Bruch's membrane	Yes	—
Retinal pigment epithelium	No	Pigment epithelial cells and their junctional complexes
Vessels of iris and ciliary body	Yes	—
Ciliary epithelium	Yes	—
Vitreoretinal barrier	Yes	—
Optic nerve head vessels		
Superficial retinal capillaries	No	Endothelial cells and their junctional complexes
Prelaminar capillaries	No	Endothelial cells and their junctional complexes

manifested on late angiography as a peripheral rim of fluorescence along the larger retinal veins (Fig. 2-5D). Under normal conditions there is no discernible permeation of dye beyond the lumen of the retinal arterioles or capillaries.

2. *Vitreoretinal Barrier.* There is experimental evidence to suggest an active transport mechanism for removing fluorescein entering the retina from the vitreous.[43] The sites of active transference appear to be the endothelial cells of the retinal vessels and possibly the retinal pigment epithelium.[13] Thus the retina has the ability to eliminate fluorescein entering it by a vitreous pathway or from defective retinal vessels.

3. *Choriocapillaris.* These capillaries have a more tenuous endothelial lining with less secure junctional complexes. They also possess multiple fenestrations and pores [14] (Fig. 2-2B). Fluorescein freely permeates the choriocapillaris layer and accumulates in the extravascular spaces of the choroid, becoming loosely bound to the connective tissue of this layer. Also, by posterior diffusion, fluorescein reaches the inner sclera and becomes loosely bound to it. This staining of the inner sclera and connective tissue of the choroid is responsible for the background

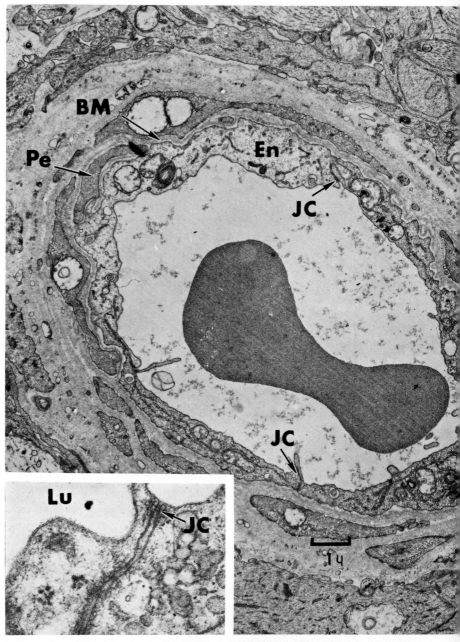

FIG. 2-2A. *Electron micrograph of a human retinal capillary. Densely packed endothelial cells* (**En**) *are surrounded by a thick basement membrane* (**BM**). *The basement membrane encloses the intramural pericytes* (**Pe**). *Junctional complexes* (**JC**) *are apparent at the intracellular spaces of the endothelial cells* (×15,000).

Inset. *High-power view of one intercellular space showing junctional complexes* (**JC**). *Note the fusion of the outer leaves of the cell membranes* (arrow) *closing the intercellular space.*

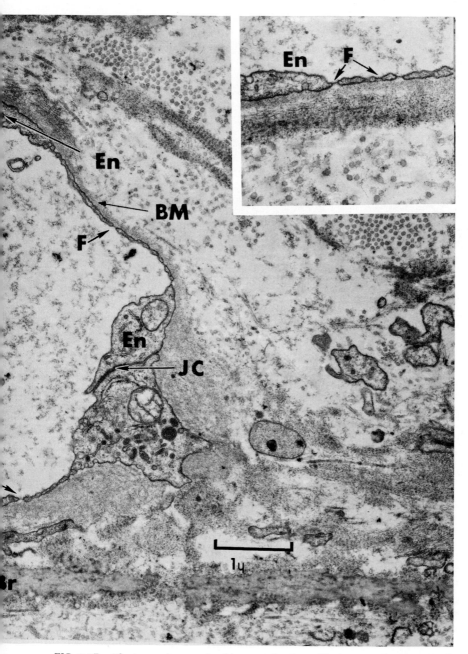

FIG. 2-2B. Electron micrograph of human choriocapillaris. Note the attenuated,
flattened endothelial cells (**En**) lying on a thin basement membrane (**BM**). Fenestrations (**F**) are obvious at the endothelial cells. A junctional complex (**JC**) is
present between two endothelial cells. Bruch's membrane is labeled **Br** (×36,000).

   Inset. High-power view of an endothelial cell (**En**) demonstrating the fenestrations (**F**). Plasma membrane is intact at these areas of cytoplasmic discontinuity.

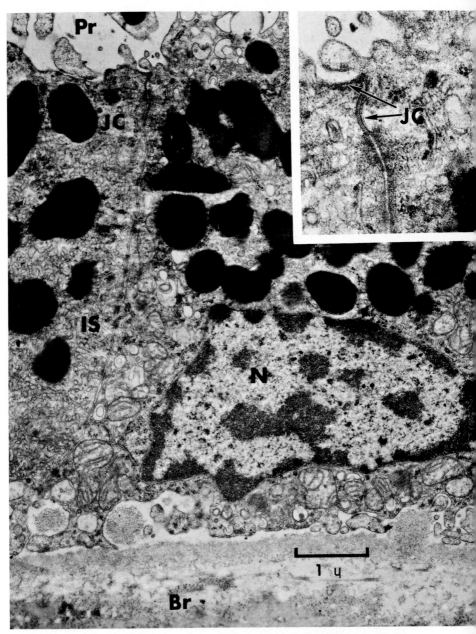

FIG. 2-3. *Electron micrograph of human retinal pigment epithelium. Bruch's membrane is denoted* **Br**. *The intercellular space between two pigment epithelial cells is labeled* **IS**, *and the nucleus of one cell* (**N**). *A junctional complex* (**JC**) *is noted at the upper portion of the intracellular space adjacent to the epithelial processes* (**Pr**) (×13,000).

Inset. *High-power view of the junctional complex* (**JC**).

fluorescence seen in the late stages of angiography. Staining of the outer layers of the sclera also occurs as a result of diffusion of dye from the orbital vessels.[21]

4. *Choroidal Arteries and Veins.* Fluorescein does not appear to permeate the major choroidal vessels in measurable amounts.

5. *Bruch's Membrane.* Diffusion of fluorescein also occurs in an anterior direction through Bruch's membrane to the level of the retinal pigment epithelium. The dye becomes loosely bound to the collagen tissue of Bruch's membrane.

6. *Retinal Pigment Epithelium.* This layer does not stain with fluorescein but presents a barrier to further anterior diffusion of the dye. The site of obstruction to the progress of dye appears to be at the level of the zonulae occludentes which seal the intercellular spaces of the pigment epithelium (Fig. 2-3). In the experimental animal the zonula occludens of the pigment epithelium obstructs small particles such as peroxidase (molecular size 25 to 30 angstroms) in their passage across the retina from the vitreous,[48] and also exerts a similar barrier effect upon fluorescein molecules reaching it from the choriocapillaris.[49] Thus, under normal circumstances, there is no fluorescein within the retina during the early stages of angiography. During the late stages of dye transit some dye may conceivably diffuse into the retina from the vitreous.

7. *Optic Nerve Head Vessels.* Fluorescein does not leak from the retinal capillaries into the superficial nerve fibers at the optic disc. The prelaminar and postlaminar capillaries of ciliary origin are also impermeable to fluorescein.[21] However, dye leaks from the choriocapillaris at the disc margin into the nerve head, staining the peripheral connective tissue of the papilla. Fluorescein does not reach the surface of the optic disc nor gain entry to the vitreous at this point. This staining of the connective tissue of the optic disc and lamina cribrosa contributes to the late fluorescence of the nerve head on angiography.

8. *Ciliary Body Vasculature.* Fluorescein is known to permeate many of the other ocular tissues. The ciliary vessels are freely permeable to dye, and the ciliary body stroma stains intensely. The dye reaches the anterior chamber by means of the ciliary vessels, via the epithelium of the ciliary body, which itself stains slightly. The iris vessels likewise are permeable to fluorescein. Several workers [40, 53] have demonstrated that fluorescein is actually secreted into the posterior chamber via the ciliary processes. Fluorescein may pass from the aqueous into the endothelium of the cornea and the lens capsule.

9. *Pathological Alterations.* Damage to the retina by trauma or disease results in drastic alteration of the physiological barriers mentioned.

Injury to the retinal blood vessels results in profuse leakage of dye across the blood-retinal barrier into the retina. Likewise, changes in the retinal pigment epithelial cells may result in staining of these cells and permeation of dye through or between the cells into the inner retina. These changes will be discussed in detail in subsequent sections. An understanding of normal fluorescent patterns of the eye is necessary before changes that result from interruptions of the normal physiological barriers can be interpreted and predictions made concerning alterations in pathological states.

TECHNIQUE

The attainment of fluorescein angiograms of high contrast is dependent upon several technical, photographic, and optic factors, and these will be discussed in order.

PREPARATION OF PATIENT

The pupil should be maximally dilated to avoid the scattering of light from the edge of the iris should the camera or eye be moved fractionally. In addition, dilatation should be complete so that the pupil size remains constant during the series of exposures. In most instances tropicamide 1% and Neo-Synephrine 10% provide excellent mydriasis for testing within 15 to 30 minutes.

For good quality angiograms, patient cooperation is mandatory. It is important to explain to the patient the nature of the test to be conducted and to insure his ability to maintain adequate fixation prior to angiography. Particular patience is required with the patient who has no central fixation in one or both eyes. The patient should be acquainted with the viewing light and flash discharge prior to angiography. For use under general anesthesia, a vertically mounted camera may be employed or the patient positioned on his side on an adjustable couch or operating table, and the camera moved toward the patient until the correct distance and orientation are obtained.

METHOD OF DYE ADMINISTRATION

Maximum fluorescein concentration in the fundal vessels is attained by a highly concentrated bolus of dye reaching the ocular circulation. Injection of small amounts of highly concentrated dye into the common carotid artery is the most favorable procedure for high-contrast angiograms.[33] However, the dangers of arterial injection or catheterization, particularly amongst elderly patients with generalized vascular disease, cannot be neglected. Catheterization of the superior vena cava has also advantages,[17] in that the injected bolus becomes less diluted before its arrival in the retinal vessels. However, in most instances this method is unsuitable for routine ophthalmic use.

The intravenous injection of fluorescein into the antecubital vein is the most convenient and effective method for routine ophthalmological procedures and is considered suitable and sufficient by most authors. If injected rapidly enough (within 1 or 2 seconds), the dye disperses relatively little during its first passage and arrives in a sufficiently high concentration in the central retinal artery to provide good angiographic conditions. A 19-gauge needle connected to the syringe by a short polyethylene catheter permits the operator to inject the dye and also to take the photographs.

DOSAGE

Sodium fluorescein is used most frequently in 5, 10, or 25 percent solutions. In general, 10 ml of the 5 percent solution, 5 ml of the 10 percent solution, or 3 ml of the 25 percent solution is the dose most commonly used in the average adult. The usual total dose is between 250 and 1,000 mg. Most workers prefer a dose level of 10 mg per kilogram of body weight. Concentrations above 25 percent solution are not advisable, as beyond this level fluorescein may crystallize out of solution.

TYPE OF CAMERA

The apparatus usually used for fluorescein angiography is a fundus camera, such as the Zeiss or some modification of it. Many of the current camera backs now available are motorized and capable of taking one or two photographs per second. Such rapid-sequence photography permits all phases of angiography to be examined in detail and the maximum data to be elicited from each angiographic series.

Polaroid cameras [1] may be used in conjunction with the Zeiss fundus camera to provide a means of immediate evaluation of the angiographic findings. However, the pictures usually show less detail than those taken with 35 mm film. The camera is also more cumbersome to use than the 35 mm camera back, and the film is more expensive than that used routinely.

For accurate reporting of retinal hemodynamics, some synchronized timing device is essential. Most automatic cameras are now equipped to print the exact time on the side of each exposed frame. Automatic timing devices may be synchronized with the flash tube, providing a printed recording of the time of each photograph. Similarly, a photo-electric cell may be used to record the time of each flash on a moving paper recorder.

EXCITOR AND BARRIER FILTERS

The quality of fluorescent photographs is greatly influenced by the choice of appropriate filters. Ideally, filter pairs should produce high contrast between fluorescent and nonfluorescent structures and still preserve a maximum yield of fluorescence at the photographic film. An excitatory filter is incorporated before the flash source of the fundus camera, and a barrier filter in the camera back just before the film plane. The excitatory filter theoretically should have a maximum transmission of between 485 and 500 nm, where fluorescein has its maximum light absorption, and likewise the barrier filter should peak close to where the fluorescein emission is at a maximum, i.e., between 525 and 530 nm. A sharp cutoff should exist between the range of

TABLE 2-2
Filter Combinations for Fluorescein Angiography

Excitor Filter	Barrier Filter
Kodak W. 47	Kodak W. 12
Kodak W. 47	Kodak W. 15
Kodak W. 47	Kodak W. 15 G
Kodak W. 47	Kodak W. 56
Kodak W. 47	Kodak W. 58
Kodak W. 47 A	Kodak W. 15
Kodak W. 47 A	Ilford 109
Kodak W. 47 A	Schott GG 14
Kodak W. 47 B	Kodak W. 56
Kodak W. 47 B	Kodak W. 58
Kodak W. 75	Kodak W. 56
Baird-Atomic B4	Ilford 109
Baird-Atomic B4	Baird-Atomic B5
Schott BG 1	Schott GG 14
Schott BG 12	Schott GG 14
Fugi 18	Ilford 109
Fugi 18	Fugi 12
Ilford 622	Kodak W. 15

transmission of excitor and barrier filters, so that exciting light re-flected from the fundus through the barrier filter does not diminish the contrast on the photographic film. However, wavelength transmissions overlap considerably in most filter pairs so that the ultimate choice of filters is usually a compromise.

Experience has shown that there are many effective combinations of both interference and absorption filters,[60] and some of the established pairs are shown in Table 2-2. Gelatin absorption filters are considerably cheaper than the interference filters. We find that a Baird-Atomic B4 filter in the excitatory pathway and a Baird-Atomic B5 as the barrier filter permit critical resolution of the retinal and choroidal vessels.[22]

As indicated previously, with most filter combinations and using moderately high flash intensities, a very faint image of the fundus may be discernible in the control photographs — i.e., the photographs taken prior to the injection of dye (Fig. 2-4).

TYPE OF FILM AND DEVELOPING TECHNIQUE

Absorption and interference filters have a maximum transmis-sion in the region of 70 to 80 percent, so that some light intensity

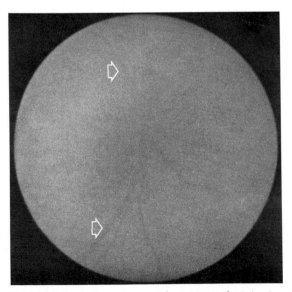

FIG. 2-4. Control angiogram taken prior to the injection of dye. The faint negative figures (arrows) corresponding to the major retinal vessels result from some transmission overlap of the filter pairs. There is no significant autofluorescence of the optic disc.

is unavoidably lost. The optimal conditions for high contrast created by interference filters have the additional disadvantage of yielding little fluorescence at the film plane, so that in general one is working with a very faint image, requiring a very fast film and special forced developing techniques to attain sufficient photographic detail.[61] Colored fluorescein angiography is technically feasible but, in our opinion, offers little or no advantage over black and white photography as yet.

FREQUENCY OF PHOTOGRAPHS

With our technique,[3] fundus photographs are started 5 seconds following injection of dye, and taken thereafter at 1-second intervals for 20 seconds. Pictures are then taken at 5 and 10 minutes after injection and thereafter at selected intervals up to 1 hour. Most angiographic data are gained during the initial dye transit, and by 10 minutes almost all angiographic abnormalities have become manifest. On occasion, however, as in cystoid macular edema, the defect may not assume its characteristic fluorescent appearance until 1 hour after injection. Should rapid-sequence photography not be available, angiograms taken during the arteriovenous or late venous phases and 3 minutes after injection usually suffice for most diagnostic problems.

OFFICE FLUORESCEIN ANGIOGRAPHY

As an office procedure, considerable data may be gleaned by inspection of the fundus using an ophthalmoscope combined with a cobalt blue filter. This is particularly useful when macular leakage or optic nerve disease is suspected (see discussions under these sections). A binocular view may be obtained using a similarly equipped indirect ophthalmoscope or biomicroscope.

COMPLICATIONS OF FLUORESCEIN INJECTION

Sodium fluorescein is a relatively nontoxic substance. Remarkably few side effects have been reported following its intravenous use, and those that do occur are mostly harmless. Its low toxicity is probably related to its negligible tissue-binding properties.

EXTRAVASATION AT INJECTION SITE

This is an infrequent complication which can be rather disturbing to the patient. The local extravasation of dye into the tissues is highly irritant, and venous thrombosis may occur. Should extravasation occur, the infiltration of 3 to 4 ml of a local anesthetic, such as 1% Xylocaine, is usually sufficient to dilute the dye and relieve any pain.

GASTROINTESTINAL COMPLICATIONS

Vertigo, nausea, and vomiting are the most frequent general side effects. The incidence appears to be related to the volume and rapidity with which the dye is injected. In our experience, there is less nausea with 5 ml of 10% dye than with 10 ml of 5% dye. These side effects occur more commonly in younger patients, particularly those in the second and third decades. There is some evidence that sodium fluorescein solution may have some parasympathomimetic action; however, this effect must certainly be mild.

ALLERGIC REACTIONS

Allergic reactions, although infrequent, do occur following intravenous administrations of fluorescein, and several reports of serious reactions have appeared in the more recent literature.

1. Mild reactions: Urticaria, pruritis, and edema of the face and arms are the most common reactions to the dye. Intramuscular injection of an antihistamine usually effects rapid relief of the symptoms.
2. Severe reactions: Although less common, instances of bronchospasm, leading to apnea, have been recorded. Severe cardiovascular aberrations, including myocardial arrythmias and infarction leading to severe shock and cardiac arrest, have occurred.

The immunological mechanism for these reactions is far from clear. As fluorescein forms no stable bond with plasma proteins, it is unlikely to have any important antigenic action. Also, the fact that it is excreted unchanged in the urine eliminates the possibility of degradation products combining with plasma proteins to form an antigenic molecule (hapten). Furthermore, in patients manifesting allergic responses following injection of fluorescein, little in the way of antibodies to the dye has been found.[58]

In some cases a vagovasal reaction obviously occurs, and such an attack may cause sufficient systemic hypotension to produce ischemia of already compromised vital organs.

It is important that the physician be aware of these reactions, particularly in patients suffering from eczema, asthma, or hay fever. In such cases, we recommend that a small test dose of fluorescein be administered prior to the full injection necessary for angiography. It is also important that the investigator be prepared to treat any anaphylactoid reaction should it occur. The angiography room should have a bed or couch available and an emergency tray immediately at hand. The tray should contain epinephrine hydrochloride solution 1:1,000, hydrocortisone succinate, diphenylhydramine hydrochloride (Benadryl) parenteral, aminophylline, and metaraminal bitartrate (Aramine).

ACHROMATOPSIA

Following angiography, the patient may report temporary achromatopsia. Usually a yellow or a blue-purple hue is superimposed on objects in the field of vision; this phenomenon is usually short-lived. However, should the patient have retinal edema, this visual aberration may persist for several hours.

RECENT TECHNICAL ADVANCES

STEREOSCOPIC ANGIOGRAPHY

Stereoscopic angiography,[1] now made practical by the introduction of the Allen separator, provides valuable three-dimensional information concerning the retinal vasculature. This technique is somewhat limited in the early stages of angiography because of the rapid changes in dye perfusion occurring at this time. However, considerable stereoscopic data can be obtained in the later stages of angiography when there is little discrepancy in successive exposures. In the absence of a stereo camera capable of simultaneous exposures or an image separator, adequate stereo angiograms can be simply achieved by moving the incident light beam of the fundus camera from one side of the widely dilated pupil to the other—i.e., from the three o'clock to nine o'clock position. Photographs are taken at each position, and the positive prints are mounted with careful attention paid to the horizontal, vertical, and torsional alignment. Small hand stereo viewers, in general, provide excellent visualization and sufficient magnification for routine clinical practice.

By using suitable stereo pairs it is possible to construct a three-dimensional model of fundal lesions.[12] This technique is referred to as stereophotogrammetry, and permits the ophthalmologist to assess the degree of papilledema or the rate of growth of an ocular tumor in precise quantitative terms. In a similar fashion an exact volumetric assessment may be made of the optic disc in glaucoma. These procedures, however, require sophisticated photographic and mathematical equipment, and are confined to a few specialized centers as yet.

CINEMATOGRAPHY

For the study of retinal and choroidal hemodynamics in detail, cinematographic techniques are needed to keep pace with the rapidly advancing dye front in the retinal arterioles. These techniques for the most part require intense light sources, provided by powerful generators or rapidly discharging stroboscopes.[9] Image intensification techniques have permitted the use of less intense light sources for cinephotography,[16] but in general such procedures are confined to laboratory investigation. The question of how much light is safe for either the normal or diseased eye is still unresolved, but this problem should not be ignored, particularly where continuous high-intensity light sources are used.

TELEVISION FLUORESCEIN ANGIOGRAPHY

Television fluorescein angiography is now a practical proposition both in color and in black and white.[59] Much less intense light sources are required compared with cinephotography, and instant replay on videotape is of obvious consultation and conference value. The main advantages are the close and repeated perusal of the retinal hemodynamics. To date the resolution is inferior to that obtained with 35 mm film and is therefore less rewarding for the scrutiny of the retinal microvasculature.

OTHER DYES

Indocyanine

Indocyanine (Cardio-green), a dye used routinely by cardiologists for the assessment of cardiac output, has been used to provide angiographic data of the retinal and choroidal vasculature in animals.[29, 30] This dye has a peak spectral absorption at 800 mμ, and contrast angiograms of good quality can be obtained using an infrared sensitive film (Kodak Ektachrome, infrared aero film type 8443). An orange filter can be utilized over the camera lens to exclude shorter wavelengths. The dye is almost completely removed from the circulation by the liver during its first passage, and recirculation is negligible. As a result, repeated angiograms can be executed without confusion from background dye. An additional advantage is that the emitted wavelengths from the dye are not materially absorbed by the retinal pigment epithelium. This permits an almost unobstructed view of the choroidal vasculature. To provide satisfactory contrast angiography in man, the dye has to be administered intraarterially, and this so far has proven an unsurmountable obstacle.

Lissamine Rhodamine B

Lissamine Rhodamine B (RB 200),[41] a dye somewhat like fluorescein in structure, has also provided high-quality angiograms in animals. This dye maximally absorbs light at 310, 350, and 575 mμ and reaches an excitation peak at 595 and 710 mμ. A Kodak Wratten 47 is used as the exciting filter, and Kodak 13 as the barrier filter. About twice the quantity of dye and twice the flash intensity are required to produce angiograms of equivalent quality to those obtained by sodium fluorescein. The toxicity of this drug has not been determined for the human, and at this time its use is confined to animals.

Conjugated Fluorescein

Conjugated fluorescein with albumin has likewise been employed experimentally to obtain fluorescent angiograms.[57] Poorer results were obtained with the conjugated molecule as compared with the aqueous solution as a result of the modified intensity of the fluorescence.

TERMINOLOGY

FLUORESCENCE

Fluorescence is that physical property of certain substances which, upon exposure to light of short wavelength, emit light of longer wavelengths in a characteristic spectral range.

AUTOFLUORESCENCE

Certain of the ocular tissues and refracting media themselves possess the property of fluorescence. The lens of the eye, yellowing with age, has an emission peak in the yellow-green range when stimulated with a light in the blue or violet range. The cornea and intraocular fluids also have a certain autofluorescence. However, under most conditions the effect is slight and does not interfere materially with the fluorescent patterns of the fundus on angiography. The term "autofluorescence" has also been loosely used to encompass highly reflectile intraocular structures—for example, drusen of the optic disc and hypertrophic scars, which reflect sufficient light to cause a striking image on the photographic film prior to the injection of dye. This phenomenon is exaggerated by the use of high-intensity light sources and reduced by incorporating filter pairs with small overlap in wavelength transmission. In order to avoid misinterpretation in such instances, it is necessary to obtain control photographs of the fundus prior to the injection of dye.

Figure 2-5 shows one such example of autofluorescence. The black and white picture shown in Figure 2-5A demonstrates drusen of the optic disc in a patient with angioid streaks. Figure 2-5B is a control photograph taken prior to fluorescein angiography. Note the markedly fluorescent quality of the drusen outlining the retinal blood vessels at the disc as negative figures. The intensity of fluorescence of the drusen changed little throughout the different stages of fluorescein angiography, indicating that they absorbed little or no fluorescein themselves. Figure 2-5C, taken during the midretinal phase of angiography, and Figure 2-5D, taken two minutes after injection of dye, show negligible fluorescence of the drusen compared with the hyperfluorescent areas of the adjacent pigment epithelial atrophy. Control photographs thus obviate the error of attributing fluorescent characteristics to structures where there is no true localization of fluorescein.

PSEUDOFLUORESCENCE

Pseudofluorescence refers to secondary light emitted by intraocular fluorescein.[42] This characteristically occurs with highly reflectile fundal structures during the *late stages* of angiography when fluorescein has penetrated in quantity into the aqueous and vitreous humors of the eye. Light reflected from white structures, such as confluent waxy exudates and hypertrophic scars, excites the residual fluorescein in the aqueous and vitreous humors of the eye, thus causing an image on the photographic plate. This should be distinguished from true fluorescence of fundal tissues that actually contain or absorb fluorescein onto their surfaces. However, with the exception of exceedingly white areas, pseudofluorescence is only a minor problem in interpretation of angiograms. Again, as in autofluorescence, by the use of a uniform light source and filter pairs with a sharp cutoff, pseudofluorescence can be kept to a minimum.

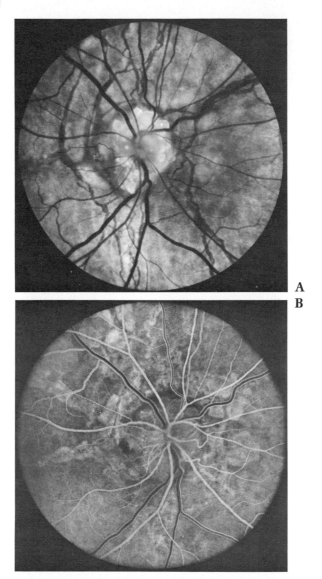

A

B

FIG. 2-5A. Right posterior fundus demonstrating angioid streaks and prominent drusen of the optic disc. B. Control photograph prior to dye injection. The major retinal vessels are faintly outlined. Drusen of the nerve head demonstrate striking autofluorescence. C. Midretinal venous phase angiogram showing homogeneous fluorescence at the disc equal in intensity to the background fluorescence. D. One-minute angiogram. Fluorescence has faded at the optic disc and sharply contrasts with hyperfluorescent areas adjacent to the papilla at sites of pigment epithelial atrophy. These latter regions represent true fluorescence emanating from dye within the choroid and sclera.

(continued)

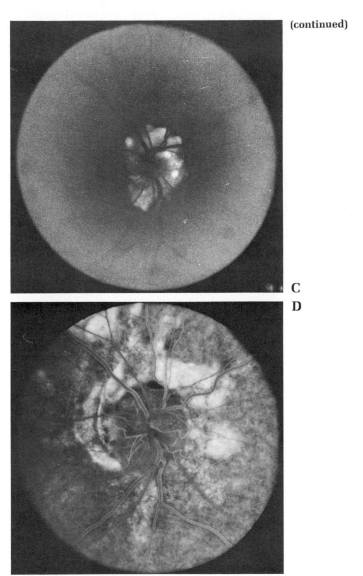

C
D

RETROFLUORESCENCE

Retrofluorescence is a phenomenon whereby nonfluorescent structures are strikingly silhouetted against a background fluorescence.[51] An example is shown in Figure 2-6, an angiogram taken in the late stages of dye transit. The empty choroidal vessels, in particular

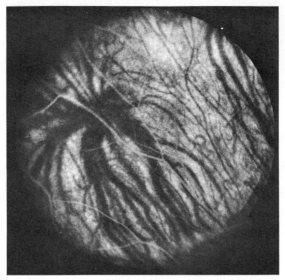

FIG. 2-6. Two-minute angiogram of right superotemporal fundus. A vena vorticosa complex is strikingly silhouetted against the background fluorescence. (From Archer, D., et al. Amer. J. Ophthal. 69:543, 1970.)

one vena vorticosa system, stand out in negative relief against the densely uniform and fluorescent background of the choroid and sclera.

CHOROIDAL FLUSH AND BACKGROUND FLUORESCENCE

The choroidal flush represents the rapid filling of the choriocapillaris with fluorescein and is appreciated by the photographer as a sudden diffuse illumination of the photographic field. This fluorescence rapidly fades over the next few seconds. Background fluorescence in the early stages of angiography refers to the intense and uniform fluorescence of the perfused choriocapillaris (Figs. 2-7F and G). In the late stages of angiography, background fluorescence is maintained by the loose binding of fluorescein to the sclera and to the collagen of the choroidal stroma and Bruch's membrane (Fig. 2-6).

FLUORESCEIN STAINING

Fluorescein becomes loosely bound and annexed to various structures within the eye for short periods of time in both physiological and pathological conditions. Under normal conditions, fluorescein becomes joined to scleral and choroidal collagen and to Bruch's membrane.

There is some adherence of dye to the endothelium of the major retinal vessels. These structures fluoresce for some time after dye has left the retinal and choroidal circulations. In disease states of the retinal vasculature, intense fluorescein staining of the vessel walls occurs and persists long after the late stages of angiography.

HYPERFLUORESCENCE

An increase in the intensity of fluorescence of any portion of the fundus is referred to as hyperfluorescence. Three main factors contribute toward the production of this angiographic phenomenon.

1. An increased density of fluorescein at a particular site. The extravasation of dye from defective retinal vessels, and its accumulation within the retina, will produce such a hyperfluorescent area.
2. Enhanced visibility of the choroidal fluorescence. Reduction in the pigment content or changes in the orientation of pigment granules within the retinal pigment epithelial cells permit a clearer view of the underlying choroidal fluorescence. Such areas appear hyperfluorescent in comparison with the adjoining areas with normal pigment epithelium.
3. Localization of fluorescein at sites of tissue pathology. Fluorescein may become localized at sites of tissue destruction and repair as a result of its loose binding to the damaged structures. Such tissues retain their hyperfluorescent character for some time after dye has left the retinal and choroidal circulations.

HYPOFLUORESCENCE

This phenomenon may result from reduced density of fluorescein at any part of the fundus, as in retinal vascular obstruction, or from absorption of fluorescent wavelengths from tissues with normal density of dye — e.g., by overlying pigment or hemorrhage.

FLUORESCEIN LEAKAGE

Any permeation of dye beyond the physiological barriers just mentioned is interpreted as "leakage of dye." Leakage sites are generally characterized by an initial hyperfluorescent point corresponding to the site of barrier breakdown, but expand later in the angiographic series as dye becomes distributed throughout extracellular spaces produced by the disease. Such hyperfluorescent areas remain obvious for some time following angiography, often for periods of up to one hour.

PERFUSION PRESSURE

This is a measurement of the hydrostatic or intraluminal pressure at any point within the retinal or choroidal vasculature. It may be conveniently measured by the combined technique of fluorescein angiography and ophthalmodynamometry. The perfusion pressure within any vessel is that level of intraocular pressure (IOP) that just permits dye to enter it.

NORMAL FLUORESCEIN ANGIOGRAPHY

INTENSITY OF FLUORESCENCE

The intensity of fluorescence in the fundus varies with (1) the quantity and concentration of dye injected, (2) the rate at which the dye is injected, (3) the site of injection, (4) the circulatory status of the patient (cardiac output, viscosity of blood, hemoglobin concentration), and (5) the transparency of the retinal and choroidal vessel walls.

ARM-TO-RETINA CIRCULATION TIME

Fluorescein appears in the major retinal arteries at the optic disc some 8 to 14 seconds after intravenous injection of dye into the antecubital vein. The time interval between the injection of dye and its appearance at the optic disc is called the arm-to-retina circulation time. This time is dependent upon such factors as cardiac output, blood volume, viscosity of blood, caliber of the carotid vessels, and peripheral resistance of the cerebral circulation. Thus, in most individuals, this value is a highly variable one, and may even differ in the same patient with repeated testing. Variables such as the speed at which fluorescein is injected and subjective errors in evaluating the appearance of dye in both eyes make accurate assessments difficult. Large discrepancies in the time required for the dye to appear at the optic disc suggest unilateral internal carotid artery obstruction. A difference of 20 percent or more in the time needed for the dye to reach the optic discs is considered to be significant. However, a normal arm-to-retina circulation time on both sides does not exclude unilateral carotid artery disease, as a normal time interval may occur because of a well-developed collateral circulation.

Retinal Arterial Phase

Filling of the central retinal artery and its branches with fluorescein takes place very rapidly. Peak fluorescence of the arteries is generally attained within one to two seconds. This is termed the arterial phase of dye transit (Fig. 2-7B). The temporal retinal arteries fill slightly in advance of the nasal retinal arteries. The macular arteries fill very rapidly, and are generally the first to complete perfusion. During the earliest stage of arterial filling, the leading edge of the dye front occupies only the axial part of the bloodstream. The luminal diameter of dye-filled retinal arteries exceeds that of those measured by color photography by some 10 to 15 percent (compare Figs. 2-7A and 2-7B).[55] This discrepancy is attributed to the mixing of fluorescein with the peripheral plasma column, which is not obvious on color photography or direct ophthalmoscopic examination. Fluorescein angiography thus provides a more accurate estimation of luminal diameter.

Retinal Capillary Phase

Filling of the retinal capillaries immediately follows the retinal arterial phase of angiography. Fluorescence of the capillary bed is first noted at the posterior pole of the eye, in the region of the arterioles. Peak fluorescence of the capillary bed occurs during the midretinal venous phase of angiography (Fig. 2-7C) and fades rapidly during the late venous stage. Under optimal conditions, the fine network of capillaries can be photographed (Fig. 2-7D). The best capillary definition is attained in darkly pigmented subjects where the heavily pigmented epithelium strikingly contrasts with the fluorescent capillaries. In these instances the underlying choroidal fluorescence is also effectively screened and does not mask the retinal capillary architecture.

A variety of capillary patterns can be identified throughout the fundus of the eye:

1. Papillary capillaries: Radially arranged capillaries ramify over the surface of the optic disc, being particularly noticeable on the temporal aspect of the papilla (Fig. 2-7E). Many capillaries branch

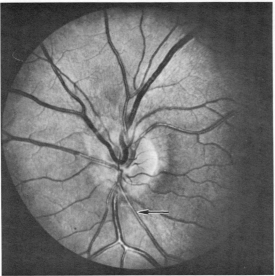

A

FIG. 2-7A. *Black and white photograph of normal left posterior eyegrounds. B. Retinal arterial phase of angiography. Arteries are vividly outlined with dye. Note the difference in arterial caliber as seen in fluorescein angiography and black and white photograph, especially the inferotemporal artery (compare arrows in Fig. 2-7A and Fig. 2-7B). The background fluorescence is due to filling of the choriocapillaris. The segmental, nonfluorescent areas represent segments of choriocapillaris as yet unfilled. C. Capillary phase of angiography. Midretinal venous phase angiogram demonstrating peak capillary fluorescence. The capillaries at the optic disc (D), peripapillary plexus (P), and macula (F) can be identified. D. The macular capillaries. The macular and perimacular capillaries are arranged in a concentric fashion about the fovea (F), merging peripherally into the peripapillary network. Small dilations or microaneurysmal-like malformations are occasionally noted as a result of photographing the capillaries end-on as they pass between the superficial and deep plexuses. E. Capillaries at the optic disc and peripapillary region. The peripapillary vessels continuous with the superficial capillary plexus of the papilla radiate from the temporal (T) and nasal (N) aspects of the disc. F. Early retinal venous phase of angiography, indicated by the commencement of laminar flow. Small nonfluorescent areas represent zones of choriocapillaris which have failed to fill with dye (arrows). G. Midretinal venous phase of angiography, showing multiple laminar columns in the major veins. The background fluorescence is now homogeneous. H. Late retinal venous phase of angiography. The retinal arteries have largely emptied of dye, although a small peripheral rim of fluorescence represents some adherence of fluorescein to the endothelial cells (arrow). The vacant choroidal vessels produce a mottled background fluorescence. Note the discrepancy in caliber between the veins, as demonstrated in angiography, and those shown in the black and white control photograph (Fig. 2-7A).*

(continued)

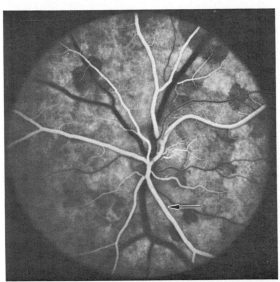

B

C

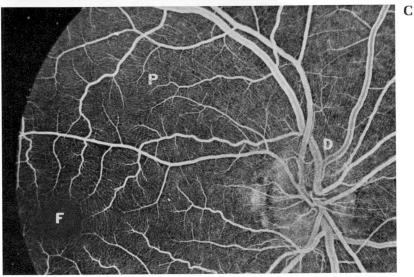

(continued)

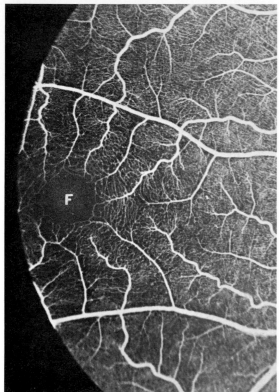

D

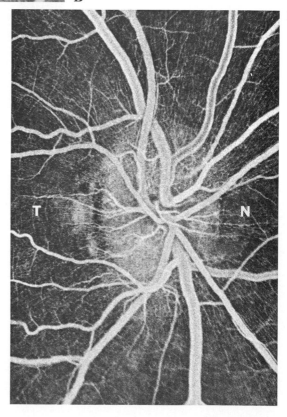

E

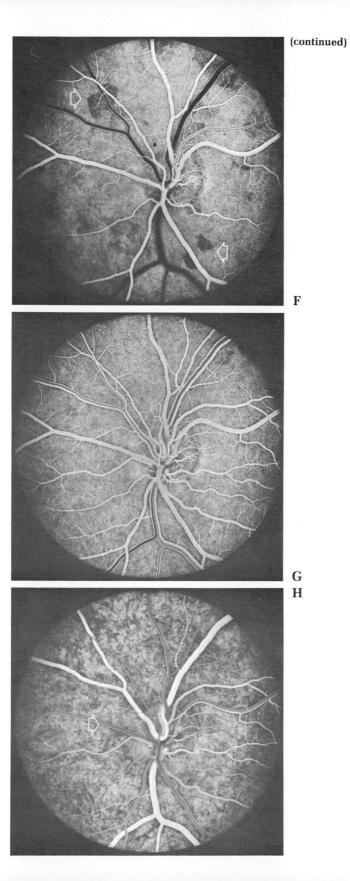

F

G
H

directly from the larger arterioles and cross the surface of the optic disc to supply the peripapillary retina.

2. Peripapillary capillaries: Adjacent to the optic disc, the radially arranged capillaries, with their branches diverting at right angles, extend in an arcuate fashion along the major superior and inferior temporal vessels above and below the macula (Fig. 2-7E). Similar vascular arcades are distributed along the superior and inferior nasal borders of the optic disc and directly nasal to the optic disc for a short distance.

3. Macular capillaries: At the macula, the capillaries form concentric vascular loops surrounding a central avascular area (Fig. 2-7D). The individual vascular loops can be identified in the perifoveal region and for a short distance beyond. On venturing farther into the macula, these loops become more numerous and intermingle with the arborizations of the peripapillary plexus, forming a dense network (Fig. 2-7D).

4. Peripheral capillaries: In the periphery the network is less well circumscribed, and a well-defined avascular space exists between the arterioles and the capillary loops. Toward the extreme periphery the capillary loops become less dense, and small areas of nonperfused capillary bed are visible. Microaneurysms and small vascular aberrations are uniformly found in the normal periphery.

Retinal Venous Phase

The smaller venous radicles at the macula fill first, followed by the larger branches of the posterior eyegrounds. Venous filling in the larger vessels is characterized by a laminar type of flow, which persists until the late stage of venous filling. In the early stages of retinal venous filling, the blood containing fluorescein is close to the vascular wall as it enters the main branches, and shows little tendency to mix with the axial stream of nonfluorescent blood. This laminar pattern exists along the entire length of the vessel (Fig. 2-7F). As the more distal branches of the retinal veins empty fluorescent blood into the main channel, new fluorescent zones continue to form which are located more toward the center of the bloodstream (Fig. 2-7G). As many as seven laminar zones may be noted in the bloodstream of a major retinal vein. The *early retinal venous stage* is characterized by a single layer of fluorescein, whereas the presence of several laminar columns in the major veins denotes the *midretinal venous phase*. With the *late phase* of filling, the veins become uniformly fluorescent and no longer demonstrate the laminar pattern of flow. This stage is usually well developed within five seconds after the earliest appearance of dye in the retinal veins and is accompanied by decreasing arterial fluorescence (Fig. 2-7H). A gradual decrease in fluorescence of the retinal vessels follows, although with the recirculation of dye some minor fluctuation in fluorescence occurs. In health there is no leakage of dye beyond the lumens of any of the retinal vessels.

Recirculation of Dye and Residual Fluorescence

Recirculation of fluorescein in a much diluted form occurs about half a minute following injection. This is observed as a mild exacerbation of fluorescence within the retinal vasculature. Gradual diminution in intensity of fluorescence of the major retinal vessels is apparent for several minutes. Some slight staining of the intima of the major retinal arteries (Fig. 2-7H — arrow) and veins may be detected near the optic disc. As a rule the veins stain more vividly than the arteries. There is, however, no permeation of dye beyond the vessel walls in health.

CHOROIDAL CIRCULATION

The choroidal circulation is difficult to visualize on two counts. First, much of the fluorescence from the choroidal vessels is absorbed by the retinal pigment epithelium. Second, the rapidly filling choriocapillaris produces a dense blanket of fluorescence that precludes any view of the underlying choroidal vasculature in the later phases of angiography.

Considerable information has been obtained on the normal choroidal circulation from the study of albinos and patients with defective retinal pigment epithelium.[3,4]

Choroidal Artery Filling

Fluorescein appears in the choroidal circulation at the posterior pole, approximately half to one second prior to its arrival at the major retinal vessels at the optic disc (Fig. 2-8A — arrow). The choroidal vessels at the macula are the first to fill, and the temporal choroidal vessels fill slightly before the nasal choroidal vessels. When a cilioretinal vessel is present, it fills in advance of the major retinal arteries (Fig. 2-8B). Fluorescein appears in peripheral choroidal arteries about the same time as it does in peripheral retinal arteries (Fig. 2-8C). There is little difference between the size of the choroidal vessels as compared by fluorescein and color slides.[3]

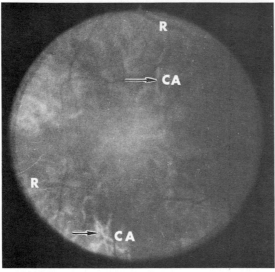

A

FIG. 2-8A.   Left posterior eyegrounds of a patient with ocular albinism photographed eight seconds following injection, prior to the appearance of dye in the
major retinal arteries. Note early filling of the choroidal arterioles at the macular
and perimacular area (arrows, **CA**). The unfilled retinal arteries (**R**) are outlined
as negative figures against the evolving choroidal fluorescence. B. Early arterial
phase of angiogram of right posterior fundus, normal eye. Dye has just presented
in the proximal portion of the major retinal vessels. A cilioretinal complex is
already in an advanced stage of filling. The background fluorescence denotes
filling of the choriocapillaris. The temporal choroid fills slightly in advance of
that on the nasal side. Note the sharp demarcation between areas of perfused
choriocapillaris and areas of nonperfused choriocapillaris (arrows). (From
Archer, D., et al.   Amer. J. Ophthal. 69:543, 1970.)   C. Right superior temporal
equatorial retina. There is coincident filling of the retinal arteries (**R**) and the
choroidal arteries (**C**). No measurable filling of the retinal capillaries has occurred
at this stage. (From Archer, D., et al.   Amer. J. Ophthal. 69:543, 1970.)   D. Right
inferotemporal fundus of patient with pigment epithelial and choriocapillaris
atrophy. The major choroidal arteries arise from point sources coincident with
their origin from the posterior ciliary arteries (arrow). Second- and third-order
arterioles (precapillary arterioles) feed into small areas of residual choriocapillaris (**Ch**). The choroidal venules (**V**) likewise can be seen to drain blood into a
vortex system inferotemporal to the right macula. This picture was taken during
the midretinal venous phase of angiography. (From Archer, D., et al.   Amer. J.
Ophthal. 71:266, 1971.)

(continued)

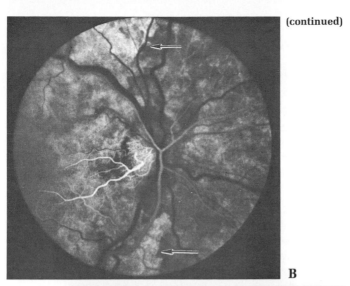

B

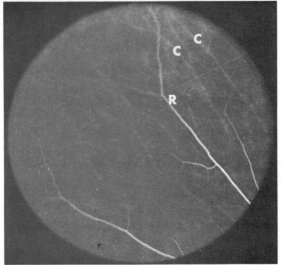

C

D

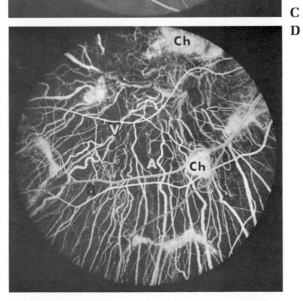

Filling of the second or third order branches from the choroidal arteries (termed precapillary arterioles [4]) cannot be viewed adequately under normal circumstances as a result of the masking effect of the perfusing choriocapillaris. However, in circumstances where there is localized disappearance of the choriocapillaris, these vessels can be readily identified (Fig. 2-8D). Persistent islets of choriocapillaris fill centrifugally from these precapillary arterioles.

Choriocapillaris Filling

Filling of the choriocapillaris is first apparent early in the retinal arterial phase of angiography. It is usually complete by the end of the retinal arterial phase or the beginning of the retinal venous phase of angiography. In the posterior fundus, the choriocapillaris perfuses before the retinal capillaries, although in the equatorial fundus there is little difference in the sequence of filling of the two systems. The earliest appearance of dye and most rapid filling occurs in the choriocapillaris at the macular area. Filling of the choriocapillaris in the temporal fundus usually occurs before it does in the nasal fundus (Fig. 2-8B). In the early stages of angiography the choriocapillaris fills in a mosaic pattern (Fig. 2-8B). The mosaics remain discrete for a short period of time, but eventually become confluence as neighboring segments of choriocapillaris perfuse. By the midretinal venous phase of angiography, dye in the choriocapillaris is seen as a dense homogeneous background fluorescence, which obscures visualization of most or all of the underlying larger choroidal vessels (Fig. 2-7G). This homogeneous fluorescence is particularly dense at the posterior pole of the eye, where it reflects the density of the choriocapillaris.

On occasion, isolated segments of choriocapillaris may not fill with dye until several seconds after the adjoining capillaries have perfused. These are conspicuous as sharply outlined areas of negative fluorescence (Figs. 2-7B, 2-7F—arrows). Such areas eventually perfuse and merge with the background fluorescence. These patterns of irregular choriocapillaris perfusion are reproducible on repeated testing.

Dye has largely left the choriocapillaris by the late retinal venous phase of angiography. The homogeneous intense choriocapillaris fluorescence is replaced by a mottled background fluorescence from dye in the intravascular choroidal spaces. A mild exacerbation of choroidal fluorescence may be evident concurrent with recirculation of dye.

Choroidal Venous Filling

The exact sequence of perfusion of the choroidal veins is difficult to assess in normal subjects because of the superimposed dye-filled choriocapillaris. However, it is presumed that this choroidal venous filling occurs during the midretinal venous phase of dye transit, as the choroidal veins are unfilled during the early retinal venous phase of angiography, and have emptied of dye in the late retinal venous phase. In patients with localized choriocapillaris atrophy,[4] filling of the choroidal veins can be visualized (Fig. 2-8D). It is then noted that they fill during the midretinal venous phase of angiography.

Dye Leakage and Background Fluorescence

The larger choroidal vessels and precapillary arterioles do not appear to leak fluorescein. Dye leaks freely, however, from the normal choriocapillaris, as it does from capillaries elsewhere in the body, excepting those of the retinal and cerebral circulations. The loose binding of the extravasated dye to collagen in the choroid, sclera, and Bruch's membrane provides a prolonged background fluorescence which silhouettes the major choroidal vessels as negative figures after they have emptied of dye. This background fluorescence is maximum at about five minutes after dye injection, and then slowly diminishes in intensity after that time. It may be seen six hours after dye injection.

OPTIC DISC CIRCULATION

Fluorescein angiography strikingly demonstrates the blood supply to the optic nerve head and peripapillary region. Three separate vascular complexes contribute to the fluorescence of the optic papilla during angiography. These plexuses cannot be readily differentiated during routine angiography. However, they may be separated by artificially raising the intraocular pressure, so that one vascular bed may perfuse while the others remain obstructed.

Postlaminar Capillaries

A deep complex of capillaries lies behind the lamina cribrosa and contributes to the background fluorescence of the optic disc. These vessels are not influenced by pressure changes within the globe and are seen to fluoresce during angiography when the vessels supplying the papilla are occluded by artificially raising the IOP above central retinal artery systolic pressure. Under these circumstances of induced ocular hypertension, fluorescein becomes apparent in these vessels some 8 to 14 seconds after injection, concomitant with the arrival of dye at the optic disc. The fluorescence reaches a maximum within 4 to 7 seconds, is homogeneous, and occupies the full area of the optic nerve head, outlining the empty major retinal vessels at the optic disc as negative figures (Fig. 2-9B). The individual capillaries of this com-

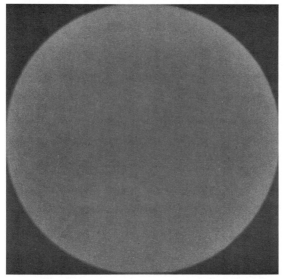

A

FIG. 2-9A. *Control angiogram of normal optic disc. There is no evidence of autofluorescence or dye in the posterior fundus. B. Angiogram taken 15 seconds after the injection of dye with the intraocular pressure elevated to 75 mm Hg. There is homogeneous fluorescence at the optic disc. The major retinal vessels contain no dye and are silhouetted against the disc fluorescence. C. Angiogram of normal optic disc with large physiological cup. The angiogram was taken 13 seconds after the injection of dye with the intraocular pressure elevated to 78 mm Hg. Note that the area of the physiological cup fluoresces intensely. D. Early venous angiogram of normal left optic disc. The deep homogeneous background fluorescence at the optic disc is equivalent to that in the adjoining choriocapillaris. It is easily observed on the nasal side of the disc (N), where it is unobscured by filling of the retinal capillaries. On the temporal side of the disc (T) the retinal capillaries have already filled. The nonfluorescent border tissue of the optic disc is indicated by arrow. E. Left optic disc. Midretinal venous phase of angiography. Filling of the nasal and temporal capillaries (arrow) of the disc has occurred. The optic disc has a discrete edge and is sharply demarcated from the surrounding retinal and choroidal fluorescence. The nasal aspect of the disc is denoted (N) and the temporal aspect (T).*

plex cannot be identified. This fluorescence cannot be attributed to autofluorescence, as the control angiogram shows no fluorescence (Fig. 2-9A); and likewise it cannot be a pseudofluorescent phenomenon, as dye has not reached the anterior chamber or vitreous in any quantity at this stage of angiography. Fluorescence of this group of vessels is most obvious when a large physiological cup is present. Under these

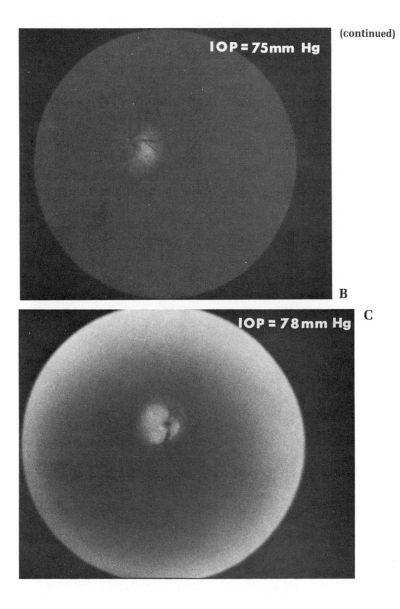

(continued)

IOP = 75mm Hg

B

IOP = 78mm Hg

C

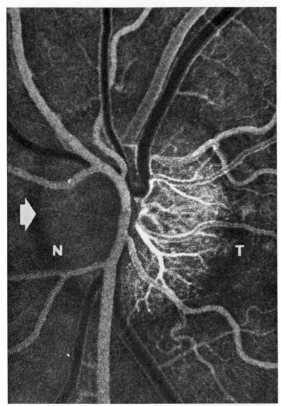

N

T

D

E

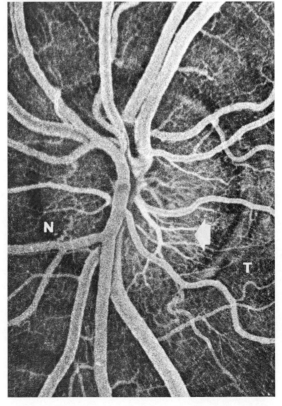

N

T

circumstances, an unobstructed view of the lamina cribrosa is obtained (Fig. 2-9C), and fluorescence from the postlaminar capillaries is less absorbed by blood in the overlying papillary vasculature.

Prelaminar Capillaries

A second set of capillaries, also of ciliary origin, lies more anteriorly in the prelaminar area of the optic nerve head.[24, 25] The perfusion of these vessels is dependent on the level of IOP, and they do not fill when the IOP is above systolic retinal artery pressure. During routine angiography, these vessels fill simultaneously with the larger choroidal vessles (Fig. 2-9D). The fluorescence is homogeneous and increases in intensity throughout the early stages of angiography. It is accentuated by transmitted fluorescence from the above-described posterior plexus of capillaries. The fluorescence from this plexus of vessels is best appreciated before dye has filled the overlying retinal capillaries. The fluorescence is usually sharply demarcated from that of adjacent choroidal vasculature by a nonfluorescent rim, corresponding to the connective tissue border of the papilla and posterior limit of the choroidal vasculature (Fig. 2-9D–*arrow*). When a cilioretinal vessel is present, the two plexuses fill simultaneously.

This plexus is derived largely from the short posterior ciliary vessels and the circle of Zinn and Haller, with substantial contributions from the peripapillary choroidal vasculature. These capillaries fill normally in the presence of a central artery occlusion.[24]

Retinal Capillaries

The most anterior capillary plexus of the optic nerve head is derived from the retinal circulation, apparent as a network of vessels lying in the superficial nerve fibers of the optic disc (Fig. 2-9E–*arrow*). The individual vascular radicles are delineated in high-contrast angiograms. Some of these capillaries arise from branches of the central retinal artery at the optic disc (Fig. 2-9E) and ramify in a stratified arrangement in the nerve fiber layer of the papilla, gradually merging into the peripapillary vessels of the retina. Others have their origin from the peripapillary retinal arterioles, and then traverse the disc edge in retrograde fashion in the nerve fiber layer to supply the superficial papilla. These vessels attain peak fluorescence during the mid-retinal venous phase of angiography in sequence with the filling of the retinal capillaries at the posterior pole of the eye. The capillaries drain into the central retinal vein. They are especially dense in the temporal papilla, and perfuse first in this region (Fig. 2-9D). It is this plexus of vessels that becomes dramatically dilated in papilledema and central retinal vein obstruction.

Under normal circumstances, the fluorescence apparent at the optic disc in the early stages of angiography is a reflection of dye in the various capillary networks. There is no leakage of dye from the retinal capillaries at the nerve head, nor from the deeper capillaries of posterior ciliary origin. However, some dye does penetrate the peripapillary choriocapillaris to reach the peripheral tissues of the papilla, becoming loosely bound to the connective tissue of the lamina cribrosa. This accounts for the prolonged fluorescence of the optic disc still obvious 10 to 15 minutes following injection of dye. Pseudofluorescence of the disc may be apparent in the late stages of angiography, particularly if high intensities of illumination, overlapping filter pairs, and an abnormally pale optic disc are present. The normal fluorescence of the optic disc may be masked to a variable degree by pigment accumulation on or adjacent to the disc. Absence or retraction of the retinal pigment epithelium (e.g., crescents) results in hyperfluorescence, owing to the unmasking of the choroidal fluorescence. Excessive deposition of pigment results in absence or diminution of fluorescence. As pigment variations are common at the edge of the optic disc, these factors are important in the interpretation of the angiograms.

RETINAL HEMODYNAMICS

Angiography has provided the first practical method of recording changes in retinal and choroidal hemodynamics in man. Intracarotid injection of dye is necessary to provide a sharp edge to the dye front in the retinal vessels and to facilitate precise tracking of the leading edge on photographs as the dye passes along the retinal arteries. However, using high concentrations of dye and rapid intravenous injections, some assessment can be made of the retinal circulation time by studying the dye transit time between different points in the retinal arterial and venous circulations. Detection of peak fluorescence in the retinal artery and then in the retinal veins can be achieved by applying densitometric techniques to the fluorescein film negatives. Hickam and Frayser,[26] using a time concentration curve of fluorescein from successive photographs, derived a mean (4.7 sec ± 1.1 sec) for dye to pass arterial and venous points in the circulation at the posterior pole of the eye.

The circulation time varies widely between the rapidly filling macular circulation (an average of 3 seconds) and the more slowly filling peripheral retinal circulation (an average of 9 seconds).

To assess the velocity of flow in the arterioles, cinematographic techniques of recording are necessary. Using such techniques, the velocity of the axial stream in the largest retinal arteries was found to be between 20 and 40 mm per second. Dollery,[16] using arterial injection and cinephotography with image intensification, introduced a quantitative method to measure flow in the retinal circulation. He calculated the volume flow rate to the superior temporal retinal artery in man to be approximately 7 microliters per minute. It is important when assessing transit time of fluorescein in the retinal circulation that the two points to which the transit time refers be quoted. However, for practical purposes, detection of defects in retinal hemodynamics remains approximate. Because of the difficulty in visualizing the choroidal circulation by fluorescein angiography, no accurate measurements of circulation time within these vessels have yet been achieved.

EFFECTS OF INDUCED OCULAR HYPERTENSION ON NORMAL RETINAL, CHOROIDAL, AND OPTIC DISC CIRCULATION

By means of suction ophthalmodynamometry, it is possible to effect an acute rise in intraocular pressure. This technique, in combination with fluorescein angiography, presents a convenient method of measuring the intraocular pressures at which the retinal and choroidal vessels fill with dye.[11] The intraocular pressure is raised to just above central retinal artery pressure, the end point registered as cessation of retinal arterial pulsation at the optic disc, as observed through the fundus camera. An injection of 5 ml of 10% fluorescein is then given intravenously, and 15 seconds later, when the dye is judged to have reached the eye, angiograms are recorded while the intraocular pressure is reduced at a constant rate. No untoward side effects have been reported with the use of this technique, but considerable caution should be exercised with older patients, particularly in the length of time the intraocular pressure is maintained above central retinal artery pressure. This test is not advocated in patients with retinopathy of any nature, as considerable stress may occur within the microvasculature.

The intraocular pressures corresponding to the negative pressure exerted by the suction cup may be calculated from previously established charts or by repeating the experiment, correlating each level of suction cup pressure with an applanation tonometric reading.

Table 2-3 shows the sequence of dye appearance in the various radicles of the ocular circulation as the IOP is reduced. In general, the retinal and choroidal circulations appear to fill at almost identical levels of intraocular pressure.

TABLE 2-3

Sequence of Fluorescein Appearance in the Retinal, Choroidal, and Papillary Circulations with Reductions in Intraocular Pressure from Levels above Central Retinal Artery Systolic Pressure

	Retinal Vessels	Choroidal Vessels	Comment
Decreasing IOP	First-order arteries	First-order arteries	Fill at equivalent levels of intraocular pressure (IOP).
	Branch arteries	Branch arteries	Fill at equivalent levels of intraocular pressure. Temporal retinal and choroidal vessels fill at higher levels of IOP than their nasal counterparts.
	Capillaries	Choriocapillaris	Earliest filling of the choriocapillaris occurs at slightly higher levels of IOP than the retinal capillaries. Completion of filling occurs at equivalent levels of IOP. The temporal choriocapillaris and retinal capillaries fill at higher levels of IOP than their nasal counterparts.
	Superficial papillary vessels		Fill at slightly lower levels of IOP than the retinal capillaries at the posterior pole.

At levels above the retinal systolic pressure, no dye is visible in either retinal or choroidal vessels. The papilla, however, may fluoresce because of dye in the postlaminar capillaries, which are unaffected by the induced intraocular hypertension. As the IOP falls below the central retinal artery systolic pressure, dye appears in the central retinal artery, corresponding with the first pulsations of this vessel. As the IOP is decreased (to 71 mm Hg, in this case, Figs. 2-10A and B), dye slowly advances along the retinal arteries, characterized by a conoid edge to the dye front. Filling of the larger choroidal vessels from the perforating short posterior ciliary vessels can also be identified at this stage (Fig. 2-10B — *arrow*). There is, however, no capillary filling in either the retinal or choroidal circulations at this pressure. Cilioretinal arterioles, if present, likewise perfuse with dye at this level of intraocular pressure. The fluorescence of the optic disc at this stage represents dye posterior to the lamina cribrosa.

Further reduction in intraocular pressure (to 66 mm Hg) permits filling of the smaller retinal arteries and second-order choroidal

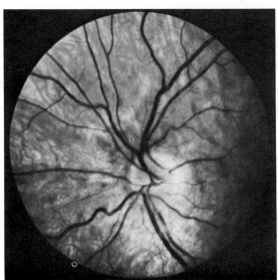

A

(continued)

FIG. 2-10A. Left optic disc and posterior pole of a universal albino. The choroidal vasculature is visible. B. Angiogram of same area as Fig. 2-10A taken 18 seconds after fluorescein injection and with IOP at 71 mm Hg. Dye has entered the central retinal artery trunk and progressed to the area of its major branches. Dye is present in one of the major choroidal arteries (arrow). Fluorescence of the disc is visible. C. Angiogram with IOP at 66 mm Hg. Dye fills second-order branches of the major retinal and choroidal arteries. The fluorescence at the optic disc has intensified. D. Angiogram taken with IOP at 61 mm Hg. Dye perfuses the terminal retinal arterioles. Early filling of the choriocapillaris (Ch) is evident superotemporal to the optic disc (arrow). Further filling of large and intermediate-sized choroidal vessels occurs at the posterior pole. E. Angiogram taken with intraocular pressure at 58 mm Hg. The retinal capillary phase is complete, and dye is now apparent in the major retinal veins on the temporal aspect of the fundus. Note that the choriocapillaris and retinal capillaries on the temporal aspect of the fundus fill at higher levels of IOP than those situated nasally. F. Angiogram taken with intraocular pressure at 52 mm Hg. Dye is now apparent in the major retinal veins and homogeneous filling of the choriocapillaris is present at macular and perimacular areas. There is still a marked difference in the extent of choroidal filling at the nasal and temporal aspects of the fundus.

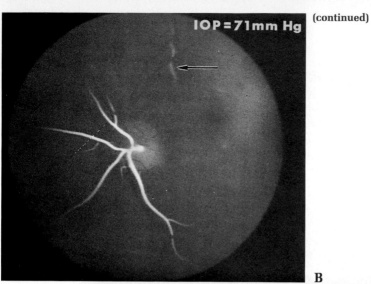

(continued)

B

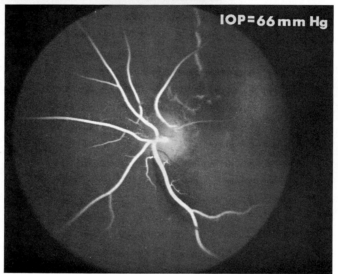

C

D

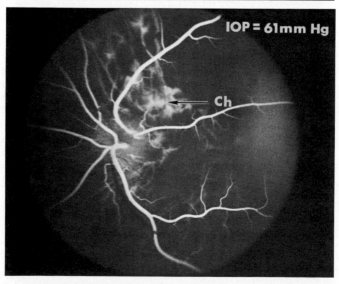

(continued)

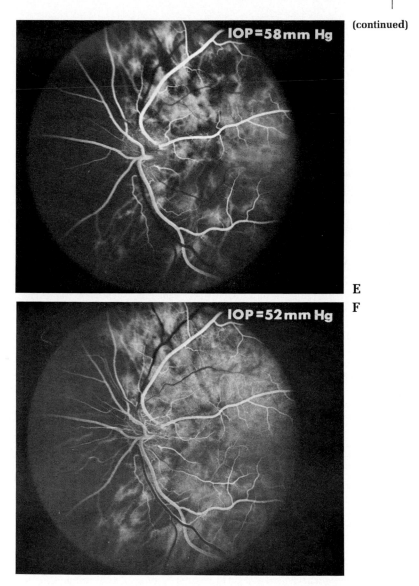

IOP=58mm Hg

IOP=52mm Hg

E

F

vessels (Fig. 2-10C). Subsequent reduction in pressure (to 61 mm Hg) permits choriocapillaris perfusion, seen initially as isolated patches of fluorescence at the posterior pole (Fig. 2-10D). There is coincident perfusion of scattered retinal capillary beds, especially at the posterior pole and optic disc. Heightened fluorescence of the papilla at this time is caused by filling of the prelaminar and retinal capillary network of the papilla (Fig. 2-10D). With additional reduction in intraocular pressure (to 58 mm Hg), choriocapillaris filling proceeds centrifugally (Fig. 2-10E). The larger choroidal vessels and choriocapillaris perfuse at a higher pressure level in the temporal fundus compared with the nasal fundus (Fig. 2-10E). Eventually these patches of dye-filled chorio-capillaris coalesce, forming a uniform fluorescent background (at 52 mm Hg) (Fig. 2-10F). The retinal capillaries are likewise filled, and some dye is apparent in the retinal veins.

FIG. 2-11A. *Midretinal venous phase angiogram of left macula of a patient with diabetic retinopathy. Note gross alteration in structural organization of the small capillaries at this area (compare with the normal macula, Fig. 2-7D). Capillaries show marked variation in caliber and distortion of their form. In some areas fusion of adjacent capillaries occurs (arrow). Multiple microaneurysms (M) are present throughout the angiographic field. Some are highly fluorescent and leak dye beyond their lumens. In some areas there is complete absence of capillaries. B. Black and white photograph of the left posterior eyegrounds of a 28-year-old diabetic female. Small hemorrhages, occasional microaneurysms, and hard exudates are evident. Little is seen of the retinal microvasculature. C. Midretinal venous phase angiogram of same area as in Fig. 2-11B. Note the myriad micro-aneurysms, defects of capillary architecture, dilated hairpinlike capillaries (arrow), and areas of defective capillary circulation (D). (From Krill, A. E., et al. Amer. J. Ophthal. 72:299, 1971.) D. Left fovea (F) and macular region of a patient with left inferotemporal branch vein obstruction. Note the dilated capil-laries and collaterals (C) transferring venous blood from the area of impaired drainage across the macula to the unimpaired superotemporal retina. Capillary disorganization and microaneurysms are apparent. Widespread areas of non-perfused (NP) retina are evident in the inferior macula. E. Late retinal venous angiogram of patient with left superotemporal branch vein obstruction (bottom arrow at site of obstruction). The highly developed collateral circulation is suffi-cient to overcome the circulatory embarrassment. There is no significant delay in circulation time in the obstructed quadrant. A large shunt directly connects the dilated capillary complexes with an unobstructed branch of the superotem-poral vein (S). F. Late venous phase angiogram of patient with Leber's miliary aneurysms involving right macula. Note the telangiectatic arrangement of vessels at the right posterior eyegrounds. Multiple microaneurysms are outlined and stain with dye. Some of the major retinal vessels also show extensive staining of their walls (arrow). A large preretinal hemorrhage (H) along the superotemporal veins is seen as an area of non-fluorescence. G. Leber's miliary aneurysms of the left inferotemporal peripheral retina with abnormal telangiectatic vessels and microaneurysms adjacent to an area of nonperfused retina. The peripheral fluorescent choroid outlines the nonperfused retinal capillaries as negative figures (NP). H. Left posterior eyegrounds of a patient with diabetic retinopathy illustrated in Fig. 2-11C. This patient has had extensive photocoagulation. Note the changes that have occurred in the microvasculature of the eye. There is less congestion of the capillary network. Many of the hairpinlike capillaries have become attenuated (compare arrows, Fig. 2-11C and Fig. 2-11H), although there are still substantial capillary structural defects throughout the posterior eyegrounds. (From Krill, A. E., et al. Amer. J. Ophthal. 72:299, 1971).*

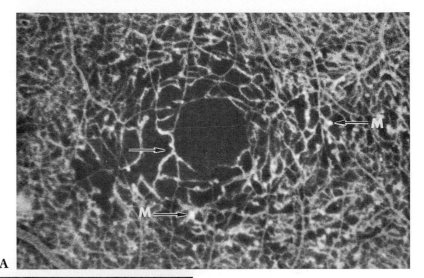

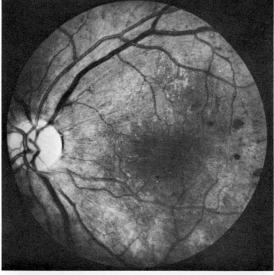

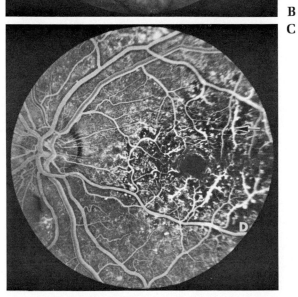

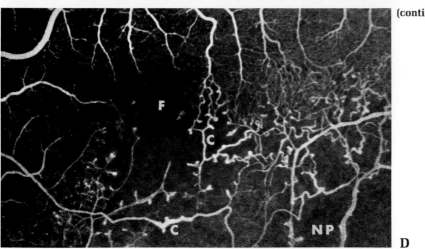

D

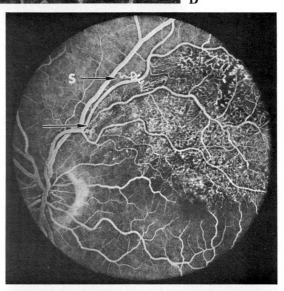

E

F

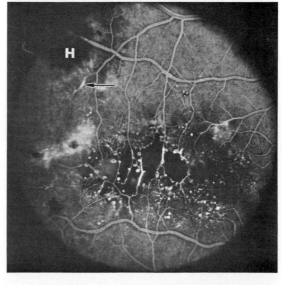

(continued)

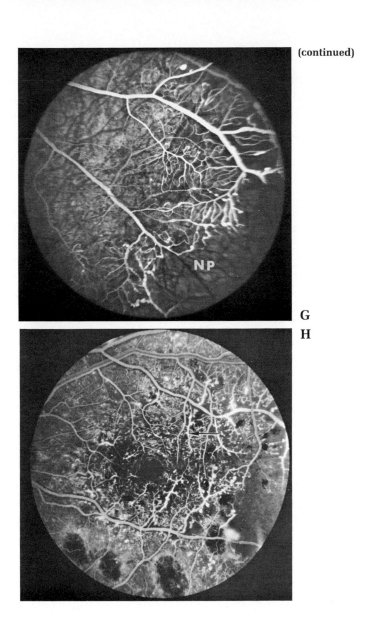

G

H

ABNORMALITIES OF THE RETINAL VASCULATURE AND CIRCULATION

IDENTIFICATION OF STRUCTURAL ABNORMALITIES

Because of their tight endothelial junctions, the retinal capillaries do not leak measurable amounts of fluorescein. The contrast afforded thus permits high angiographic resolution of these vessels. Indeed, under optimal optical conditions the smallest retinal capillaries (5 to 10 μ diameter) can be seen. These vessels are well beyond the optical resolution of the ophthalmoscope or biomicroscope and cannot be seen on color photography. It is therefore not surprising that fluorescein angiography has been of particular diagnostic value in elucidating those diseases which primarily affect the small retinal vessels, particularly the capillaries.

In diabetic retinopathy [31] fluorescein angiography reveals multiple microstructural vascular alterations that would otherwise elude conventional methods of examination. Irregularities within the capillary framework at the posterior pole become obvious. Tortuosity, kinking, dilatation, fusing, and stunting of the microvasculature are vividly displayed (Fig. 2-11A). These microangiographic aberrations as seen on fluorescein angiography closely correlate with those observed in trypsin digest specimens in diabetic retinopathy.[34]

Microaneurysms

Microaneurysms appear dramatically, scattered throughout the posterior pole as myriads of small saccular outpouchings from dilated capillaries (Fig. 2-11A). Occasionally small afferent and efferent vessels are visible, leading to and from the microaneurysms. Microaneurysms fill with dye during the late arterial phase of angiography and empty during the late retinal venous stage. Some, however, retain dye well into the residual stages of angiography. In general, microaneurysms can be easily differentiated from small round hemorrhages situated deeply within the retina. The latter do not fluoresce and present as negative figures in striking contrast with the adjacent fluorescent retina. The underlying choroidal fluorescence is also quenched by the absorption of these fluorescent wavelengths by the hemoglobin molecules. Occasionally microaneurysms become thrombosed and do not fill with dye. These are difficult to differentiate from small intraretinal hemorrhages. Less frequently the afferent vessel to the microaneurysm becomes occluded, and both radicles appear as negative figures against the fluorescent choriocapillaris.

Dilated Capillaries and Shunt Vessels

The development and evolution of dilated, hairpinlike capillaries (Figs. 2-11B and C) and shunt vessels occurring in diabetic retinopathy or other retinal vascular diseases can be clearly defined by fluorescein angiography, and their close relationship to deficient areas of capillary perfusion demonstrated. These vessels fluoresce vividly as their defective endothelium stains with dye. Leakage of dye from these vessels into the adjacent retina is frequently noted.

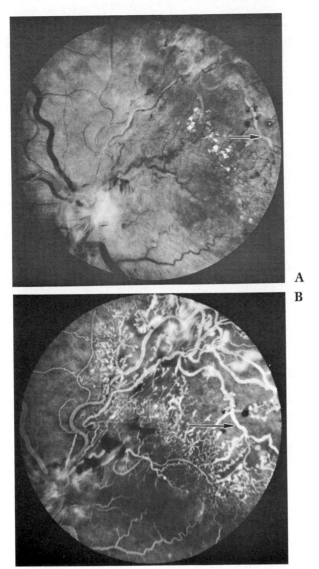

A

B

FIG. 2-12A. Black and white picture of left superotemporal fundus of patient with hypertension and superotemporal branch vein obstruction. Many of the arterioles and veins in the affected quadrant appear to be occluded (arrow). (From Krill, A. E., et al. Arch. Ophthal. 85:48, 1971.) B. Venous phase angiogram of the same patient as in Fig. 2-12A. Many of the apparently occluded vessels are perfused with fluorescein (compare arrows). (From Krill, A. E., et al. Arch. Ophthal. 85:48, 1971.)

Surface Neovascularization

Developing sites of surface neovascularization are easily identified by their irregular architecture, preretinal location, and incompetence to dye (Figs. 2-14C and 2-17A). New retinal vessels are best appreciated during the early retinal venous phase of angiography, before profuse leakage of dye masks their fine structure. In some instances of extensive neovascularization, the feeding arterioles may be identified, facilitating their subsequent occlusion by photocoagulation.

Collateral Vessels and Congenital Malformations

In instances of branch arterial or venous obstruction, the dilated capillary bed can be displayed dramatically (Fig. 2-11D). The development of the collateral circulation can be traced with ease and some determination made of the efficacy of these vessels in bypassing the obstruction (Fig. 2-11E). Congenital malformations of the retinal vascular bed are particularly amenable to study by fluorescein angiography. The extent of telangiectatic patterns in Leber's miliary aneurysms (Figs. 2-11F and G), Coats' disease, and von Hippel's disease can be clearly demarcated.

Aberrations of Larger Retinal Vessels

Aberrations of the larger retinal vessels, such as beading, outpouchings, and loops, may also be outlined by angiography. Staining of the vessel walls at these sites is characteristic due to injury of the endothelial cells. Advance lesions may feature frank leakage of dye into the retina.

ASSESSMENT OF PATENCY OF RETINAL VESSELS

Angiography provides an accurate estimation of the vascular lumen diameter. Fluorescein mixes freely with plasma, including that peripheral to the axial red-cell column. Thus, most vessels appear wider on fluorescein angiography (approximately 15 percent) as compared with direct observation. In a large variety of retinal vascular diseases, sclerosis of the vessel wall occurs. This may obstruct, to varying degrees, the ophthalmoscopic vision of the red-cell column; indeed, at times such vessels appear occluded. Fluorescein, because of its high contrast, can be visualized in these vessels, clearly outlining the lumen and indicating the true status of vascular patency (Figs.

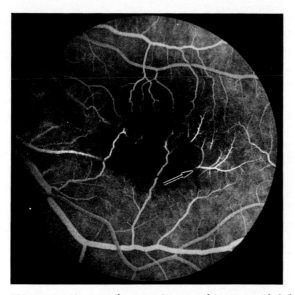

FIG. 2-13. Venous phase angiogram of patient with left inferotemporal branch artery occlusion. A small complex of dilated collaterals attempting to bypass the obstruction is outlined. Note the hyperfluorescent and granular column of dye proximal to the obstruction. Retrograde flow of dye is noted in the peripheral portions of the obstructed vessel (arrow).

2-12A and B—arrows). In benign and malignant hypertensive retinopathy and in retinal degeneration, e.g., retinitis pigmentosa,[36] angiography gives a more valid indication of the degree of vascular attenuation and the degree to which the retinal blood supply is impoverished.

DETERMINATION OF ARTERIAL, VENOUS, AND CAPILLARY OBSTRUCTION

Large Vessel Obstruction

Angiography is used to accurately delineate and pinpoint sites of obstruction within the retinal arteries and veins.[15] As the majority of vascular occlusions within the eye are transitory or incomplete, it is unusual to see total obstruction of a major retinal vessel on angiography. Also, on account of the high diffusion properties of fluorescein, vascular obstruction must be virtually complete before the fluorescent column is interrupted. The actual site of occlusion is often characterized by an area of hyperfluorescence, resulting from stasis and concentration of fluorescein at that point (Fig. 2-13). Gross sluggishness of dye circulation occurs at and beyond sites of incomplete obstruction. When sufficiently severe, the fluorescent column becomes fractionated, with alternating areas of hyperfluorescent and nonfluorescent blood (Fig. 2-13). This phenomenon indicates severe stasis of the bloodstream with clumping of the red blood cells. The aggregations of red blood cells absorb the fluorescent wavelengths and appear nonfluorescent,

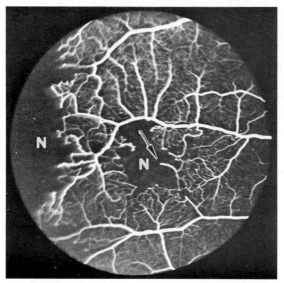

A

FIG. 2-14A. *Right temporal periphery of patient with SC (sickle-cell) disease. Note points of arteriolar and capillary obstruction (arrow). The nonperfused capillary bed corresponding to the obstructed arteriole and capillaries is denoted* **N**. *Background choroidal fluorescence can be seen in this area.* B. *Right super- otemporal eyegrounds of patient with advanced diabetic retinopathy. Areas of neovascularization along superotemporal vein and a large preretinal hemorrhage along the superior branch of the superotemporal vein are apparent. Microaneu- rysms, hard exudates, and intraretinal hemorrhages are evident at the right macula. Several areas of infarcted retina (cotton wool spots) are noted superior to the macula. (From Krill, A. E., et al. Arch. Ophthal. 85:48, 1971.)* C. *Mid- venous phase angiogram of area described in Fig. 2-14A. Arrow points to area of capillary nonperfusion, corresponding to sites of cotton wool spots. Note com- plete absence of background fluorescence at this point due to intraretinal edema. Superior to this zone are further areas of nonperfused retina; however, in these areas the choroidal fluorescence is apparent due to the absence of intraretinal edema. Retinal neovascularization* (**NV**) *is outlined superior to the optic disc. (From Krill, A. E., et al. Arch. Ophthal. 85:48, 1971.)* D. *Midretinal venous phase angiogram of same area shown in previous photograph, following photo- coagulation. Reperfusion of the retina in the region of the cotton wool spots has taken place. Disappearance of most of the new vessels at the optic disc and in the superotemporal retina has occurred. Compare identical arrow sites in Fig. 2-14C and Fig. 2-14D. (From Krill, A. E., et al. Arch. Ophthal. 85:48, 1971.)*

(continued)

B

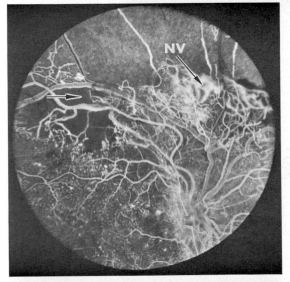

NV

C

D

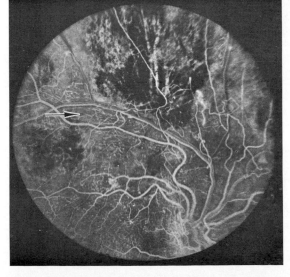

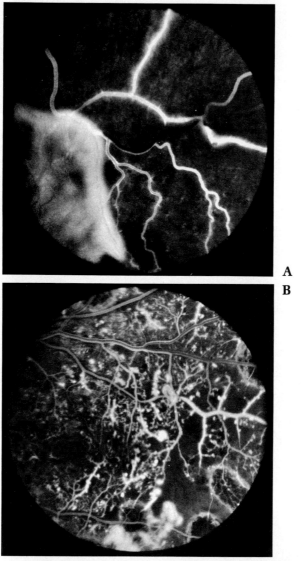

A

B

FIG. 2-15A. *Superotemporal eyegrounds of a patient with branch retinal vein obstruction. New retinal vessels overlying the optic disc fluoresce brightly. Note absence of capillary network and marked staining of retinal vessels with leakage of dye beyond their lumens, particularly in the superior vessels. B. Posterior pole of patient with diabetic retinopathy. Note widespread leakage of dye from the smaller retinal vessels. (From Krill, A. E., et al. Arch. Ophthal. 85:48, 1971.)*

and conversely the intervening plasma column fluoresces brightly (Fig. 2-13). Retrograde filling of the obstructed artery may be easily demonstrated (Fig. 2-13 — *arrow*).

Capillary Obstruction and Nonperfusion

In many vascular diseases, obstruction occurs at a precapillary and capillary level – e.g., diabetic retinopathy, malignant hypertension, collagen diseases and sickle-cell retinopathy. Fluorescein angiography dramatically indicates the obstructed vessels (Fig. 2-14A) as well as accurately depicting areas of capillary closure and nonperfusion (indicated as N in Fig. 2-14A). Nonperfused areas of the retinal capillary bed are sharply outlined by the surrounding fluorescent capillary bed (Fig. 2-14A). The choroidal background fluorescence is usually visible through these areas of nonperfusion, silhouetting the empty capillary bed as negative figures. However, in the acute stage of retinal infarction (evident as a cotton wool spot), the extensive intraretinal edema provides an effective barrier to the underlying choroidal fluorescence, and the nonperfused retina is represented by completely nonfluorescent areas (Figs. 2-14B and C).

EVALUATION OF COMPETENCE OF RETINAL VESSELS AND CAPILLARIES

Under normal circumstances, fluorescein does not permeate beyond the lumen of the retinal vessels, although there is some adherence to, or slight staining of, the endothelial cells by fluorescein, particularly on the venous side of the circulation. Exaggerated staining of the endothelium occurs as a result of circulatory stasis, as in venous obstruction, diabetes, and malignant hypertension. In mild cases the staining occurs without leakage of dye beyond the vessel walls and is manifested on angiography as a fluorescent rim to the vessels, which remain apparent long after dye has left the retinal circulation (Fig. 2-15A).

The identification of fluorescein leakage beyond the vascular lumen indicates a breakdown of the blood-retinal barrier. This occurs in a wide variety of traumatic, inflammatory, and degenerative diseases of the retinal vasculature at arterial, arteriolar, and capillary levels (Figs. 2-15A and B).

Cystoid Macular Edema

Sudden or prolonged lowering of the intraocular pressure, e.g., following trauma or surgery to the eye or chronic inflammatory disease of the choroid, often results in altered permeability of the retinal capillaries, particularly at the macula. Fluid extravasating from these vessels accumulates in the inner plexiform and nerve fiber layer and is often referred to as cystoid macular edema.

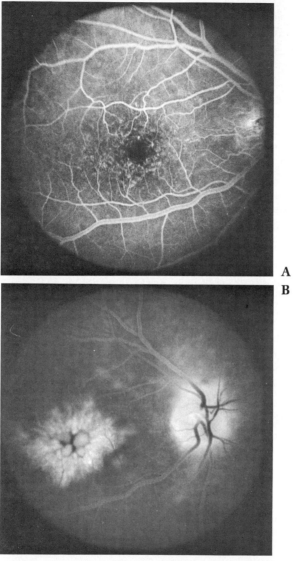

A

B

FIG. 2-16. *Patient with right cystoid macular edema following cataract extraction. A. Midretinal venous phase of angiogram showing pinpoint areas of dye leakage from defective retinal capillaries at the macula. Note concentric arrangement of dye spots corresponding to the architecture of the microvasculature at this point. B. Ten-minute angiogram. Note widespread accumulation of dye within the plexiform and nerve fiber layers of the retina. The characteristic petaloid areas of dye pooling are seen. Hyperfluorescence of the papilla with extension of dye beyond the disc edges signifies disc edema.*

In this disease characteristic angiographic findings occur and may be particularly helpful in diagnosis. Small foci of dye leakage from the perifoveal and macular capillaries become apparent during the mid-retinal phase of angiography (Fig. 2-16A). During the later stages of angiography these areas of dye leakage expand, resulting in a characteristic mottled fluorescence of the macula. The central areas of fluorescence in the residual stages of angiography (often up to one hour) frequently assume circular or hexagonal forms, demarcated from their neighbors by thin nonfluorescent borders (Fig. 2-16B). This pattern probably represents the accumulation and concentration of dye within the cystoid spaces of the retina. Such accumulation of fluid at the macula is present to some degree after many cataract extractions. However, in the majority of cases there is rapid recovery, and return to normal capillary permeability. Angiography is of considerable help in identifying macular edema as the cause of impaired vision following cataract extraction, particularly where the edema is subtle in nature.

Neovascularization

Newly formed retinal vessels, both on the surface of the retina and proliferating into the vitreous, characteristically leak fluorescein into the adjoining retinal tissue or vitreous. This is probably due to the poorly developed junctional complexes between the newly formed endothelial cells which fail to contain the dye. The characteristic lack of pericytes in these vessels may also contribute to their permeability to fluorescein. Angiography therefore provides a valuable method for identification of such vessels in diabetes, sickle-cell disease (Figs. 2-17B and C), branch vein obstruction (Fig. 2-17A), Eales' disease, and polycythemia. Angiography also provides a convenient means to assess the efficacy of treatment aimed at the attenuation or obliteration of these vessels—i.e., photocoagulation (Figs. 2-17B, C, and D) or hypophysectomy.

Hemorrhages

Retinal hemorrhages produce a negative fluorescent pattern, having a profound filtering effect on the retinal and choroidal fluorescence. Preretinal hemorrhages quench both the retinal and choroidal fluorescence (Figs. 2-18A and B). The fluorescent pattern is analogous to the cotton wool spot, although the borders are usually more sharply demarcated. Intraretinal hemorrhages are apparent on angiography as small circular areas of nonfluorescence; an occasional dye-filled capillary may be observed on its surface. Subretinal hemorrhages mask the choroidal fluorescence, but interfere little with the retinal fluorescence.

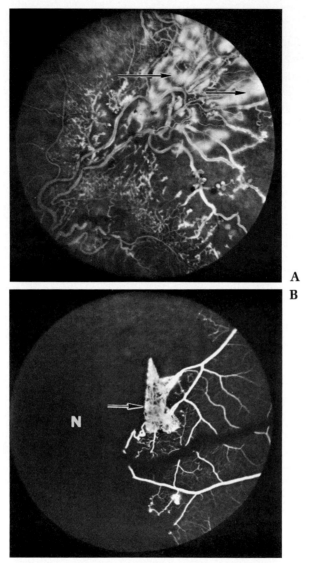

A

B

FIG. 2-17A. *Late venous angiogram of a patient with left superotemporal branch vein obstruction. Areas of retinal neovascularization fluoresce brightly (arrows). These vessels border ischemic retina which is demarcated by microaneurysms and dilated capillaries. Large-vessel disease is indicated by staining of the vessel walls. B. Temporal periphery of patient with SC (sickle-cell) disease during late venous phase angiography. Area of neovascularization is indicated by arrow. Dye leaks from these abnormal vessels. Widespread areas of nonperfused retina (N) are present temporal to the abnormal microvasculature. C. Two-minute angiogram of same area as in Fig. 2-17B. Widespread leakage of dye from areas of neovascularization. D. Same area of fundus as shown in Fig. 2-17B and Fig. 2-17C, six months after photocoagulation. Note complete disappearance of neovascularization, together with its feeding arteriole (arrow).*

(continued)

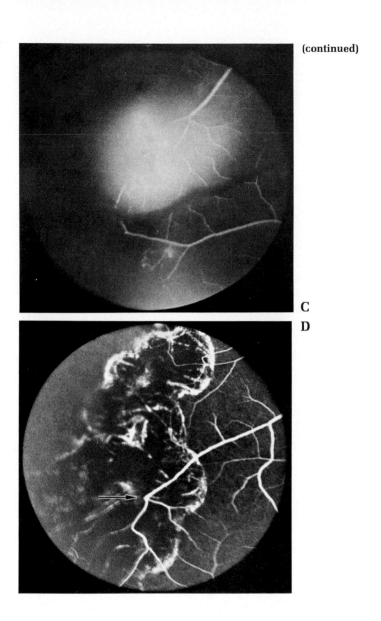

C

D

DETECTION OF ALTERATIONS IN RETINAL HEMODYNAMICS

Change in Circulation Times

A number of retinal vascular diseases, characterized by venous stasis, show significant changes in the retinal circulation times on angiography—e.g., central retinal vein obstruction, polycythemia, and

133

macroglobulinemia. Return of circulation times to normal levels may also be documented following therapy or resolution of the obstructive process. When disease of the retina is sectorial, an accurate comparison of the circulation time in abnormal and normal retinal vessels can be conveniently made (Figs. 2-18A and B).

Changes at Arteriovenous Junctions

Alterations in retinal hemodynamics at arteriovenous junctions can be well elucidated by the study of fluorescein flow patterns in the retinal vessels at these sites. Sclerosis of the retinal arteries and compression of the adjacent veins are reflected in changes in width and direction of the fluorescent columns. In advanced disease with marked constriction of the venous lumen, the characteristic laminar pattern of venous flow becomes turbulent in nature. This is manifested by premature coalescence of the dye lamellae with the formation of a homogeneous fluorescent column. Occasionally complete obstruction of the venous lumen results in interruption of the fluorescent column at the arteriovenous junction. The evolution of these changes can be precisely documented by fluorescein angiography.

1. *Normal Arteriovenous Junction* (Fig. 2-18C). The fluorescent columns in both the retinal artery and vein are of uniform width, and show little change in direction before and after the crossing. The laminar flow pattern is maintained throughout the region of the arteriovenous junction.

2. *Moderate Changes at the Arteriovenous Junction* (Fig. 2-18D). Alterations in caliber of the retinal arteries and veins are evident on angiography as irregular attenuations of the fluorescein column. The dye column also accurately reflects directional changes in the vein at the arteriovenous junction. The laminar pattern of dye flow is frequently preserved despite significant tortuosity of the vein and constriction of its lumen (Fig. 2-18D — arrow). Dilated capillaries and venules in the vicinity of an arteriovenous crossing often signify vascular stasis, and occasionally herald venous thrombosis at this point.

3. *Marked Changes at the Arteriovenous Junction* (Fig. 2-18E). In addition to the aforementioned findings, significant alterations in venous hemodynamics are evident at the crossing sites, as a result of critical narrowing of the retinal vein. The laminar flow pattern, which is present up to the site of the crossing, is lost for a short distance beyond, where turbulent flow produces a homogeneous

fluorescence occupying the entire width of the vessel. Laminar flow, however, is often reinstituted farther along the retinal vein.

4. *Occlusion of the Retinal Vein at the Arteriovenous Junction* (Fig. 2-18F). The arterial caliber is usually grossly attenuated at the region of the arteriovenous junction. The fluorescent column in the retinal vein is interrupted at the crossing. Dilated collateral vessels attempt to bridge the venous obstruction. No laminar flow is present in the obstructed vein due to the marked venous stasis.

CALCULATION OF PERFUSION PRESSURES WITHIN THE RETINAL CIRCULATION

By means of suction cup ophthalmodynamometry, estimations can be made of filling, at varying intraocular pressures, of the major retinal vessels at the optic disc and posterior eyegrounds. Gross discrepancies in the perfusion pressure of the major retinal vessels can often be elicited when segmental disease of the retinal vasculature is suspected. In patients with branch artery obstruction or branch vein obstruction (Fig. 2-19), low perfusion pressures can be readily discerned using this technique. Filling pressures can likewise be calculated for the retinal microvasculature, and areas of poor perfusion accentuated and identified. In general, the quality of angiograms during suction cup ophthalmodynamometry is inferior to those obtained by routine angiography, and the retinal capillary architecture is poorly defined. This technique also affords precise measurement of the central retinal artery systolic and diastolic pressures.

DOCUMENTING THE COURSE OF A DISEASE

Some quantitative evaluation of small vessel disease can be made by comparing sequential angiograms. This has been particularly useful in assessing the natural course of diabetic retinopathy,[32] especially with regard to the fate of microaneurysms and cotton wool spots. Fluorescein angiography has likewise been proved a valuable tool in monitoring the course of branch retinal vein obstruction, notably with regard to the formation of the collateral plexuses and the emergence of new blood vessels.[37] In sickle-cell retinopathy, fluorescein angiography is valuable in closely following the growth of new retinal blood vessels, as well as identifying small and new bleeding sites.

The response of the retina to ischemic insults both acute and chronic can be followed in detail by angiography. The extension of areas of nonperfused retina can be accurately recorded in diabetic retinopathy,

FIG. 2-18A. *Inferotemporal branch vein obstruction, at a site of arteriovenous crossing, marked by large preretinal hemorrhage.* B. *Midretinal to late-retinal venous angiogram indicates gross delay in venous return distal to the obstructed vessel, as compared with normal circulation in the major inferotemporal vein. Early formation of collateral vessels is evident adjacent to the obstruction. Well-formed collaterals are present in the superior macula at the site of another branch vein obstruction. (From Krill, A. E., et al. Arch. Ophthal. 85:48, 1971.)* C. *Normal arteriovenous crossing in the inferotemporal quadrant of retina. The photograph was taken during the midretinal venous phase of angiography. The retinal artery and vein are of uniform diameter. There is only slight displacement of the retinal vein at the arteriovenous crossing.* D. *Arteriovenous junction of hypertensive patient with long-standing hypertension. The retinal artery is markedly attenuated and of irregular caliber particularly at the crossing. Note the segmental narrowing of the retinal vein at the site of the crossing, together with significant displacement (arrow). Despite these changes, however, the laminar flow pattern is not interrupted. The dilated capillaries and venules in the vicinity of the arteriovenous crossing are markedly dilated, signifying local venous stasis.* E. *Inferotemporal arteriovenous crossing in a patient with long-standing hypertension. The retinal artery is somewhat attenuated. Note that the laminar pattern of dye flow is interrupted beyond the first crossing. The homogeneous fluorescent dye column (arrow) represents turbulent dye flow. Beyond the second crossing the lamellar pattern of dye flow is reinstituted.* F. *Inferotemporal arteriovenous crossing in patient with extensive arteriosclerosis. The retinal vein is grossly attenuated on both sides of the crossing. There is loss of continuity of the dye column at the arteriovenous junction (arrow). Blood is diverted around the obstructed vein by collaterals and shunts. The capillary bed of the obstructed vein is widely dilated.*

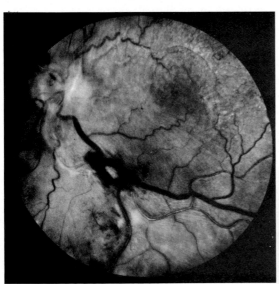

A B

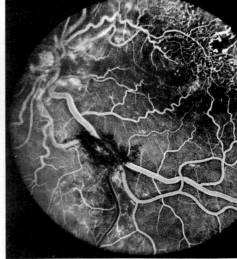

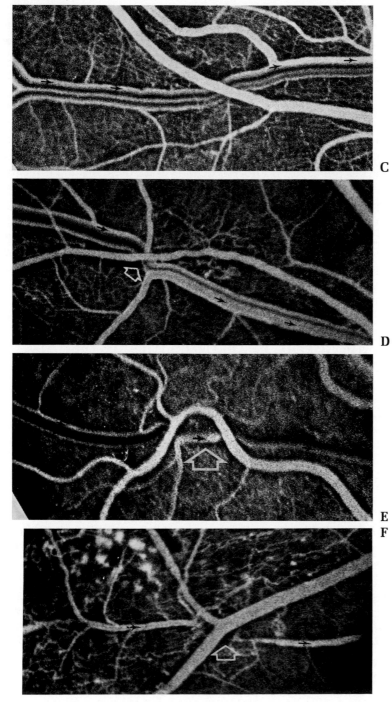

C

D

E

F

malignant hypertension, and Leber's miliary aneurysms. Likewise, reperfusion of ischemic retina, in diabetic retinopathy and following treatment in malignant hypertension, may be documented (compare Figs. 2-14C and D).

STUDYING THE EFFECTS OF TREATMENT

In many of the conditions mentioned, angiography serves as an invaluable aid in assessing the effects of treatment, particularly in controlling the use of photocoagulation in diabetic retinopathy, sickle-cell disease, and branch vein obstruction.[5]

Alterations in the number and distribution of microaneurysms and changes in the development and ramifications of hairpin capillaries and shunt vessels can all be documented with accuracy after treatment (compare Figs. 2-11C and 2-11H). The extent of the destruction of new retinal blood vessels can likewise be carefully visualized and recorded.[38] Angiography occasionally may also indicate revascularization of areas of ischemic retina.

ANGIOGRAPHY IN ABNORMALITIES OF THE CHOROIDAL VASCULATURE AND CIRCULATION

STRUCTURAL ABNORMALITIES OF THE CHOROIDAL VESSELS

Choriocapillaris

According to current knowledge, atrophy or destruction of the choriocapillaris is always associated with retinal pigment epithelial atrophy and creates a characteristic pattern on fluorescein angiography. The uniform background fluorescence is absent at the sites of choriocapillaris atrophy, and the major choroidal arteries and veins become visible throughout all phases of fluorescein angiography (Figs. 2-20A and B). Normally, these vessels are not apparent beyond the early retinal venous phase of angiography when they become obscured by dye in the choriocapillaris. The intermediate-sized choroidal vessels likewise become obvious when the choriocapillaris is absent (Fig. 2-20B).[4] These vessels can be seen to supply residual islets of choriocapillaris, which leak dye around their circumference into the neighboring choroid. This imparts a halolike appearance in the latter stages of angiography, when dye has departed from the central area of choriocapillaris.

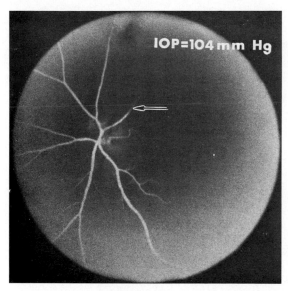

FIG. 2-19. *Angiogram taken with IOP at 104 millimeters of mercury. At this stage there is good retinal arterial filling except in the area of the vascular obstruction. Dye perfuses to the point of obstruction in the superotemporal vessel (arrow).*

Larger Choroidal Vessels

Defects of the larger choroidal vessels, in addition to choriocapillaris loss, result in total absence of choroidal fluorescence. This is the characteristic finding in choroideremia and total choroidal atrophy, of degenerative, traumatic, or inflammatory etiology. However, the denuded sclera often fluoresces in the later stages of angiography because of the loose binding of fluorescein that reaches it from the small islets of residual choriocapillaris which are invariably present, and also as a result of pseudofluorescence (Figs. 2-21A and B).

PATENCY OF THE CHOROIDAL VESSELS

Angiography provides considerable information concerning the patency of the larger and intermediate-sized choroidal vessels. In a wide variety of degenerative and atrophic diseases of the choroidal vessels, often categorized as "choroidal sclerosis," the large choroidal vessels appear narrowed on ophthalmoscopic examination. Partial or complete loss of the red-cell column is a common finding, with the vessel finally apparent as only a white or yellow cord. These blood vessels are found to be quite patent on angiography and correlate exactly with the histological studies that have been carried out in these eyes (Figs. 2-22A and B).[6]

139

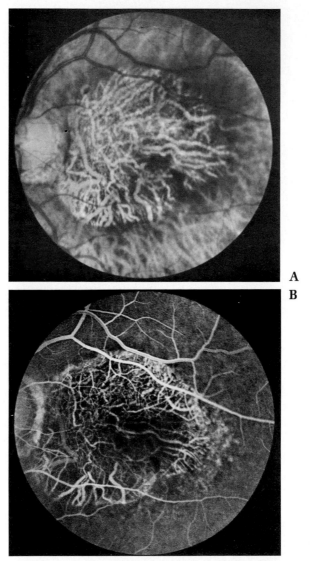

A
B

FIG. 2-20A. *Black and white photograph of posterior fundus of a patient with choriocapillaris and pigment epithelial atrophy. (From Archer, D., et al. Amer. J. Ophthal. 71:266, 1971.) B. Midretinal venous phase angiogram of same area. The larger choroidal vessels are visible throughout the angiographic series. Absence of fluorescence is apparent at sites of retinal pigment aggregation. (From Archer, D., et al. Amer. J. Ophthal. 71:266, 1971.)*

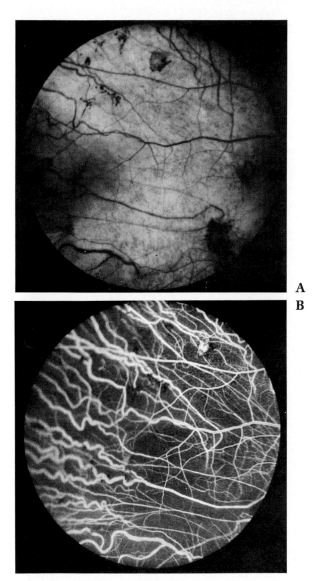

A
B

FIG. 2-21A. *Black and white photograph of the right temporal fundus of patient with subtotal choroidal atrophy. Note the almost total absence of larger choroidal vessels. Pigment is scattered throughout the fundus. (From Archer, D., et al. Amer. J. Ophthal. 71:266, 1971.) B. Midretinal venous phase angiogram of same area. Note absence of many of the larger choroidal vessels, although many more are seen than would be expected from ophthalmoscopic appearances. There is almost a total absence of choriocapillaris. The retinal capillaries fill normally. (From Archer, D., et al. Amer. J. Ophthal. 71:266, 1971.)*

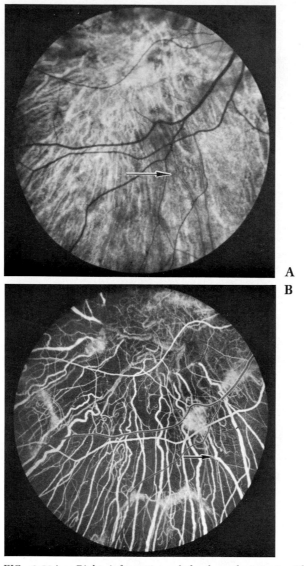

FIG. 2-22A. *Right inferotemporal fundus of patient with diffuse choroidal sclerosis. Many of the choroidal vessels appear to be completely sclerosed or obliterated (arrow). (From Archer, D., et al. Amer. J. Ophthal. 71:266, 1971.) B. Midvenous phase angiogram of an equivalent area to Fig. 2-22A, demonstrating that the majority of these vessels are patent and of near normal caliber (compare arrows). (From Archer, D., et al. Amer. J. Ophthal. 71:266, 1971.)*

FIG. 2-23A. *Right macular area of patient with multifocal choroiditis (presumed histoplasmin). The lesion is just temporal to the fovea and associated with intraretinal edema. B. Early retinal venous phase of angiography (taken at same site as in Fig. 2-23A) demonstrates areas of choroidal neovascularization. These vessels are of a larger caliber than the retinal capillaries and arranged in a net-worklike pattern. C. Three-minute angiogram indicates that these vessels profusely leak dye into the subretinal space, completely masking the vascular architecture. Note that other areas of choroidal disease now become apparent on angiography as small fluorescent spots (arrows).*

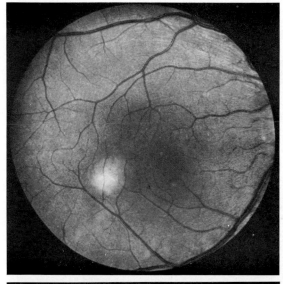

A

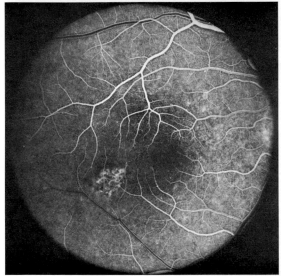

B

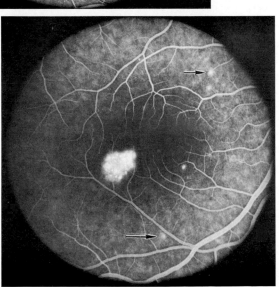

C

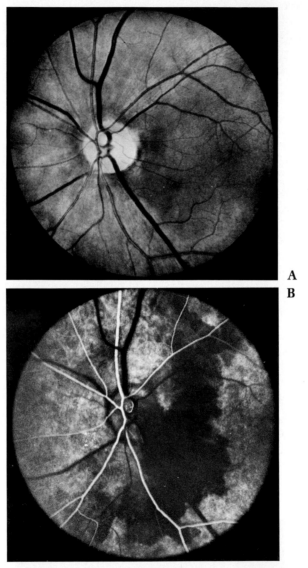

A
B

FIG. 2-24A. *Black and white photograph of left posterior eyegrounds of patient with optic atrophy. Note attenuated retinal arteries and pale optic discs, particularly the temporal portion. B. Early arterial phase angiogram demonstrates a large sector of choriocapillaris failing to perfuse with dye. A sector of the optic disc corresponding to the segment of nonperfused choriocapillaris likewise fails to fluoresce.*

CHOROIDAL NEOVASCULARIZATION

New vessels originating from the choriocapillaris frequently penetrate defects in Bruch's membrane to lie beneath the retinal pigment epithelium or within the subretinal space. These vessels are rarely obvious on routine ophthalmoscopic examination, but can be vividly demonstrated on angiography, e.g., in early multifocal (presumed histoplasmin) choroiditis. Such vessels present early in the disease process [35] and are a frequent cause of subretinal and intraretinal hemorrhage. Details of these new vessels are readily visualized only during early angiography, before profuse leakage of dye from the choriocapillaris and areas of neovascularization obscure them. They typically present as a fine interlacing network situated at the level of the retinal pigment epithelium deep to the retinal vessels. These vessels are larger than the retinal capillaries and are outlined some time before dye reaches the retinal capillary circulation (Figs. 2-23A, B, and C).

Fluorescein angiography fulfills two important clinical needs with regard to these vessels: firstly, to identify the sites and delineate the area of the vascular abnormality; secondly, to monitor the effectiveness of photocoagulation in obliterating these vessels.[35]

CHOROIDAL VASCULAR OBSTRUCTION

Obstruction of the short posterior ciliary vessels or their tributaries is an uncommon finding in ophthalmology. However, with the application of fluorescein angiography, frequent aberrations of the posterior ciliary and choroidal hemodynamics have been observed. Obstructions within the choriocapillaris itself are probably of little moment because of the freely anastomosing nature of this layer. Major defects of the larger choroidal vessels or short posterior ciliary arteries can, however, be detected as segments of choroid failing to perfuse in the early stages of angiography. Such an area is clearly demarcated by the surrounding perfused and fluorescent choriocapillaris (Figs. 2-24A and B). In the latter stages of angiography the defective zone becomes slowly perfused from the adjoining choriocapillaris and assumes a uniform fluorescence, undistinguishable from the background fluorescence elsewhere. Absence of the ciliary component of the optic nerve head circulation in early stages of angiography is a frequent finding in posterior ciliary artery obstruction.

CHOROIDAL VASCULAR PERFUSION PRESSURES

As with the retinal circulation, suction cup ophthalmodynamometry enables determination of the perfusion pressure of the choroidal bed. Precise perfusion pressure measurements of the major choroidal arteries can be obtained only in albinos, lightly pigmented subjects, and individuals with defective or absent retinal pigment epithelium — i.e., when these vessels are visible. Studies in patients with diffuse choriocapillaris atrophy indicate that there is little alteration in the perfusion pressure of the larger choroidal vessels. Perfusion of the choriocapillaris is easily identified as multiple points of fluorescence that expand centrifugally to form a uniform background fluorescence; and filling pressures can be accurately measured. There is some evidence at present suggesting a lower perfusion pressure of the peripapillary and papillary capillaries of ciliary origin in glaucomatous eyes, as compared with the normal.[10] The results, however, are not conclusive.

DISEASES OF THE RETINAL PIGMENT EPITHELIUM

As indicated previously, fluorescein passes freely from the choriocapillaris into the intravascular spaces of the choroid, and then diffuses through Bruch's membrane to the level of the pigment epithelium. Fluorescein does not appear to pass, at least in measurable quantities, anterior to the pigment epithelium in health (Table 2-1). The pigment granules of the pigment epithelium have an absorption spectrum in the same region as the emitted wavelength of fluorescein, and thus exert a filter effect on the fluorescent dye in the choriocapillaris and intravascular spaces. Changes in the pigment content or reorientation of pigment within the pigment epithelium will therefore modify the underlying fluorescence.

It is important to appreciate that not all fluorescent abnormalities of the pigment epithelium are necessarily associated with dysfunction of the pigment epithelial cell layer. In rubella retinitis, gross changes in the fluorescent pattern correspond to the depigmented and hyperpigmented areas of retina, yet there appears to be little change in the functional integrity of the epithelial cells, as assessed by vision and electrophysiological tests (see Chapter 4, *Electroretinogram*). On the other hand, in vitelliruptive macular degeneration, where a diffuse abnormality of pigment epithelial function is present, a fluorescent aberration appears only in the macular area. Thus, angiography, although a sensitive index of changes in pigment within the epithelial cells, may provide little insight into the viability or functional capacity of this layer.

Nevertheless, angiography does accurately define and accentuate characteristic patterns of pigment deficiency, e.g., the "bull's-eye" appearance of chloroquine retinopathy, as well as facilitating early diagnosis in certain situations, e.g., chloroquine retinopathy, juvenile macular degeneration, or choroidal folds, before ophthalmoscopic changes are evident. Also, in patients with retinitis pigmentosa with preservation of central vision, and where electrophysiological evaluation and often ophthalmoscopic appearance provide little prognostic insight as to macular function, angiography may reveal changes within the pigment epithelial layer indicating early involvement of this area in the disease process.[36]

CHANGES IN PIGMENT CONTENT OF THE PIGMENT EPITHELIAL CELL

Blond individuals and albinos demonstrate a benign reduction of pigment within normal cells. Likewise, in myopic and aging eyes depigmentation may occur without detectable alteration in the function of the cells. These latter changes have been labeled "depigmentation in situ" by Klien.[28] In such cases, the choroidal fluorescence is less obstructed and the background choroidal fluorescence may be intense.

Depigmentation and atrophy of the pigment epithelium as a result of trauma, inflammatory or degenerative conditions shows areas of hyperfluorescence corresponding to the affected areas. These hyperfluorescent areas demonstrate characteristic patterns on angiography (Figs. 2-25A–D). They are first apparent during the early arterial phase of angiography as the choriocapillaris becomes perfused with dye (Fig. 2-25B). The fluorescence increases in intensity, reaching a maximum during the midretinal venous phase of angiography, coincident with peak choroidal fluorescence (Fig. 2-25C). A more uniform pattern is apparent during the late venous and residual phases of angiography (Fig. 2-25D). The area of hyperfluorescence corresponds precisely with the dimensions of the pigment epithelial defect and shows no centrifugal expansion throughout angiography. During the latter stages of angiography the intensity of fluorescence diminishes, but is often detectable up to one hour after injection (Fig. 2-25D).[39] Accumulations of pigment within the pigment epithelium or retina produce areas of hypofluorescence or absence of fluorescence on angiography.

CHANGES IN ALIGNMENT OF THE PIGMENT EPITHELIAL CELLS

Changes in the alignment of the pigment epithelial cells also cause characteristic alterations in the transmission of fluorescence

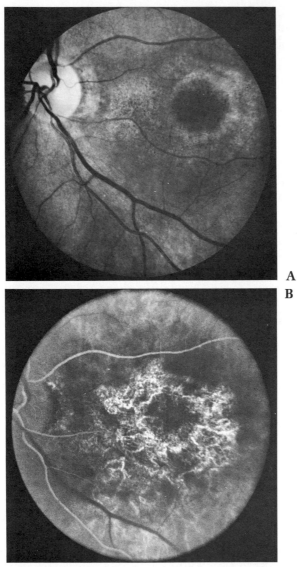

A
B

FIG. 2-25A. Black and white photograph of left macula of patient with chloroquine retinopathy. Pigmentary changes at the macula and perimacular areas, as
well as atrophy of temporal optic disc, are evident. B. Early arterial angiogram
of area described in Fig. 2-25A. Hyperfluorescence corresponding to the area of the
pigment epithelial atrophy is noted during the early arterial phase. C. Early
venous angiogram demonstrates increasing intensity of the pigmentary defect
as filling of the choriocapillaris continues. D. Late venous phase angiogram
demonstrates the pigment epithelial defect as a discrete hyperfluorescent area.
There is no spread of dye beyond the anatomical limits of the pigment epithelial
defect.

(continued)

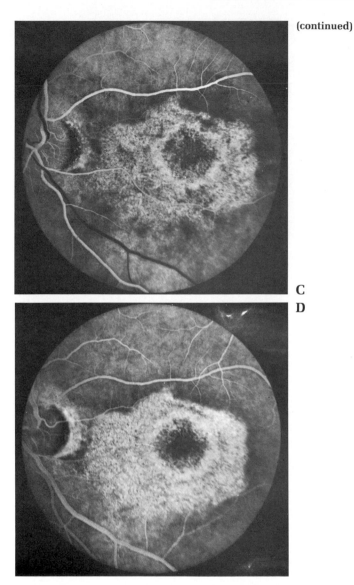

C
D

through this layer. Folds and wrinkles of the choroid and retinal pigment epithelium — e.g., in hyperthyroidism, ocular hypotony, and retrobulbar tumors — show peculiar patterns.[45] An enhanced view of the
underlying choroidal fluorescence is attained at the elevated portion
or crest of the folds, due to the attenuated pigment epithelium in this
region. This is manifested as a hyperfluorescent streak, extending the
length of the fold. The troughs of the folds appear as hypofluorescent

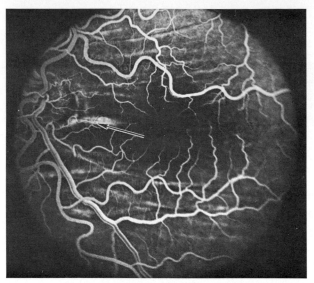

FIG. 2-26. *Midvenous phase angiogram of patient with orbital tumor and choroidal folds. The fluorescent pattern is characteristic. The crests of the folds are outlined as hyperfluorescent bands, and the troughs as hypofluorescent areas. These alternate as oblique or horizontal stripes across the posterior eyegrounds. Structural defects within Bruch's membrane or pigment epithelium fluoresce much more intensely, owing to staining with fluorescein (arrow).*

streaks, reflecting the relative increase in density of the pigment where the pigment epithelial cells are compressed in the depths of the folds, as well as the longer course taken by the fluorescent wavelengths from the choriocapillaris through the obliquely arranged pigment epithelial cells. The hyperfluorescent crests and hypofluorescent troughs alternate as horizontal or oblique striae across the posterior eyegrounds (Fig. 2-26). Staining of the pigment epithelium may occur at sites of undue stress, producing hyperfluorescent zones that persist long after dye has left the choriocapillaris. The overlying retinal vessels show no evidence of increased permeability or structural change. Folds of the internal limiting membrane of the retina—e.g., resulting from papilledema or vitreous retraction—on the contrary, demonstrate no fluorescent aberrations on angiography.

DETACHMENT OF THE PIGMENT EPITHELIUM

The pigment epithelium may become dislodged from Bruch's membrane in a wide variety of diseases, and the intervening space occupied by a consortium of pathological materials, e.g., serous fluid exudate, blood, new vessels, drusen material, and tumor. Changes in the arrangement and concentration of pigment granules within the pigment epithelial cells is a common counterpart to disturbance in the relationship between this layer and Bruch's membrane. Therefore, hyperfluorescence results from both depigmentation of the retinal pigment epithelium and alteration in the alignment of the pigment granules.

Serous Fluid

The accumulation of serous fluid beneath the retinal pigment epithelium is one of the more common disorders affecting this region and is frequently referred to as disciform detachment of the pigment epithelium or serous detachment of the pigment epithelium.[20] The fluid collecting beneath the retinal pigment epithelium originates from the choriocapillaris. The facility with which it accumulates is undoubtedly related to the high perfusion pressure in these vessels as a result of their wide diameters, sinusoidal arrangement, and direct branching from the larger choroidal arterioles. The appearance of serous fluid beneath the pigment epithelium may be idiopathic (central-serous choroidopathy) or be the forerunner of more advanced changes in the retina, as in Khunt-Junius disease or multifocal (presumed histoplasmin) inner choroiditis. Two physical barriers limit the spread of fluid at this site. The junctional complexes (zonula occludens) of the pigment epithelium cells resist anterior movement of the serous fluid; and the firm adherence of the basement membrane of the pigment epithelial cells to the inner collagenous portion of Bruch's membrane limits lateral diffusion. Serous detachments of the pigment epithelium are largely confined to the macular area, although they may be found in a variety of regions at the posterior pole, where predisposing factors exist—e.g., pits of the optic disc and chorioretinal scars.

The angiographic features are characteristic (Figs. 2-27A–D). A uniform area of hyperfluorescence, precisely related to the configuration of the detached pigment epithelium, develops in the arterial phase of angiography, simultaneous with filling of the choriocapillaris with dye (Fig. 2-27B). This area of hyperfluorescence intensifies during the dye transit (Fig. 2-27C), reaching a maximum by the late retinal venous stage of angiography (Fig. 2-27D). The zone of hyperfluorescence is usually circular, with well-defined margins, and shows little or no tendency to expand beyond the limits noted during early angiography or as defined clinically. Fluorescence gradually fades after one or two minutes, but is often discernible for as long as one hour after injection. Staining of the pigment epithelial cells probably contributes in part to this prolonged fluorescence.

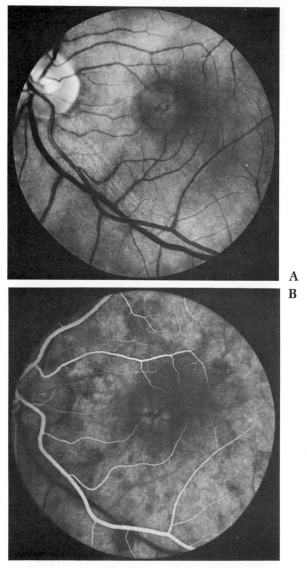

A
B

FIG. 2-27A. *Black and white photograph of left macula of patient with disciform detachment of the pigment epithelium. The lesion is outlined as a discrete elevated circular area at the left fovea. B. Early arterial angiogram shows a faint, but diffuse, accumulation of dye at the lesion concurrent with the appearance of dye in the choriocapillaris. The total lesion is fluorescent, although somewhat mottled because of overlying aggregations of pigment. C. Midretinal venous angiogram of same patient. Increasing intensity of fluorescence is apparent, discretely localized to the area of detachment. D. Two-minute angiogram shows the hyperfluorescent detached area of pigment epithelium, discretely outlined.*

(continued)

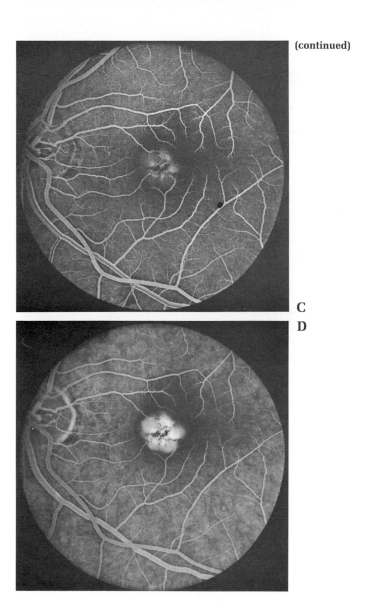

C

D

Choroidal Neovascularization and Hemorrhage

New vessels from the choriocapillaris on occasion penetrate Bruch's membrane to lie beneath the retinal pigment epithelium. Such vessels are invariably associated with detachment of the retinal pigment and changes within the overlying retinal pigment epithelial cells. Such vascular invasion occurs in the early stages of multifocal inner choroiditis and Khunt-Junius disease, and may be the precursor of extensive subretinal hemorrhage.[35] The exact stimulus initiating neovascularization from the choroid is as yet unclear; however, defects in

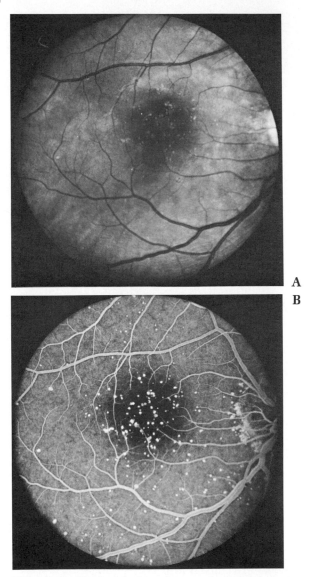

A
B

FIG. 2-28A. *Black and white photograph of right posterior eyegrounds of patient with drusen of the fundus. B. Late venous angiogram of patient in Fig. 2-28A, showing discrete hyperfluorescent spots identifying localized sites of drusen formation. They remain discrete and dye does not leak beyond their borders. There are more hyperfluorescent spots than drusen on white-light examination.*

Bruch's membrane and perhaps a hypoxic environment created by chronic serous fluid formation underneath the pigment epithelium may produce favorable conditions for the propagation of such vessels underneath and into the retina. As indicated previously (Fig. 2-23), these vessels can often be vividly demonstrated by angiography, although once hemorrhage has occurred, identification becomes difficult.

Drusen

Drusen deposits accumulate between the retinal pigment epithelium and Bruch's membrane. In the early stages of formation the drusen elevate the pigment epithelium and cause changes in the pigment content of the cell. In later stages of development, there is atrophy of the pigment epithelial cells, which is replaced by drusen material. These alterations permit an unobstructed view of the underlying choroidal fluorescence, visualized as discrete areas of hyperfluorescence on angiography, which demonstrate the sequence of changes common to any pigment epithelial defect (Figs. 2-28A and B).

BREAKDOWN OF THE RETINAL PIGMENT EPITHELIAL BARRIER

A wide variety of conditions exist where there is focal or widespread breakdown of the pigment epithelial barrier. In such instances, serous fluid traverses the pigment epithelial cell, or penetrates the tight junctions, and accumulates in the subretinal space between the pigment epithelium and the retinal receptors. This may occur as a sequel to long-standing detachment of the retinal pigment epithelium, or spontaneously without prior evidence of fluid beneath the retinal pigment epithelium. New choroidal vessels and hemorrhage likewise may gain access to the subretinal space via similar dehiscences in the pigment epithelial layer. Fluid in this region is less limited in its lateral spread and may occupy a sizable area of the embryonic vesicular space. Anterior permeation into the layers of the retina may also take place, although the compact structure of the intertwining neural cells, with almost complete absence of extracellular space, limits accumulation of fluid here.

Fluorescein angiography is of immense value in eliciting the site or sites of breakdown and delineating the extent of the subretinal fluid. Angiography is also indispensable in deciding upon the advisability of photocoagulation and assessing its effectiveness when employed.

With a focal defect, a bright fluorescent spot corresponding to the defect becomes apparent during the retinal arterial phase of angiography. As a rule, this area is small, circular, and discrete (Figs. 2-29A and B). Accumulation of dye within the subretinal space becomes ob-

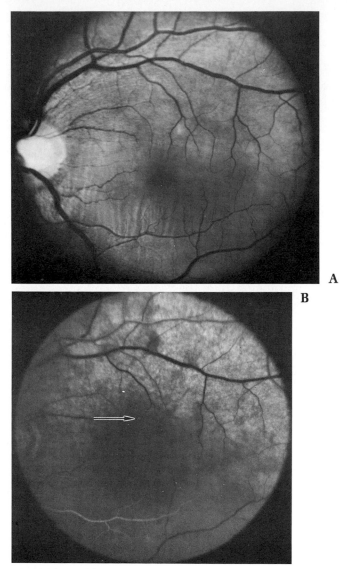

A

B

FIG. 2-29A. *Left posterior eyegrounds of patient with macular edema (black and white photograph). There is an extensive accumulation of subretinal and intra-retinal fluid at and inferior to the fovea. Vertical folds in the internal limiting membrane are present, inferior to the fovea. B. Early arterial phase angiogram of area described in Fig. 2-29A. Small hyperfluorescent spot (arrow) indicates the site of defective pigment epithelium by which dye gains access to the subretinal space. Note that this hyperfluorescent area forms simultaneously with the appearance of dye in the choriocapillaris and before any fluorescein has reached the retinal arterioles in this region. C. Midretinal venous phase angiogram. The densely fluorescent spot expands as dye enters the subretinal space. D. Three-minute angiogram shows diffusion of dye within the subretinal space. Expansion of dye occurs in all directions. E. Twenty-minute angiogram. There is widespread diffusion of dye within the subretinal space. Note that the folds in the internal limiting membrane in Fig. 2-29A show no fluorescent abnormality.*

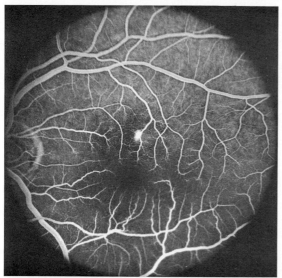

C

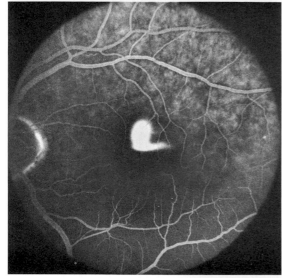

D

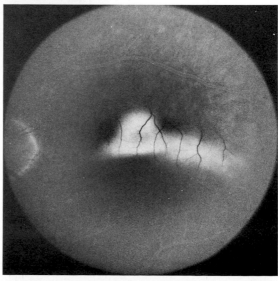

E

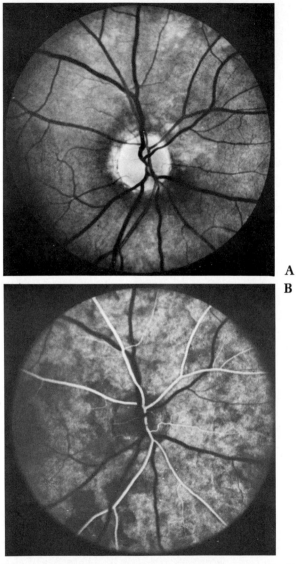

A

B

Fig. 2-30A. Black and white photograph of right optic disc of patient with pri-mary optic atrophy. B. Arterial phase angiogram of same areas as Fig. 2-30A. There is absence of fluorescence of retinal and ciliary capillary networks at the temporal aspect of the optic disc. There is some filling of the prelaminar plexus inferiorly and nasally at the papilla. C. Midretinal venous angiogram of same patient now demonstrates minimal filling of the retinal and ciliary capillary network at the optic disc. D. Late venous phase angiogram shows generalized absence of fluorescence at the disc, compared with the adjacent background fluorescence. E. Midretinal venous phase angiogram of left optic disc with optic pit. The area of optic pit is hypofluorescent (arrow).

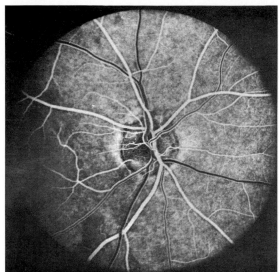

C

D

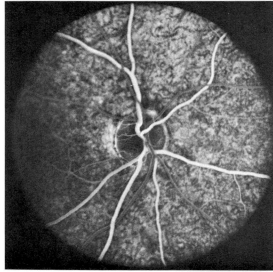

E

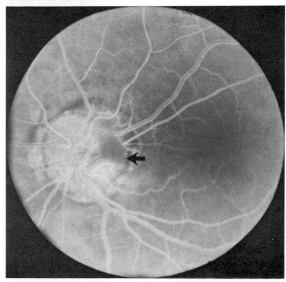

vious during the later stages of angiography as a diffuse hyperfluorescence which expands centrifugally (Fig. 2-29B). Diffusion of dye within this space is modified by gravity and possibly convection currents as a result of the temperature differential between the choroid posteriorly and inner retina anteriorly,[19] and dye may be observed tracking from an inferior leakage point to a superior position within the subretinal space. The lateral limits of dye extension are diffuse and poorly defined. Fluorescence persists for some time after dye injection, often up to one hour.

The complete spectrum of changes, beginning with alterations in Bruch's membrane, detachment of the pigment epithelium, and accumulation of fluid in the subretinal space, may be observed in a variety of diseases involving inner choroidal vasculature, as in disciform degeneration of the macula, angioid streaks, and multifocal inner choroiditis. Such changes frequently set the stage for the invasion of Bruch's membrane and inner retina by new vessels. Such vessels can be identified by fluorescein angiography; however, once hemorrhage and intraretinal scar tissue form, their presence is often difficult to detect.

ABNORMALITIES OF THE OPTIC DISC AND PAPILLARY CIRCULATION

The various vascular plexuses of the optic nerve head tend to show similar responses to disease processes involving this region. In general, there is a reduction in the number of capillaries of both retinal and ciliary origin in optic atrophy and engorgement of both capillary beds in papilledema, although in some instances of optic atrophy secondary to retinal lesions—e.g., central retinal artery obstruction—the superficial retinal capillaries are more severely affected than the prelaminar vessels of ciliary origin.

OPTIC ATROPHY

Primary Atrophy

The disappearance of vessels in both the superficial and deep networks of the papilla in optic atrophy is apparent on fluorescein angiography. The absence of the deep network of ciliary and choroidal capillaries is manifested as loss of the uniform background fluorescence during the arterial phase of angiography (Figs. 2-30A and B), and loss of the superficial retinal capillaries is indicated by failure of these radicles to fluoresce in the arteriovenous phases of dye transit (Fig. 2-30C). In the late venous phase of angiography the fluorescence at the disc is much less intense than that of the peripapillary choroid (Fig. 2-30D), whereas in normal circumstances the reverse is true (Fig. 2-7H). In the residual stages of angiography some weak fluorescence of the disc is often appreciated. This is attributed to some diffusion of fluorescein from the adjoining choriocapillaris into the substance of the nerve head and its loose binding to the connective tissue of the lamina cribrosa. Some fluorescence is also derived from recirculating dye in the small vessels supplying the lamina cribrosa and anterior optic nerve. In exceptional optic disc pallor, pseudofluorescence must be taken into account in the late residual stages of angiography.

Glaucomatous Atrophy

A peripapillary zone of compromised choroidal microvasculature is frequently noted, in association with severe glaucomatous atrophy.[25] These vessels fill sluggishly or occasionally not at all, which is evident on angiography as a hypofluorescent or nonfluorescent ring around the optic disc. This defect can be exaggerated by performing angiography under conditions of induced ocular hypertension. The peripapillary choroidal vessels, which are particularly sensitive to rises in intraocular pressure,[10] fill at much lower levels of intraocular pressure as compared with similar-sized vessels at the posterior pole.

Sectorial Atrophy

The vascular changes producing or associated with sectorial atrophy of the nerve head can likewise be fully amplified during angiography. Infarction of the optic nerve head, either partial or complete as a result of embolic or thrombotic processes within the ophthalmic or ciliary vessels, may show characteristic features on angiography. Absence or gross impairment of the capillary circulation in either the upper or lower portions of the optic disc is a common finding, often in conjunction with retarded retinal circulation times. Obstruction of one or more of the posterior ciliary vessels produces particularly striking changes during filling of the choriocapillaris. There is no fluorescence of the involved segment of choroid, which is clearly demonstrated by the surrounding dye-filled choriocapillaris (Fig. 2-24). The sector of optic disc supplied by this short posterior ciliary vessel likewise fails to fluoresce during early angiography. During the latter stages of angiography fluorescence does occur in both these deficient regions, as dye reaches these zones from the partially obstructed channels or by various collateral pathways.

OPTIC PITS

Unsuspected pits of the nerve head may become evident on angiography due to the contrast between the avascular papillary defect and the surrounding fluorescent papilla (Fig. 2-30E). Both retinal and ciliary plexuses of vessels are absent at the pit. In the late stages of angiography some faint fluorescence is apparent at the pit due to permeation of dye into the defect from the adjoining choriocapillaris. An adjoining serous detachment of the retina extending to the macula is not an uncommon associated finding. It is unusual, though, for dye to reach the subretinal space in detectable concentrations.

EDEMA OF THE OPTIC NERVE HEAD

The anatomical peculiarities of the optic nerve head, including the loose arrangement of its tissues, account for the rapid and widespread accumulation of fluid that occurs with alteration in the delicately balanced capillary perfusion pressures in this area. Edema and capillary dilatation of the various plexuses are constant counterparts of papillary swellings. Fluorescein angiography provides a convenient tool for outlining these dilated vessels, detecting even minimum amounts of fluid leakage into the nerve head, and estimating any retardation in venous filling.

In many instances — e.g., optic neuritis and ischemic optic neuropathy — edema precedes and contributes to the vascular stasis by compression of these thin-walled vessels. Most of the retinal capillaries on the surface of the disc are venous and represent the terminal portion of the peripapillary capillary plexus proximal to entering the central retinal vein. Obstruction of these vessels produces dramatic dilatation and further edema, which extends frequently several disc diameters along the peripapillary network.[8, 44]

In certain instances the primary pathological process is in the blood vessels, and edema of the nerve head is secondary — e.g., in central retinal vein obstruction. In ocular hypotony, fluid accumulates at the disc as the result of a disturbance between the hydrostatic and intraocular pressures. The mechanism of disc edema secondary to severe uveitis or pars planitis is uncertain, but may represent increased permeability of the papillary vessels to toxic by-products of the inflammatory process, or perhaps participation of the vessel walls in antigen-antibody reaction as part of a generalized vasculitis.

Papilledema

Acute optic disc swelling secondary to raised intracranial pressure (papilledema) shows characteristic features on angiography. The dilated retinal capillaries on the surface of the disc are especially conspicuous as they ramify over the disc surface and merge into the peripapillary network (Fig. 2-31A). Frequently these capillaries are photographed end-on, as they pass from one layer to another within the nerve fiber layer, giving the appearance of microaneurysmal dilatations. True microaneurysms probably are uncommon at the optic disc in papilledema. Dilatation of the prelaminar ciliary capillaries also occurs and can be best appreciated using stereo techniques; however, in the latter stages of angiography they are difficult to visualize through the dilated retinal capillary bed and extravasated fluorescein.

The dilated capillaries permit considerable extravasation of dye into the substance of the optic nerve head, and for some distance beyond the disc margin. Dye tends to spread preferentially along the major retinal vessels following the course of the peripapillary capillaries. Extension of fluid into the macular area may cause changes in the pigment epithelium, producing a mottled hyperfluorescent pattern at this site. The hyperfluorescence resulting from dye extravasation and binding to the lamina cribrosa is noticeable several hours following injection. Staining of the major retinal vessels at the optic disc, particularly the retinal veins, is common with extensive disc edema. Hemorrhages and exudates at the disc and peripapillary retina are seen as negative figures (Fig. 2-31A). Retinal circulation times in papilledema are generally within normal limits or only slightly delayed, in contradistinction to their marked delay in central retinal vein obstructions. There is no significant alteration in the filling pressures of the retinal and choroidal circulations under conditions of induced ocular hypertension.

Resolution of disc edema—as, for example, following removal of a cerebral tumor—may be accurately documented by fluorescein angiography (Fig. 2-31B). Absorption of edema is rapid, and the permeability of the retinal vessels to fluorescein is strikingly reduced. The retinal capillaries return to near normal caliber, and the margins of the optic disc again become discrete.

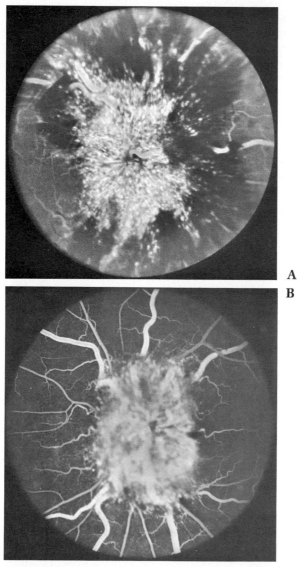

A
B

FIG. 2-31A. *Midretinal venous phase angiogram of patient with right papilledema due to sphenoidal ridge meningioma. Widely dilated incompetent capillaries are arrayed over the surface of the optic disc and for some distance beyond. Many of these capillaries photographed end-on give the appearance of microaneurysms. At the site of juxtapapillary hemorrhages, there is absence of fluorescence. B. Late venous phase angiogram of a patient with resolving papilledema. Widespread leakage of dye from the region of dilated capillaries is still evident, although the fluorescent pattern is more discrete, with less involvement of the peripapillary network.*

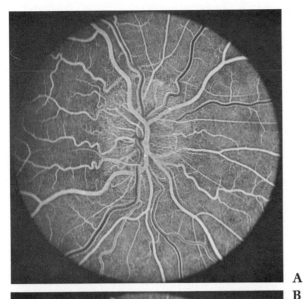

A

B

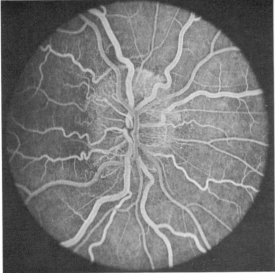

FIG. 2-32A. *Midretinal venous angiogram of patient with long-standing papil-ledema due to benign intracranial hypertension. Note that the disc fluorescence extends well beyond the normal anatomical margins. The retinal capillaries are dilated, but remain competent to dye. They merge subtly with the peripapillary network of vessels. There is little dilation of the major retinal arterioles. B. Three-minute angiogram in the same patient. The capillaries are dilated and quite obvious, although they do not leak dye even at this stage. The optic disc still has a fairly discrete, although expanded, margin.*

Chronic Papilledema

Chronic disc swelling may evolve as a result of prolonged or intermittent elevation of intracranial pressure, as in pseudotumor cerebri (Figs. 2-32A and B). Hyperfluorescence persists circumferentially for some distance beyond the disc margin, although the peripheral edge becomes more discrete with time. There are absence of dye leakage along the major retinal vessels, diminution in retinal venous staining, and little change in the retinal circulation times. The retinal capillaries remain obvious and dilated, but seem to be competent to dye, as though some equilibrium has been established in venous return from the disc by means of collateral flow to the ciliary circulation. Chronic disc swelling may result from a variety of lesions at the nerve head, but in general there are uniform fluorescein findings.

Retrobulbar Neuritis and Papillitis

Swelling of the optic disc that is mild or occasionally not even noted on ophthalmological examination may be readily recognized by fluorescein angiography. Edema of the disc is the predominant finding in the majority of cases and may exist without any obvious capillary dilatation. In retrobulbar neuritis a mild hyperfluorescence of the disc, with or without leakage of dye beyond the disc margin, may be the only ocular finding. The fluorescence develops in the venous stage of angiography, becoming most obvious in the later residual phases, particularly when compared with the fellow eye (Fig. 2-33A).

Posterior Ciliary Vessel Occlusion

Occlusion of the posterior ciliary vessels or their branches may result in *infarction of the optic nerve head* — e.g., as in temporal arteritis or arteriosclerosis. Frequently only one altitudinal half of the disc may be involved. In recent cases associated with swelling, fluorescein freely permeates the ischemic portion of the optic disc and is easily identified in the early stages of angiography before diffusion occurs beyond this area (Figs. 2-34A and B). In advanced disease of the posterior ciliary vessels, segments of peripapillary choriocapillaris show irregularity of perfusion. Concomitant retinal vascular aberrations may be also revealed on angiography. These include caliber changes in the larger vessels and localized areas of capillary nonperfusion at the posterior pole.

Central Retinal Vein Obstruction

Considerable swelling of the optic disc, often clinically indistinguishable from papilledema, may occur in this condition. Fluorescein angiography, however, is of considerable diagnostic help in such instances by demonstrating grossly impaired circulation times in central retinal vein obstruction, but normal transit times in papilledema. Similarly, in central vein obstruction, particularly of inflammatory origin, peripheral sites of vasculitis often become obvious because of the permeation of dye at these sites with striking segmental staining of the vessel wall (Figs. 2-35A and B). In papilledema the florid venous changes are largely confined to the papillary and peripapillary areas. In central venous obstruction, the retinal capillaries are predominantly involved, although in the immediate postocclusion period, little is seen of their fine structure because of the widespread hemorrhage at the disc. The sparing of the prelaminar ciliary capillaries accounts for the usual mild degree of edema at the nerve head in vein occlusions, as compared with papilledema. Likewise, the preservation of this plexus of vessels provides a potential and often realized collateral pathway from the retinal to the ciliary vessels (Fig. 2-36A). Such large collaterals can be traced from the retinal arterioles to the edge of the optic disc, and flow demonstrated to occur in a posterior direction. Improvement in retinal circulation times, due to relief of the venous obstruction, formation of collaterals, or following therapy, can be adequately documented.

Edema with Posterior Uveitis or Pars Planitis

Disc edema associated with these conditions is often subtle and is frequently associated with peripheral retinal vascular changes and macular edema. Leakage of dye occurs at the surface of the disc and perfuses into the adjoining retina. Accumulation of fluorescein at the macula in a characteristic petaloid distribution and staining of the peripheral retinal vessels may provide additional diagnostic clues.

Ocular Hypotony

In ocular hypotension the reduction in tissue pressure at the papilla promotes an effusion of fluid from the ciliary and retinal capillaries due to the unopposed hydrostatic pressure within these vessels. These and similar changes at the macula can be demonstrated by

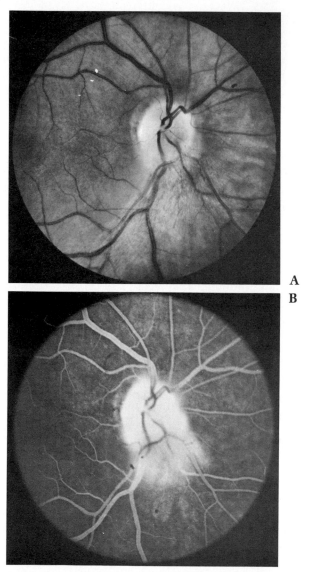

A
B

FIG. 2-33A. *Black and white photograph of right posterior eyegrounds of patient with papillitis. B. Late venous angiogram shows widespread leakage of dye in a sectorial fashion from the inferior aspect of the optic disc. There is overall hyperfluorescence of the disc with some leakage of dye beyond the upper and nasal aspects of the disc. The temporal margin remains reasonably discrete.*

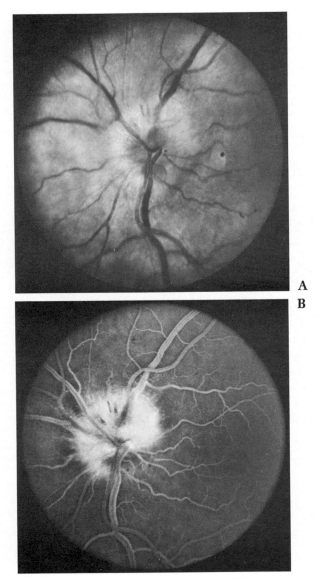

FIG. 2-34A. *Black and white photograph of left posterior eyegrounds of a patient with ischemic optic neuropathy (temporal arteritis). The patient had an inferior altitudinal field defect. B. Late venous phase angiogram of same patient demonstrating that the leakage from the optic disc is largely confined to the upper half of the disc, indicating predominant ischemia of the upper half of the papilla.*

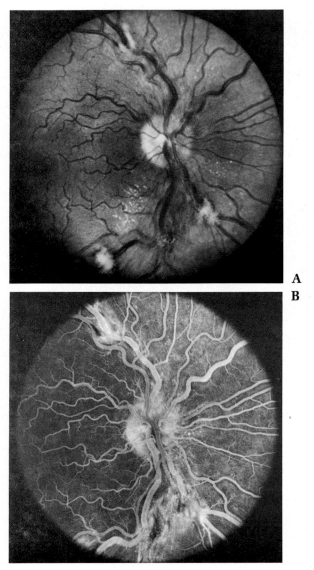

A
B

FIG. 2-35A. *Right posterior eyegrounds of patient with central retinal vasculitis and disc edema (black and white photography). Exudates and hemorrhages are noted along the major retinal veins. B. Late retinal venous angiogram shows mild edema of the optic disc with some leakage of dye beyond the margins. The dilated vessels show widespread leakage of dye at focal points along the major retinal veins. There is considerable staining of the endothelium of the major veins.*

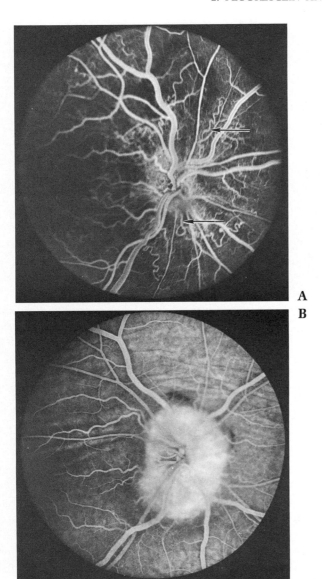

A

B

FIG. 2-36A. Venous phase angiogram of patient who had a right central retinal vein obstruction one year previously. The retinal vessels are slightly dilated, and slight permeation of dye beyond the disc margin is evident. Large shunts from the retinal arterioles drain into the choroidal veins via the disc circulation (arrows). B. Venous phase angiogram of a patient with a right orbital hemangioma. Note the widespread leakage of dye from the optic disc and the presence of choroidal folds indicating the presence of a retrobulbar mass.

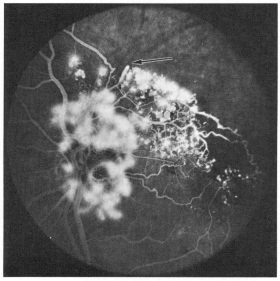

FIG. 2-37. Late retinal venous angiogram of patient with branch retinal vein and artery obstruction (arrow) and neovascularization at the optic disc. Note the characteristic variegated appearance of the new vessels overlying the optic disc.

fluorescein angiography, especially the later phases (Figs. 2-16A and B).

Sectorial Disc Edema

Certain diseases of the optic nerve head—e.g., papillitis, ischemic optic neuropathy, and juxtapapillary choroiditis—may produce localized edema of the disc. Their segmental nature, although not obvious on direct ophthalmoscopy, is dramatically borne out on fluorescein angiography. In *papillitis* the area of maximum swelling may be seen to profusely leak dye eccentrically across the disc margin. This zone of hyperfluorescence presumably correlates with a plaque of demyelinization or inflammatory focus àt the distal optic nerve. When the edema is marked, dilatation of the retinal capillaries, in the area of the disease, can be seen (Figs. 2-33A and B).

Disc Edema and Orbital Disease

Occasional clues as to the origin of papillary swelling may be yielded by angiographic findings at other areas of the fundus. The presence of choroidal and retinal folds, displayed dramatically on angiography, may provide important information as to the presence of a retrobulbar tumor (Fig. 2-36B).

PSEUDOPAPILLEDEMA

Certain optic discs, as in high hyperopia, are characterized by small or absent optic cups with blurring of the entire disc margin, and a false impression of disc edema may be gained. Angiography is helpful in such instances by demonstrating normal retinal and ciliary capillary networks with no extravasation of dye beyond the disc margins.[8, 44] Buried drusen of the optic nerve head likewise may mimic swelling of the nerve head; but again, on angiography, the disc margins, although irregular and associated with pigment epithelial changes, are discrete with no demonstrable leakage of fluorescein beyond them. A mottled fluorescence of the optic disc occurs as a result of the drusen deposits within the papilla. Drusen deposits on the surface of the optic disc demonstrate striking autofluorescence but, during the various stages of angiography, appear to have little affinity for the dye (Fig. 2-5).

NEOVASCULARIZATION AT THE OPTIC DISC

New vessels on and before the surface of the optic disc, in conjunction with their supporting connective tissue, may give the appearance of disc swelling. Angiography graphically outlines these new vessels, which first become obvious during the arterial phase of angiography. In the later stages of dye transit, localized leakage of dye from these new capillary tufts forms a characteristic variegated pattern (Fig. 2-37). The underlying condition responsible for the formation of these vessels is usually apparent on angiography—e.g., diabetic retinopathy, branch retinal vein obstruction, or polycythemia. Disappearance of these vessels following photocoagulation likewise can be carefully monitored by dye studies.[37]

TUMORS OF THE RETINA, CHOROID, AND OPTIC DISC

The investigation of tumors of the retina and choroid has undoubtedly been facilitated by fluorescein angiography, although in certain circumstances, where tumors display similar vascular arrangements and pigment disturbances, fluorescein angiography is of limited value in reaching a specific diagnosis.

TABLE 2-4
Angiographic Features of Choroidal Tumors and Their Differential Diagnosis

	Arterial Phase	Late Venous Phase	Special Features
Choroidal nevus	Localized area of hypofluorescence corresponding to the contour of the lesion	Nevus distinctly outlined by background fluorescence; some faint fluorescence occasionally apparent at nevus	Drusen in the overlying pigment epithelium fluoresce owing to dye in the choriocapillaris not totally masked by the choroidal pigment; no intrinsic vasculature
Malignant melanoma			
(i) Pigmented	Prominent blotchy fluorescence over surface of tumor; small bright fluorescent points correspond to drusen and foci of pigment epithelial degeneration	Diffuse leakage of dye, tumor staining, and hyperfluorescence	Dense surface pigmentation, subretinal hemorrhage, or extensive infarction may preclude any view of the underlying fluorescence
(ii) Amelanotic or lightly pigmented	Diffuse blotchy fluorescence; sinusoidal nutritive vessels become apparent	Almost uniformly intense hyperfluorescence	Vascular malformations in overlying retina; dilated capillaries, microaneurysms, stasis
Hemangioma	Early arterial filling of tumor vascular complexes, even prior to arterial phase; blotchy fluorescence develops with intense staining	Diffuse mottled hyperfluorescence	Effects of therapy by photocoagulation can be monitored by angiography
Metastases	Only subtle fluorescent changes; often related to pigment epithelial defects	Increasing patchy fluorescence, contrasting with pigment aggregates	Hemorrhage may mask fluorescence; often multiple lesions
Choroidal hemorrhage	Nonfluorescent area with sharply demarcated edges	Contrast heightens with dense background fluorescence	
Disciform degeneration of the macula	Networks of choroidal neovascularization apparent; spotty fluorescence at drusen sites	Blotchy fluorescence of lesion with dye leakage and tissue staining, leading to confluent intense fluorescence	
Granuloma choroid	No fluorescence	Slowly developing mottled fluorescence with intense tissue staining	

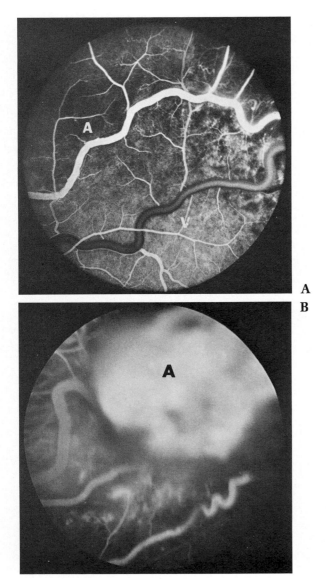

FIG. 2-38A. *Midvenous angiogram of the superior temporal fundus of patient with retinal angiomatosis. The widely dilated afferent* (**A**) *and efferent* (**V**) *vessels are obvious. Vascular stasis is indicated by the slow permeation of dye down the efferent vein. Note the telangiectatic vessels and microaneurysms. B. Late venous phase angiogram demonstrating the homogeneous and intense fluorescence of the angioma* (**A**) *itself.*

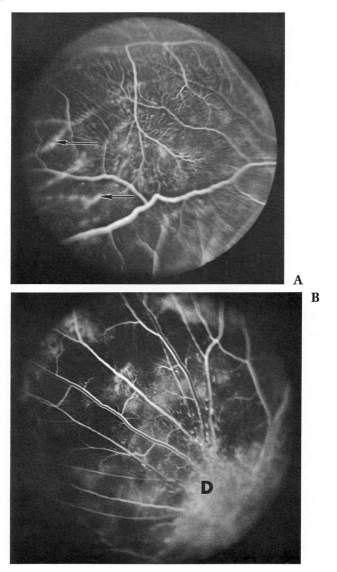

FIG. 2-39A. Right posterior fundus of a patient with an amelanotic malignant melanoma of the choroid taken during the retinal arteriovenous phase of dye transit. Widely dilated retinal capillaries and microaneurysms occur in the retina, elevated by the tumor. Large nutrient vessels from the choroidal system are seen (arrows). B. Right superonasal eyegrounds of a patient with a juxtapapillary malignant melanoma of the choroid, taken during the midretinal venous phase of angiography. Note the diffuse, blotchy fluorescence of the tumor vessels in this patient, as well as the markedly dilated vessels at the optic disc (**D**). There is extensive leakage of dye beyond the margins of the disc.

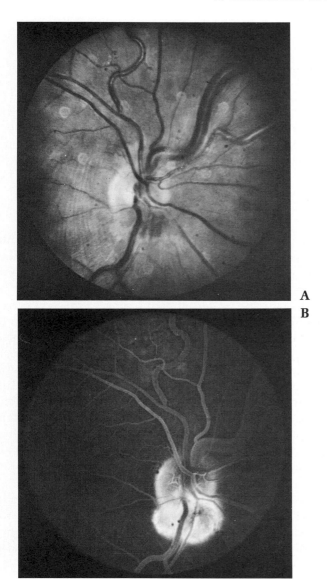

A

B

FIG. 2-40A. *Black and white photograph of posterior fundus of patient with angiomatosis retinae. The dilated nutrient arterioles course toward the tumor, situated in the peripheral temporal fundus. A small angioma is barely evident at the inferior aspect of the optic disc. (Courtesy of Mr. P. J. Holmes-Sellors.) B. Late phase angiogram of patient in Fig. 2-40A. The tumor is a hyperfluorescent area with discrete margins.*

RETINAL TUMORS

Nevus of the Pigment Epithelium and Benign Pigment Epithelium Hyperplasia

The dense accumulation of pigment within the deeper layers of the retina obscures visualization of the underlying choroidal fluorescence and results in absence of choroidal fluorescence throughout all stages of angiography at these sites. The overlying retinal capillaries are vividly seen owing to the contrast afforded by the nonfluorescent background.

Hemangiomas

These tumors particularly lend themselves to study by angiography. Hemangioblastomas, as found in von Hippel's disease, produce a dramatic fluorescent picture (Figs. 2-38A and B).[2,23] The grossly dilated, tortuous and engorged feeding artery and draining vein are vividly outlined. Damage to the endothelial lining of these vessels is indicated by dense fluorescein staining of the vessel walls and, on occasion, perfusion of dye into the adjacent retina. Vascular stasis is such that the fluorescent dye front may be easily followed as it progresses along the afferent and efferent vessels (Fig. 2-38A). The tumor itself is usually perceived as an intensely fluorescent mass in the retinal periphery, fluorescing from the earliest stages of angiography. There is widespread extravasation of dye from the vascular tumor, producing indistinct diffuse margins (Fig. 2-38B). Aberrations of the retinal microvasculature in the neighborhood of tumors and feeding vessels also become evident, particularly dilated capillaries, microaneurysms, and small areas of retinal telangiectasia (Fig. 2-38B).

Fluorescein angiography is also of value in detecting small satellite angiomas at the optic disc and throughout the ocular fundus of both the involved and fellow eye.[27] The destruction of the tumor mass and eradication of satellite angiomas by cryotherapy or photocoagulation can be carefully followed by dye studies.

Retinoblastomas

These tumors show some unique features on angiography, although this procedure is rarely required to elucidate their nature. Striking autofluorescence of these tumors may occur as a result of calcification and is readily appreciated on control angiograms. Hyperfluorescence of these lesions is noted during the retinal arterial phase of angiography with intensification during venous transit of dye. The fluorescence is largely due to leakage of dye from the abnormal nutrient capillaries and the destruction of the retinal pigment epithelium. Occasionally connections between the retinal and tumor circulations can be demonstrated, indicating the retinal origin of the tumor.[62]

CHOROIDAL TUMORS

The fluorescent characteristics of choroidal tumors depend on several factors:

1. The degree of elevation, disorientation, and destruction of the overlying retinal pigment epithelium. Changes within this layer greatly modify the visibility of fluorescence within the tumor.
2. The extent of choroidal pigment proliferation within the tumor. Deeply pigmented tumors produce a highly mottled appearance with lower intensities of residual fluorescence. Amelanotic tumors have a more confluent pattern of fluorescence, which is generally of high intensity.
3. The arrangement of blood vessels within the tumor. Large vascular channels leading directly from the major choroidal vessels permit rapid filling of the tumor with dye and early fluorescence; indeed such channels may be outlined with dye prior to the appearance of fluorescein in the retinal circulation. Smaller nutrient vessels are less visible and not clearly outlined by fluorescein until the arteriovenous phase of angiography (Fig. 2-39A).
4. Hemorrhage, exudation, and infarction within the tumor. These factors result in a significant reduction or total absence of fluorescence.[47]
5. The degree of embarrassment of the retinal circulation overlying the tumor. The elevated retina demonstrates marked changes in the local vasculature, such as capillary dilatation and microaneurysms, in addition to increased vascular permeability and retarded blood flow (Figs. 2-3A and B).

Table 2-4 outlines the fluorescent characteristics of the common choroidal tumors. As can be seen, there is considerable overlap in the fluorescein characteristics of most choroidal tumors, and indeed by the late stages of angiography many are indistinguishable. The subtle changes aiding differentiation mostly occur in the earliest stages of angiography, thus emphasizing the importance of close scrutiny of the early fluorescein pictures.

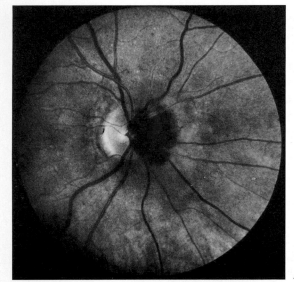

A

B

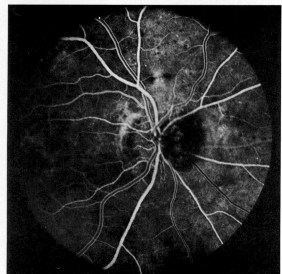

C

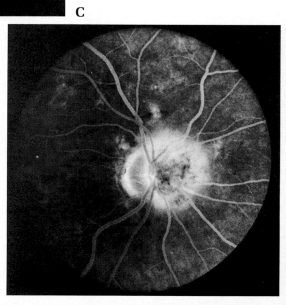

OPTIC NERVE HEAD TUMORS

The fluorescent patterns of papillary tumors are accentuated by the absence of a pigment epithelial layer but, in general, reflect the abnormal vascular networks. Associated pigment and connective tissue modify the degree of fluorescence.

Hemangiomas

These tumors fluoresce early in the retinal arterial phase, at which time individual vessels within the tumor may be discerned. In late angiography a uniform diffuse hyperfluorescence predominates, with some perfusion of dye beyond the margins of the tumor (Figs. 2-40A and B). These findings differ in no way from the fluorescent patterns of retinal hemangiomas found elsewhere.

Melanocytomas

These lesions show almost total absence of fluorescence in the early stages of angiography due to the dense accumulation of pigment within the tumor (Figs. 2-41A and B). Multiple fluorescent foci develop in the late venous phase, owing to widespread permeation of dye from the abnormal nutrient vessels into tumor substance. By the residual phase of angiography, the tumor is highly fluorescent (Fig. 2-41C). The unaffected portion of the optic disc usually is edematous, with leakage of dye within the papilla and, on occasion, beyond its margins. The striking hyperfluorescence of the tumor up to one or two hours after injection is a measure of staining of the connective tissue of the tumor with fluorescein.

Astrocytomas

Astrocytomas of the nerve head (Fig. 2-42A) (tuberous sclerosis) may show a striking autofluorescence as a result of calcium deposits within the glial proliferations. There is a general absence of fluores-

FIG. 2-41A. *Black and white photograph of melanocytoma of the right optic nerve head. B. Midretinal venous angiogram indicating a faint, mottled fluorescence of the tumor. Most of the tumor, however, is unstained at this stage. C. Five-minute angiogram indicates a diffuse staining of the tumor. There is some leakage of dye beyond the border of the lesion. The optic disc is also hyperfluorescent due to secondary pressure effects of the tumor at the papilla, causing capillaries in this area to leak.*

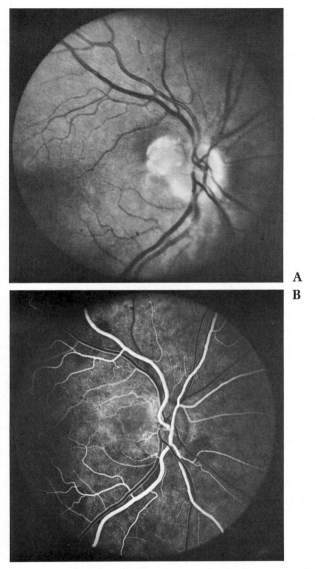

A

B

FIG. 2-42A. *Black and white photograph of right posterior fundus demonstrating an astrocytoma of the papilla in a patient with tuberous sclerosis. B. Early retinal venous phase angiogram. Dilated capillaries are present around the circumference of the tumor, but only little fluorescence of the lesion is apparent at this stage. C. Late retinal venous phase angiogram. There is considerable permeation of dye into the tumor. D. Five-minute angiogram. Dense homogeneous fluorescence of the entire tumor with some leakage of dye beyond its borders. E. Five-minute angiogram. Inferonasal fundus of same eye. Two small satellite astrocytomas are now apparent.*

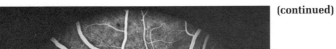

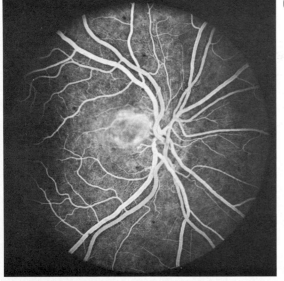

C

D

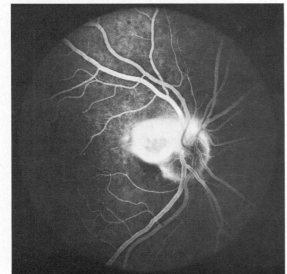

E

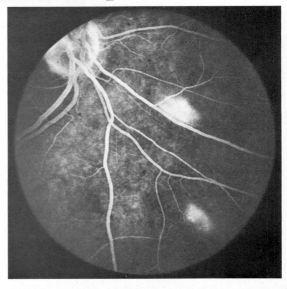

cence during the arterial phase of angiography (Fig. 2-42B), but beginning with the midretinal venous phase the tumor fluoresces brightly and uniformly and persists up to one hour or so after injection (Figs. 2-42C and D). If the tumor is large and vascularized, a unique variegated pattern may develop in the venous phase of angiography. Unsuspected astrocytomas elsewhere may be revealed by their fluorescence in the late stages of angiography (Fig. 2-42E). Rarely, the disc tumor may be associated with marked swelling of the papilla, in which case there is extensive leakage of dye for some distance beyond the disc margin. Angiography may be of help in differentiating these lesions, especially when multiple and unassociated with skin changes, from early retinoblastoma.

REFERENCES

1. Allen, L., Kirkendall, W. M., Snyder, W. B., and Frazier, O. Instant positive photographs and stereograms of ocular fundus fluorescence. *Arch. Ophthal. 75:*192, 1966.

2. Amalric, P., and Bonnin, P. L'angiographie fluorescenique. *Bull. Soc. Ophtal. France* (annual report), p. 228, 1969.

3. Archer, D. B., Krill, A. E., and Newell, F. W. Fluorescein studies of the normal choroidal circulation. *Amer. J. Ophthal. 69:*543, 1970.

4. Archer, D. B., Krill, A. E., and Newell, F. W. Fluorescein studies of choroidal sclerosis. *Amer. J. Ophthal. 71:*226, 1970.

5. Archer, D. B., Krill, A. E., and Newell, F. W. Fluorescein angiographic evaluation of the effects of photocoagulation in three retinal vascular diseases. *Trans. Ophthal. Soc. U.K. 90:*677, 1970.

6. Ashton, N. Central areolar choroidal sclerosis. A histopathological study. *Brit. J. Ophthal. 37:*140, 1953.

7. Ashton, N., and Cunha-Vaz, J. G. Effect of histamine on the permeability of the ocular vessels. *Arch. Ophthal. 73:*211, 1965.

8. Barrios, R. Fluorescein angioretinography as a diabetic method for papilledema. *Acta Neurol. Lat. Amer. 9:*213, 1963.

9. Behrendt, T. Synchronous flash motion picture camera. *Amer. J. Ophthal. 63:*946, 1967.

10. Best, M., Blumenthal, M., Galin, M., and Toyofuku, H. Fluorescein angiography during induced ocular hypertension in glaucoma. *Arch. Ophthal. 86:*31, 1971.

11. Blumenthal, M., Gitter, K. A., Best, M., and Galin, M. A. Fluorescein angiography during induced ocular hypertension in man. *Amer. J. Ophthal. 69:*39, 1970.

12. Crock, G. Stereotechnology in medicine. *Trans. Ophthal. Soc. U.K. 90:*577, 1970.

13. Cunha-Vaz, J. G., and Maurice, D. M. The active transport of fluorescein by the retinal vessels and the retina. *J. Physiol. 191:*467, 1967.

14. Cunha-Vaz, J. G., Shakib, M., and Ashton, N. Studies on the permeability of the blood-retinal barrier. I. On the existence, development, and site of a blood-retinal barrier. *Brit. J. Ophthal. 50:*441, 1966.

15. David, N. J., Gilbert, D. S., and Gass, J. D. M. Fluorescein angiography in retinal arterial branch obstructions. *Amer. J. Ophthal.* 69:43, 1970.

16. Dollery, C. T. Dynamic aspects of the retinal microcirculation. *Arch. Ophthal.* 79:536, 1968.

17. Dollery, C. T., Hodge, J. V., and Engel, M. Retinal photography using fluorescein. *Med. Biol. Illus.* 13:4, 1963.

18. Farkas, T. G., Sylvester, V., and Archer, D. B. The ultrastructure of drusen. *Amer. J. Ophthal.* 71:1196, 1971.

19. Gass, J. D. M. *Stereoscopic Atlas of Macular Diseases: A Fundoscopic and Angiographic Presentation.* St. Louis, C. V. Mosby, 1970, p. 26.

20. Gass, J. D. M., Norton, E. W. D., and Justice, J., Jr. Serous detachment of the retinal pigment epithelium. *Trans. Amer. Acad. Ophthal. Otolaryng.* 70:990, 1966.

21. Grayson, M. C., and Laties, A. M. Ocular localization of sodium fluorescein. *Arch. Ophthal.* 85:600, 1971.

22. Haining, W. M., and Lancaster, R. C. Advanced techniques for fluorescein angiography. *Arch. Ophthal.* 79:10, 1968.

23. Haining, W. M., and Zweifach, P. H. Fluorescein angiography in Von Hippel-Lindau disease. *Arch. Ophthal.* 78:475, 1967.

24. Hayreh, S. S. Blood supply of the optic nerve head and its role in optic atrophy, glaucoma, and oedema of the optic disc. *Brit. J. Ophthal.* 53:721, 1969.

25. Hayreh, S. S. Pathogenesis of visual field defects — role of ciliary circulation. *Brit. J. Ophthal.* 54:289, 1970.

26. Hickam, J. B., and Frayser, R. Photographic method for measuring the mean retinal circulation time using fluorescein. *Invest. Ophthal.* 4:876, 1965.

27. Holmes-Sellors, P. J., and Archer, D. B. The management of retinal angiomatosis. *Trans. Ophthal. Soc. U.K.* 89:529, 1969.

28. Klien, B. Diseases of the macula. *Arch. Ophthal.* 60:175, 1958.

29. Kogure, K., and Choromokos, E. Infrared absorption angiography. *J. Appl. Physiol.* 26:154, 1969.

30. Kogure, K., David, N. J., Yamanouchi, U., and Choromokos, E. Infrared absorption angiography of the fundus circulation. *Arch. Ophthal.* 83:209, 1970.

31. Kohner, E. M., and Dollery, C. T. Fluorescein angiography of the fundus in diabetic retinopathy. *Brit. Med. Bull.* 26:166, 1970.

32. Kohner, E. M., and Dollery, C. T. The rate of formation and disappearance of microaneurysms in diabetic retinopathy. *Trans. Ophthal. Soc. U.K.* 90:369, 1970.

33. Kohner, E. M., Dollery, C. T., Paterson, J. W., and Oakley, N. W. Arterial fluorescein studies in diabetic retinopathy. *Diabetes* 16:1, 1967.

34. Kohner, E. M., and Henkind, P. Correlation of fluorescein angiogram and retinal digest in diabetic retinopathy. *Amer. J. Ophthal.* 69:403, 1970.

35. Krill, A. E., and Archer, D. B. Choroidal neovascularization in multifocal (presumed histoplasmin) choroiditis. *Arch. Ophthal.* 84:595, 1970.

36. Krill, A. E., Archer, D. B., and Newell, F. W. Fluorescein angiography in retinitis pigmentosa. *Amer. J. Ophthal.* 69:1826, 1970.

37. Krill, A. E., Archer, D. B., and Newell, F. W. Photocoagulation in complications secondary to branch vein occlusion. *Arch. Ophthal.* 85:48, 1971.

38. Krill, A. E., Archer, D. B., Newell, F. W., and Chishti, M. Photocoagulation in diabetic retinopathy. *Amer. J. Ophthal. 72*:299, 1971.

39. Krill, A. E., Newell, F. W., and Chishti, M. Fluorescein studies in diseases affecting the retinal pigment epithelium. *Amer. J. Ophthal. 66*:470, 1968.

40. Linner, E., and Friedenwald, J. S. The appearance time of fluorescein as an index of aqueous flow. *Amer. J. Ophthal. 44*:225, 1957.

41. Machemer, R. Angiographic-histologic correlation of eye vessel permeability with protein-bound fluorescent dye. *Amer. J. Ophthal. 69*:27, 1970.

42. Machemer, R., Norton, E. W. D., Gass, J. D. M., and Choromokos, E. Pseudofluorescence—a problem in interpretation of fluorescein angiograms. *Amer. J. Ophthal. 70*:1, 1970.

43. Maurice, D. M. The use of fluorescein in ophthalmological research. *Invest. Ophthal. 6*:464, 1967.

44. Miller, S. J. H., Sanders, M. D., and Ffytche, T. J. Fluorescein fundus photography in the detection of early papilloedema and its differentiation from pseudopapilloedema. *Lancet 2*:651, 1965.

45. Norton, E. W. D. Characteristic fluorescein angiographic patterns in choroidal folds. *Proc. Roy. Soc. Med. 62*:119, 1969.

46. Novotny, H. R., and Alvis, D. L. A method of photographing fluorescence in circulating blood in the human retina. *Circulation 24*:82, 1961.

47. Pettit, T. H., Barton, A., Foos, R. Y., and Christensen, R. E. Fluorescein angiography of choroidal melanomas. *Arch. Ophthal. 83*:27, 1970.

48. Peyman, G. A., Spitznas, M., and Straatsma, B. R. Peroxidase diffusion in the normal and photocoagulated retina. *Invest. Ophthal. 10*:181, 1971.

49. Peyman, G. A., Spitznas, M., and Straatsma, B. R. Chorioretinal diffusion of peroxidase before and after photocoagulation. *Invest. Ophthal. 10*:489, 1971.

50. Pinkerton, R. M. H. Fluorescein angiography as a source of artifact in the investigation of hypertension. *Canad. J. Ophthal. 4*:379, 1969.

51. Rosen, E. S. *Fluorescence Photography of the Eye*. London, Butterworth & Co., 1969, p. 4.

52. Sanders, M. D., and Ffytche, T. J. Fluorescein angiography in the diagnosis of drusen of the disk. *Trans. Ophthal. Soc. U.K. 87*:457, 1967.

53. Seidel, E. Experimentelle untersuchungen ueber die quelle und den verlauf der intraokulaeren saftstroemung. *Arch. f. Ophthal. 95*:1, 1918.

54. Shakib, M., and Cunha-Vaz, J. G. Studies on the permeability of the blood-retinal barrier. IV. Junctional complexes of the retinal vessels and their role in the permeability of the blood-retinal barrier. *Exp. Eye Res. 5*:229, 1966.

55. Shikano, S., and Shimizu, K. *Atlas of Fluorescence Fundus Angiography*. Tokyo, Igaku Shoin, 1968, p. 78.

56. Sollom, A. W. Histological study of late phase fluorescence in the rabbit fundus. *Brit. J. Ophthal. 51*:821, 1967.

57. Sollom, A. W. Conjugated fluorescein for fundus photography. *Brit. J. Ophthal. 52*:691, 1968.

58. Stein, M. R., and Parker, C. C. Drug reactions following intravenous fluorescein. Presented at meeting of Association for Research in Vision and Ophthalmology, Sarasota, April 1971.

59. van Heuven, W. A. J., Schaffer, C. A., and Mehu, M.   Televised fluorescein angiography—a progress report. Presented at meeting of Association for Research in Vision and Ophthalmology, Sarasota, April 1971.

60. Wessing, A.   *Fluorescein Angiography of the Retina* (trans. by von Noorden, G. K.). St. Louis, C. V. Mosby, 1969, p. 23.

61. Wessing, A.   *Fluorescein Angiography of the Retina* (trans. by von Noorden, G. K.). St. Louis, C. V. Mosby, 1969, pp. 26–27.

62. Wessing, A.   *Fluorescein Angiography of the Retina* (trans. by von Noorden, G. K.). St. Louis, C. V. Mosby, 1969, p. 140.

3

Evaluation of Night Vision: Dark Adaptation

Most of our visual performance occurs either in daylight or in an artificially lighted environment. Only occasionally is it necessary to perform in absolute or close to absolute darkness for a prolonged period of time. The photographer developing film, the astronomer gazing through a telescope at night, and the pilot flying over the countryside at night all perform in close to absolute darkness. However, the airplane pilot, like the automobile driver, may be subject to frequent changes in illumination, sometimes of a very rapid and extensive nature. Therefore, in any discussion of everyday visual performance it is necessary to consider a wide luminance range.

PHOTOPIC, SCOTOPIC, MESOPIC

Three terms, photopic, scotopic, and mesopic (Table 3-1), define visual performance on the basis of luminance range. Photopic vision occurs in daylight. Three foot-lamberts is an average value cited as the lowest luminance for photopic vision. Cones are more sensitive in this range. Scotopic vision occurs in close to absolute darkness and is rod vision.* A luminance value cited for the upper limit of scotopic

---

* This is true except at the far red end of the visible spectrum, where rods and cones are equally sensitive.[24]

TABLE 3-1
Luminance Ranges

Designation	Luminance Limits	More Sensitive Receptors
Photopic	3 ft-lamberts and above	Cones
Scotopic	3×10^{-4} ft-lamberts and below	Rods
Mesopic	Between above values	Rods and cones

vision is 3×10^{-4} foot-lamberts.* Mesopic vision occurs in luminances between the lower value cited for photopic vision and the upper value cited for scotopic luminance. In this range, rod and cone sensitivity is similar. The precise luminance values for when either rods or cones function chiefly or when both function may vary with factors such as area of the retina stimulated, size of the stimulus, previous light experience. Examples of the type of luminance provided by various light sources are shown in Figure 3-1.

In general, much of our visual activity under reduced lighting is mesopic (Fig. 3-1). However, visual data may be easier to obtain when mainly rods or cones function in photopic or scotopic environments. Therefore, estimation of mesopic performance requires interpolation, and this may be difficult because the relative contribution of rods and cones in various mesopic environments may be impossible to predict. Usually, though, curves of data (e.g., visual acuity and minimum light detection) obtained in complete darkness after previous adaptation to a bright light are of some value in predicting mesopic as well as scotopic performance.

RODS AND CONES

It is obvious then that the human visual system is capable of functioning over a wide range of luminance (Fig. 3-1). This capability reflects the presence in our retina of two types of receptors, both rods and cones (Table 3-2). In the human retina, there are approximately 7 million cone cells and 120 million rod cells. Although fundamentally the activity of both rods and cones is initiated by the absorption of light quanta,[29] there are some basic functional differences between

* One foot-lambert equals 1.08 millilamberts.

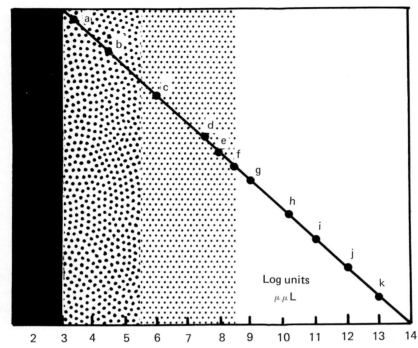

FIG. 3-1. *Graphic representation of luminance ranges. At left in black: no visual perception. Large black dots: range of scotopic vision. Small black dots: range of mesopic vision. White: range of photopic vision. The luminance values are in micromicrolamberts (log units)* a. *Night ground luminance when the weather is overcast, without moon* b. *Mean ground luminance in full moon* c. *Sky luminance in full moon* d. *Sky luminance one-half hour after sunset* e. *Mean luminance of street lighting in town* f. *Sky luminance one-quarter hour after sunset* g. *Mean weak lighting in artificial light* h. *Good reading luminance for white paper* i. *Good artificial lighting* j. *Mean diurnal lighting* k. *Snow luminance in noonday sun.* (*From Jayle, G. E., Ourgaud, A. G., Baisinger, L. F., and Holmes, W. J.* Night Vision. *Springfield, Ill., Charles C Thomas, 1950.*)

these two structures, which have been known for a considerable period of time (Table 3-2). In fact, the notion that the rods are used for seeing at night and the cones for seeing during the day, the duplicity theory, was developed during the nineteenth century.

PURKINJE SHIFT

Cones differentiate stimuli on the basis of color and brightness, but rods only on the basis of brightness. Color vision is therefore mediated by cones. Rod vision is colorless. In both rods and cones,

TABLE 3-2
Rod and Cone Differences

Rod	Cone
1. Colorless vision	Color vision
2. *Dim Light Detection*	
Excellent	Poor
3. *Greatest Concentration*	
At 15°–20° from fovea	At fovea
4. $N* = 120,000,000$	$N = 7,000,000$
5. No directional sensitivity	Directional sensitivity
6. *Most Sensitive to*	
510 nm	555 nm
7. *Flicker Fusion Frequency*	
Low	High

* N = number.

some wavelengths are much more effective in excitation than others. For rods, blue-green light near 510 nm, and for cones, yellow-green light near 555 nm, are by far more effective than all other wavelengths. Many years ago Purkinje noted a change in the relative brightness of red and blue flowers in his garden as the sunlight gradually faded in twilight. This phenomenon, now called the Purkinje shift, reflects a shift in spectral sensitivity of the eye from daylight (cone) to night (rod) vision (Fig. 3-2).

TOPOGRAPHY

Another way in which rods and cones differ is in their geographic distribution in the retina. Cone cells are of greatest concentration in the macular area (Fig. 3-3) and fall off sharply outside of this area to a rather uniform concentration. In the very center of the macula (fovea) cone density is highest and there are no rods. Rod cells, on the other hand, are of greatest density about 15 to 20 degrees outside of the fovea, with a maximum at about 15 degrees nasal to the fovea. It is understandable, then, why at very low light levels an individual may fix eccentrically for best vision (Arago's phenomenon).[31]

STILES-CRAWFORD EFFECT

Rods and cones also differ in their sensitivity to the angle of incidence of the light quanta they absorb. Rods are insensitive to the direction of the incidence of the light; but cones are much more sen-

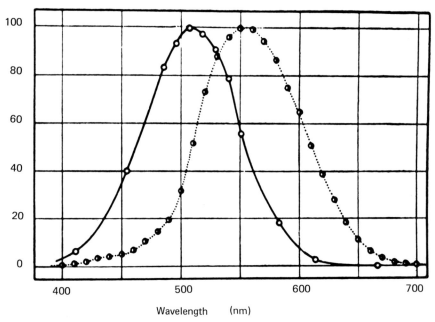

Wavelength   (nm)

FIG. 3-2. *Photopic (half-closed circles) and scotopic (open circles) relative luminosity function curves. The curves are adjusted so that the most efficient wavelength for both curves is given a value of 100. The most efficient wavelength for photopic vision is close to 555 nm and close to 510 nm for scotopic vision.* (From Wright, W. D.   Researches on Normal and Defective Color Vision. London, H. Kimpton, 1946.)

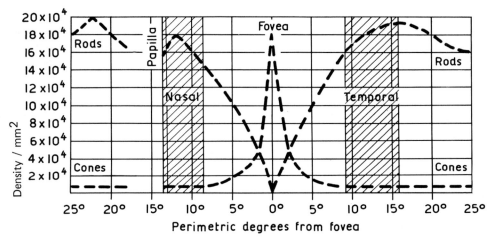

FIG. 3-3. *Distribution of rods and cones in the human retina along horizontal meridian out to 25 degrees eccentricity from fovea (X-axis). Number of receptors per square mm are plotted on Y-axis. Note greatest density of rods are close to 20 degrees nasally and 15 degrees temporally. Rod density falls off sharply as fovea is approached. Cone density is maximum at fovea and becomes uniform at 10 degrees.* (From Osterberg, G. A.   Acta Ophthal. (Suppl. VI), 1935.)

sitive to light quanta passing through the center of the pupil than to quanta passing through the pupil margin. This directional sensitivity of the retina is known as the Stiles-Crawford effect,[65] after the two scientists who first described this phenomenon in 1933.

DARK ADAPTATION

Rods and cones also differ in the rate at which they recover sensitivity in the dark after a bright exposure. Cones recover more rapidly from exposure to a bright light. Rods, although recovering more slowly, ultimately become far more sensitive light detectors. This is the process of dark adaptation, and its measurement involves the determination of the maximum sensitivity of the eye to a light stimulus (absolute threshold) at given times in the dark. In general, the greatest sensitivity of the eye is not attained until 25 to 35 minutes in the dark-adapted state, but this is dependent on many factors (Fig. 3-4). The maximum change in light detection sensitivity from a photopic to a scotopic environment may amount to as much as 100,000 times.

CLINICAL ROD-CONE SEPARATION (Table 3-3)

Flicker

Only cones respond to fast flicker.[24] Lights flickering at about 20 cycles per second or faster are seen only with cones. Rod fusion frequencies may be far below this level depending on many factors, such as area of retina tested, size of target, color of target, and background luminance.[24] With the electroretinogram (ERG), flickering stimuli above 30 flashes per second elicit only cone responses.[24, 30] Fast subjective or objective (ERG) flicker is an excellent way of evaluating cone function.

TABLE 3-3
Clinical Rod-Cone Separation

Cones
— Fast subjective or objective (ERG) flicker
— Red visual fields with photopic background luminance
— Foveal testing

Rods
— Absolute thresholds in fully dark-adapted eye away from fovea with white or blue light

---

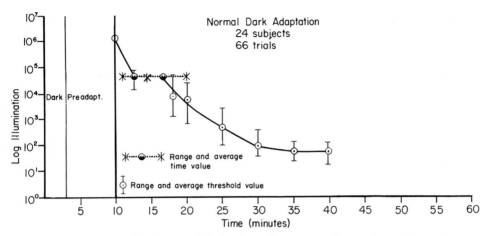

FIG. 3-4. *Normal bifunctional dark-adaptation curve with one degree target at 10 degrees superiorly showing initial cone and subsequent rod segments. Two standard deviations are shown at various segments of the curve. The most constant portion of the curve is the final rod threshold value, and next most constant is the final cone threshold value. Luminance at $10^7 = 9.4$ log micromicrolamberts.*

Luminance

At threshold levels of luminance, rods are far more sensitive, as indicated previously. Final dark-adaptation thresholds are the most sensitive index of rod function. At higher photopic levels of illumination, cones are probably far more sensitive than rods, but at lower photopic levels only slightly so.[24, 61] In the mesopic range, rod and cone sensitivities are similar. It is understandable, then, that in diseases involving only cones throughout the retina (e.g., congenital total color blindness or some cone degenerations), visual fields are normal.[61] Only receptor diseases of both rods and cones will affect visual fields, since such tests are customarily done with background luminances in a lower photopic or mesopic range.

Stimulus Color

At scotopic luminances, rod and cone sensitivity are almost the same at the long wavelength end of the spectrum.[24] However, rods are far more sensitive than cones to short wavelengths (e.g., blue and violet) at low luminance levels. At photopic luminance levels, cones are distinctly more sensitive to long wavelength stimuli than rods.[24, 60] Therefore, visual field determination done with a red stimulus in a photopic background should be a sensitive method of detecting abnormalities in conditions involving only the cones such as congenital total color blindness.[60] A basic problem greatly limiting the usefulness of a red stimulus is that most clinical visual field determinations (including those usually done with the Goldmann perimeter) are performed with background luminances in the mesopic range.

Foveal Testing

Obviously tests that measure function primarily of the fovea (e.g., foveal absolute thresholds and visual acuity) depend on cone function in this area.

PARAMETERS AFFECTING DARK ADAPTATION

PREADAPTATION

The duration, intensity, and color of light exposure prior to dark adaptation influence the rate of adaptation, and particularly the shape of the curve (Fig. 3-5). If a subject is kept in complete darkness for a sufficient period prior to testing (for example, for 30 minutes), very rapid rod adaptation will occur and only a monophasic rod curve will be obtained. Sufficient preadaptation is necessary to obtain a duplex curve with a cone as well as a rod portion.

Of practical importance is the use of red light for preadaptation for those working in reduced light levels. Preadaptation to high intensity red light results in significantly faster dark adaptation than preadaptation to the same intensity of white light.[28] However, at lower intensities of red and white light preadaptation, there is only a small difference in the rate of dark adaptation.[14] Furthermore, there is no difference in foveal recognition following preadaptation to a low-intensity level of either light.[14]

STIMULUS CHARACTERISTICS

The size, intensity, duration, and color of the stimulus are all important. A larger target produces a lower (more sensitive) absolute threshold (Fig. 3-6). However, the increase in sensitivity is more than linear, as summation, involving neural relationships, plays a greater role as target size is increased.[3, 12, 27, 54] The relationship between intensity and duration of stimulus varies with the duration of light. Of course, a test light duration that is too long will result in light adapta-

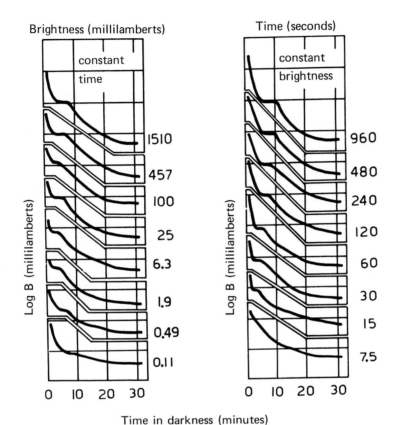

Time in darkness (minutes)

FIG. 3-5. *Dark-adaptation curves obtained monocularly with a 2° square test field presented at 6° in the lateral parafoveal area. On the left a constant preexposure time of 10 minutes is used, but preexposure brightness varies from 1,510 to 0.11 millilamberts. The final rod levels are identical in all curves, but the duration and level of the cone plateau vary with the brightness level. The cone plateau becomes less prominent and finally disappears as the brightness is decreased. The rod-cone break time decreases as the brightness is decreased. On the right the preexposure brightness is constant at 1,500 millilamberts, but preexposure time varies from 960 to 7.5 seconds. The same changes that occur when preexposure brightness (with a constant duration) is decreased occur when preexposure duration (with a constant brightness) is decreased. (From Wolf, E., and Zigler, M. J. J. Opt. Soc. Amer. 44:875, 1954.)*

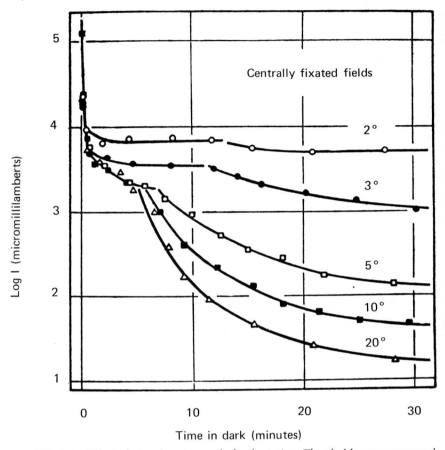

FIG. 3-6. *Effect of stimulus size on dark adaptation. Thresholds were measured with centrally fixated areas of different size. Note the geometric increase in threshold with only an arithmetic increase in size of target. (From Hecht, S., Haig, C., and Wald, G. J. Gen. Physiol. 19:321, 1935.)*

tion. In a fully dark-adapted eye, as indicated previously, rods and cones have almost equal sensitivity to red light stimuli, and therefore only a monophasic or slight bipartite curve will be obtained (Fig. 3-7). However, rods are far more sensitive to a blue light stimulus in the dark-adapted eye, so that a very large duplex curve is seen with a blue test light (Fig. 3-7).

In our experience, more consistent and reproducible results are obtained with an intermittent presentation than with a steady presentation of the light stimulus.

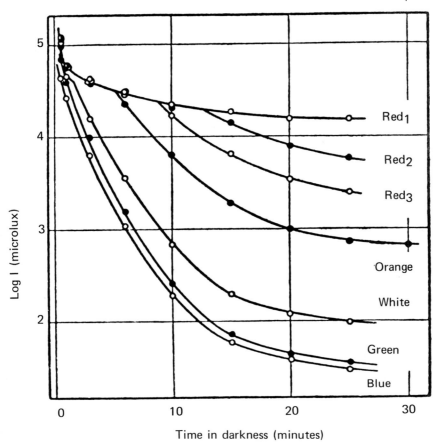

FIG. 3-7. *Dark adaptation with a 1-degree test located at 5 degrees above the fovea. With deep red (longer wavelength) only a monofunctional curve is obtained. Rods and cones have equal sensitivity for this wavelength. Rod sensitivity is greatest at the blue end of the spectrum. (From Kohlrausch, A. Pfleuger Arch. ges. Physiol. 196:113, 1922.)*

RETINAL AREA

In the fovea there is a rod-free area of about 1 degree and 40 minutes in diameter, and therefore only a monophasic cone curve is obtained upon testing this area (Fig. 3-8). The fovea is the least sensitive area in the fully dark-adapted eye. Sensitivity increases away from the fovea and reaches a maximum where rods are most heavily concentrated at 15 to 20 degrees eccentricity from the fovea (Fig. 3-9).[26, 58, 59] Thresholds become slightly higher peripheral to this area, and con-

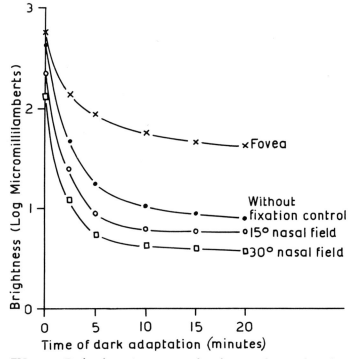

FIG. 3-8. *Dark adaptation measured at fovea and 15 and 30 degrees from the fovea. Note that the curve is highest at the fovea. Also note the importance of accurate fixation as the second curve from the top (supposedly a foveal curve) was obtained without fixation. The foveal curve is always monophasic because of the absence of rods. Peripheral curves are also monophasic here because no preadaptation was given.*

siderably higher in the far periphery. The thresholds are slightly higher from the inferior than from the superior retina (Fig. 3-10).[38] Obviously, fixation is very important when testing dark adaptation.

PUPIL SIZE

A fixed pupil size obtained by an artificial pupil or by dilation is recommended, since pupil size changes with adaptation. An artificial pupil is not practical when testing peripheral retinal areas, but is better than dilation when testing the fovea. If an artificial pupil cannot be used or dilation cannot be accomplished, pupillary size correction is particularly important if the patient has been administered a miotic

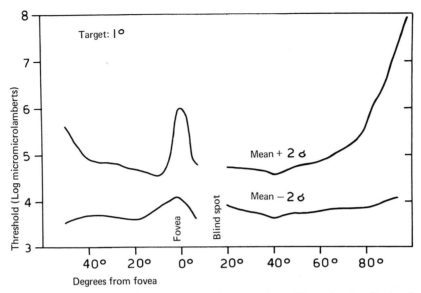

FIG. 3-9. Perimetric dark adaptation in horizontal meridian, showing final rod thresholds at each locus. Not how the rod thresholds are highest in central and far peripheral areas. (From Sloan, L. L. Amer. J. Ophthal. 30:705, 1947.)

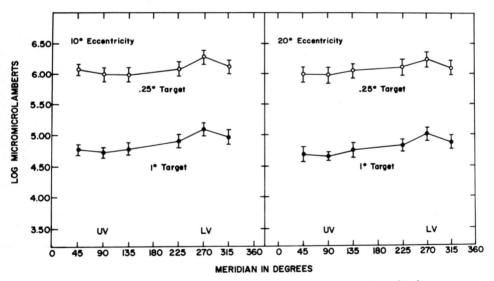

FIG. 3-10. Absolute threshold as a function of meridian for the 0.25- and 1-degree targets at 10- and 20-degree eccentricities. UV refers to upper vertical retinal meridian and LV to lower vertical retinal meridian. Note how the thresholds average higher in the inferior meridian. (From Krill, A. E., Smith, V. C., Blough, R., and Pass, A. Invest. Ophthal. 7:701, 1968.)

agent. On miotics the threshold may be elevated as much as ten times.[39, 64]

In a patient not on drugs it is questionable whether a pupillary correction factor is needed if there is interest only in the final rod threshold. Sloan [58] showed very little change in final threshold with a pupillary size of 5 millimeters or more. The pupils of most patients kept in the dark for a sufficient period of time will reach this size. However, in any dark-adaptation study in which the full curve is obtained and in which a preadapting light is used, it is essential to have a controlled pupillary size.

AGE

Sensitivity mainly to blue-violet light decreases with age [23, 43] (particularly after 40), probably reflecting the increasing yellowness of the lens nucleus, which occurs with the aging process.

VARIABILITY

Using the same test circumstances, intraindividual variability of normal final thresholds, in our experience and that of others, usually is no greater than 0.3 log unit.[48] Interindividual variability, though, may be as much as 1 log unit. The final threshold portion of the dark-adaptation curve is the least variable portion of this curve (Fig. 3-4).

TECHNIQUE

Obviously, a standardized method is necessary for useful dark-adaptation studies. We use a modified Goldmann-Weekers adaptometer (Fig. 3-11).[13, 19] (This instrument is manufactured by the Haag-Streit Company in Berne, Switzerland.) The original commercially available instrument tests only one retinal area, 15 degrees above the fovea, and uses only one target size, 11 degrees in diameter. Also, only one colored filter, red, is available with the instrument. Ideally, one

FIG. 3-11. *Goldmann-Weekers adaptometer manufactured by Haag-Streit AG of Berne, Switzerland. Side view (Fig. 3-11A) shows recording drum and intensity control apparatus. Note long tube (at top of globe) which can be inserted into four positions to project fixation light anywhere along horizontal, vertical, and oblique meridians. Front view of apparatus (Fig. 3-11B) shows aperture for one-degree target at back of globe. Perimetric fixation light tube is at side of globe. Projection device at left front of globe projects four spots of light around stimulus to give foveal testing.*

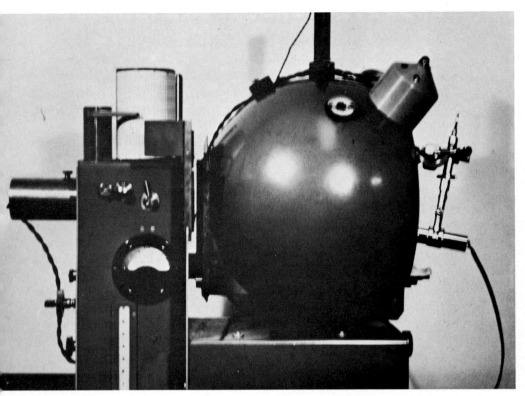

B   A

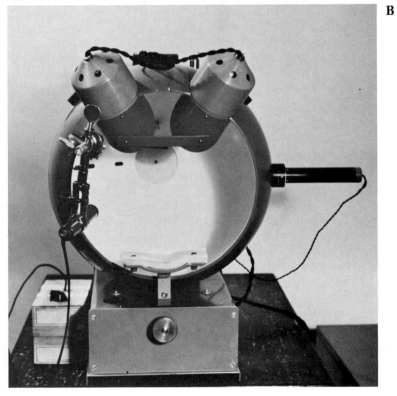

should be able to test many retinal areas, use many target sizes (a standard test size should be considerably less than 11 degrees in diameter), utilize at least two colors (preferably blue and red), and determine foveal thresholds.

The original instrument is easily modified, so that these problems can be solved without much difficulty. First of all, the Haag-Streit Company now also manufactures a globe with a movable fixation light that can be projected anywhere along the horizontal, vertical, or oblique meridians (Fig. 3-11). In addition, there are two slots in back of the old or new globe that will hold plates. A plate can be constructed for one slot with apertures for testing various-sized retinal areas. Our plates have apertures that produce test target diameters of 0.25, 0.50, 1, 2.5, and 5 degrees. In addition, we have constructed a series of plates with different-colored filters for use in the second slot. For foveal testing, a special fixation device is necessary. We use four light spots equally spaced around the test target (which is usually 0.25 degree for foveal testing). These can be obtained from a battery-powered light source placed in back of a specially constructed plate or by projection from a projector attached to the front of the globe. The subject is maintaining foveal fixation when the four light spots are simultaneously visualized. Thus, the new Goldmann-Weekers adaptometer, with proper modifications, is a versatile instrument. There are only a few other commercially available adaptometers. One manufactured in Sweden offers considerable promise.[49]

In our patients, dark-adaptation studies are performed after a careful period of instruction and an initial short trial run. The tested eye is dilated to about 7 to 8 mm with tropicamide, 1.0 percent. The patient is first placed in complete darkness for 3 minutes, and then exposed to a white preadapting illumination of 3.13 log millilamberts luminance for 7 minutes. Absolute white-light threshold measurements are started immediately at the completion of preadaptation.

The subject initially fixates on a 2 mm red light of variable brightness, located about 15 degrees above the center (the position of the fixation light in the original instrument) of the test light. In our routine testing, a retinal subtense of 1 degree is always used. The stimulus is presented in the form of light flashes of 1 second in duration; the dark interval is also 1 second. The test light is calibrated at a maximum luminance of 9.4 log micromicrolamberts and at the onset is presented at a luminance of 8.4 log micromicrolamberts, with the subsequent direction of change dependent on the response of the subject. At each test time four "on" or "ascending" and four "off" or "descending"

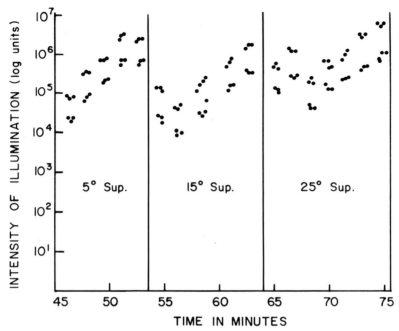

FIG. 3-12. *Raw data from patient with hysterical amblyopia after 45 minutes in the dark. The thresholds at the top are when the patient first sees the light (threshold of appearance) and those at the bottom are when the patient states the light has disappeared (threshold of disappearance). In each test period four thresholds of appearance and disappearance are obtained. These data are typical of a good subject, as the thresholds show consistency within one test period. From period to period, however, the thresholds vary but tend to shift upward, a finding typical of hysterical amblyopia. (From Krill, A. E. Amer. J. Ophthal. 63:230, 1967.)*

thresholds are noted (Fig. 3-12).* An "ascending threshold" is the intensity at which the subject first sees the test light as its luminance is increased; a "descending threshold" is the intensity at which the subject ceases to see the test light as its luminance is lowered. Each threshold intensity is mechanically plotted (on a log scale) versus time. The approximate true absolute threshold during a test time is calculated as an average of the four "on" and "off" thresholds obtained at that time. Rest periods between each test period are 0.5 minute for the first 10 minutes and then usually one minute thereafter. The sub-

---

* The reliability of a subject is determined by noting the consistency of the thresholds within each test time.

ject is notified immediately before the test light is presented and before a rest period.

Each subject is tested in the standard retinal area for a total of 40 minutes, at which time a constant final threshold value is usually obtained. The average test light luminance at the time of threshold stabilization is about 4.4 log micromicrolamberts. If threshold stabilization is not obtained by 40 minutes, it is continued until thresholds remain stabilized over three successive test periods.

After 40 minutes the movable fixation light is used and tests are made of 1-degree retinal areas at 5 and 25 degrees eccentricity in the superior meridian. Red and blue light stimuli are then used at each of the three retinal eccentricities evaluated with white light stimuli. Additional areas tested depend on the patient and the problem at hand.

ABNORMALITIES OF NIGHT VISION

As indicated previously, no one test adequately characterizes all aspects of visual performance under reduced illumination.[55] Many investigations, particularly during the Second World War,[5] searched for such a test, but were unsuccessful. Dark adaptation (the most frequently used test) for either light flashes or form could not be used to categorize normal individuals. "Not a single test could be found to categorize personnel for night duty, or for separating normal men into those with functionally inferior night vision and those with functionally adequate night vision."[5] A positive conclusion reached was that "night vision is much too complex to be assayed by any single type of test."[5]

A battery of tests might suffice for adequately evaluating scotopic and mesopic visual capabilities.[55] A possible battery of tests showing little or no correlation with each other in the normal subject (and therefore evaluating different capabilities) would include a dark-adaptation curve, visual acuity under mesopic and scotopic luminances, and a study of recovery from glare under reduced illumination. Possibly additional information might be gained from a study of contrast sensitivity (a measure that has limited correlation with clinical measurements of visual acuity) under various luminances.

In patients with organic disease, there are correlations among all visual measurements under reduced illumination. Almost any test of scotopic function will identify patients with moderate or severe organic night blindness. However, more subtle abnormalities may be revealed mainly by dark-adaptation studies—in fact, sometimes only by alterations in the rate of dark adaptation. In general, then, dark adaptation is the best single test for detecting abnormal scotopic and, to some extent, abnormal mesopic function in patients with disease. In the ensuing discussion of diseases affecting night vision (and one may presume mesopic vision to some degree as well), only the effect of the condition on dark adaptation will be mentioned.

EXTRARETINAL CAUSES OF ABNORMAL NIGHT VISION

CLINICAL VITAMIN DEFICIENCIES

Night blindness is likely to occur in diseases associated with a significant deficiency of vitamin A,[1, 2, 6, 7, 24, 25, 50, 51, 53, 67] a vitamin that plays an important role in the metabolism of rhodopsin. Vitamin A deficiency (Table 3-4) may occur because of the following: (1) Deficient intake due to starvation. Alcoholism is a frequent cause of deficient intake in this country. A greater requirement for vitamin A may exist during the last few months of pregnancy;[31] therefore, the complaint of night blindness is likely to occur during this period, particularly if dietary intake is inadequate to begin with, or a superimposed illness occurs. (2) Deficient fat absorption due to achlorhydria, sprue, celiac disease, chronic gastritis, chronic pancreatitis, chronic gastroenteritis, cystic fibrosis, giardiasis, or after gastric resection. Data on a patient with celiac disease whom we tested before and after treatment are shown in Figure 3-13. Gallbladder secretion is essential for fat absorption, and therefore obstruction of the common duct may produce a deficiency of vitamin A. (3) Deficient metabolism in the liver due

TABLE 3-4
Causes of Vitamin A Deficiency

Problem	Cause
Deficient intake	Starvation, increased need (pregnancy)
Deficient fat absorption	Sprue, celiac disease, chronic gastritis, giardiasis, chronic pancreatitis, achlorhydria, cystic fibrosis, gastric resection
Abnormal liver metabolism	Chronic disease
Massive urinary excretion	Cancer, severe acute and chronic infections, rheumatic heart disease

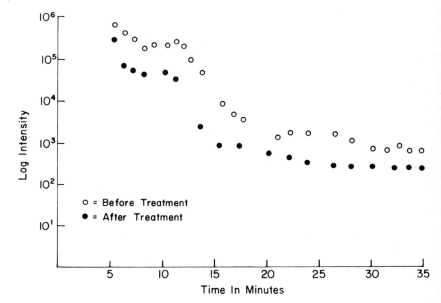

FIG. 3-13. *Absolute thresholds from patient with celiac disease before and six months after therapy was initiated. Note that after treatment final thresholds occur more rapidly and all thresholds are lower (more sensitive).*

particularly to chronic disease of this organ. And (4) massive urinary excretion of vitamin A likely to occur in cancer, severe acute infections with pyrexia, such as pneumonia, and rheumatic heart disease, or chronic infections such as tuberculosis and chronic nephritis.[46, 47, 52]

Deficient vitamin B intake probably also affects night vision, although the relationship is less clear here. It is likely that such deficiencies affect the metabolism of the protein portion, opsin, of the substance rhodopsin.[15] In deficient intake problems or in chronic liver disease, multivitamin deficiencies result, and therefore it is hard to identify which vitamin or vitamins are most important in the cause of visual problems that occur. In patients with deficient dietary intake or liver disease, it is usually just as well to assume that multiple vitamins will be needed, rather than just vitamin A. It has been shown, in fact, that treatment with proteins and vitamin B supplement alone may create additional problems. In the treatment of a starvation disease, kwashiorkor, it is necessary to supplement the treatment of patients with severe protein deficiency with vitamin A.[4] If this is not done, as dietary protein supplement is given, vitamin A requirement increases and the last reserves of this vitamin in the liver eventually are used up.[4, 53]

In general, abnormalities of both dark-adaptation rate and threshold are characteristic in patients with multivitamin deficiencies. Classically, it has been claimed that in vitamin A deficiency there is only an elevated final threshold. There are definite examples, though, in which abnormalities of both dark-adaptation rate and threshold are noted (for example, in celiac disease), in spite of what appears to be almost a pure vitamin A deficiency.

OTHER SYSTEMIC DISEASES

Elevated rod absolute thresholds have been cited in patients with hyperthyroidism.[31] In fact, normalization of dark adaptation after treatment of the thyrotoxicosis was noted in a few cases where repeated dark-adaptation studies were done. On the contrary, no conclusive abnormalities are seen in hypothyroidism.

The hemoglobin level may be significant, particularly in patients with nutritional deficiency. Someswara and Subha [62] found a higher incidence of night blindness where both nutritional deficiency and anemia were found together.

HYPOXIA

The retina is markedly susceptible to a decrease in available oxygen (termed hypoxia) because of its relatively high metabolic rate. It has been demonstrated by several workers [17, 40, 42, 45, 56] that hypoxia results in a decrease in white and colored light absolute thresholds. In experiments where hemoglobin oxygen saturations have been monitored,[17] it has been shown that hypoxia raises both cone and rod absolute visual thresholds (Fig. 3-14). Rod thresholds are elevated to a greater extent. Peripheral rod thresholds are affected more than central rod thresholds. Only the latter portions of rod and cone dark-adaptation curves are affected by hypoxia (Fig. 3-14). The first four minutes of either type of curve are unaffected.

An elevation of rod absolute threshold also occurs with increasing altitude.[41] The precise altitude at which deterioration of night vision occurs is dependent on many factors. (In one experiment first effects were detected at about 9,000 feet.) This elevation may be due to a decrease in available oxygen, but a question that has not been resolved is whether there is an independent effect of barometric pressure on threshold.

In general, it is thought that increasing the oxygen concentration received by a subject who is hypoxic will result in improved visual sen-

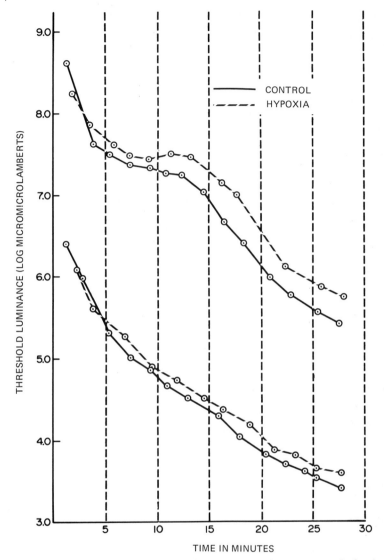

FIG. 3-14. *Effect of hypoxia on dark adaptation. The upper two dark-adaptation curves were obtained with a one-degree circular yellow target at an eccentricity of five degrees in the nasal field on the horizontal meridian. The subject's eye was preadapted with blue light having a luminance of 1,000 millilamberts. The lower two dark-adaptation curves were recorded with a one-degree circular blue target at the same five-degree eccentricity. The subject's eye was preadapted with red light having a luminance of 1,000 millilamberts. Note how the upper and lower curves were elevated by hypoxia. (From Ernest, J. T., and Krill, A. E. Invest. Ophthal. 10:323, 1971.)*

sitivity, but this improvement can in no way be extrapolated to the hyperoxic condition. In fact, breathing high concentrations of oxygen under pressure decreases various aspects of visual performance. It is also of interest to note that glucose [44] or rapid breathing (hypercapnea) may protect against the effects of increasing altitude on the dark-adaptation thresholds, whereas insulin enhances this effect.

REFRACTIVE ERRORS

In one study it was noted that myopes, particularly those with a refractive error of over 15 diopters, had higher than normal thresholds even with no associated retinal disease. However, it is not certain that a retinal pathological process was ruled out in all of these patients.[31] In another study of 10 patients with a refractive error over 20 diopters and a diagnosis of myopic degeneration, nine showed significantly elevated thresholds.[8a]

GLAUCOMA

Zuego and Drance [70] reported a selective elevation of the final rod threshold at a retinal eccentricity of 15 degrees in early open-angle glaucoma. This abnormality was best shown by comparing a ratio of the absolute threshold at 15 degrees with that at 30 degrees in glaucoma and normal patients of the same age. This abnormality was demonstrated in patients with elevated ocular tension even before visual field changes were noted.

Occasionally, a patient with untreated glaucoma will complain of some degree of night blindness and show an improvement in dark adaptation after treatment.

Patients on miotic agents experience a loss in visual sensitivity which is roughly proportional to the reduction in area of pupillary size caused by the drug (see discussion under *Pupil Size* in the section *Parameters Affecting Dark Adaptation*).

RETINAL CAUSES OF ABNORMAL DARK ADAPTATION

ABNORMALITIES OF DARK-ADAPTATION TIME

Oguchi's Disease

This is a form of congenital stationary night blindness associated with a peculiar yellowish or grayish bandlike or homogeneous discoloration of the fundus. Prolonged periods in darkness usually lead to a disappearance of the abnormal fundus coloration and marked improvement or normalization of subjective dark adaptation.

Patients with Oguchi's disease have been divided into two major types.[20] Type 1 patients are characterized by the occurrence of rod dark adaptation after a sufficient period of time in the dark. The final rod threshold may be normal or elevated. (Figure 3-15 is from a patient who took 4 to 5 hours to show a rod-cone break. Note that the final threshold is elevated about 1 log unit.) Also, after sufficient time in the dark, the abnormal fundus coloration disappears in Type 1 patients. This latter event is known as Mizuo's phenomenon. Patients in a second group, Type 2, show no rod dark adaptation. These patients have less striking abnormal fundus coloration than those classified as Type 1. Some of these patients, Type 2A, show Mizuo's phenomenon, whereas others, Type 2B, do not.

The time for complete secondary dark adaptation to occur in Type 1 patients varies from case to case and also with the degree of preadaptation. Generally, most cases take 2 to 4 hours, but as long as 24 hours has been reported. The time for complete disappearance of the ab-

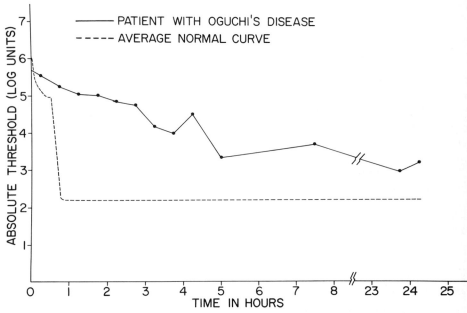

FIG. 3-15. Dark-adaptation curve from a patient with Oguchi's disease. The patient took about 4 to 5 hours to reach a final threshold. Final threshold is slightly elevated.

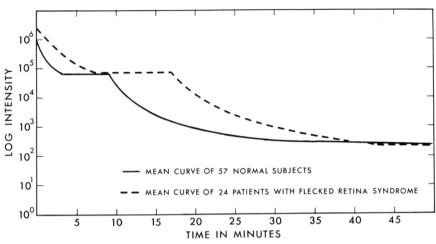

FIG. 3-16. Mean dark-adaptation curves for 57 normals and 24 patients with the "flecked-retina syndrome." Note the delay in reaching the final cone and rod thresholds and in the rod-cone break in the patient curve. The values of the final thresholds are about the same in the two groups. (From Krill, A. E., and Klien, B. A. Arch. Ophthal. 74:496, 1965.)

normal coloration is not related to the time for complete secondary dark adaptation.

Flecked Retina Syndrome

Three conditions characterized by a limited or widespread distribution of deep yellowish or white lesions of various sizes and configuration without vascular and optic nerve abnormalities or pigment migration have in common certain features designated as the flecked retina syndrome.[35] The three conditions, drusen, fundus albipunctatus, and fundus flavimaculatus, have distinct ophthalmoscopic, fluorescein, and probably pathological characteristics.* [17a,32a]

The common features include a high incidence of macular disease, normal peripheral visual fields, a usual abnormal electrooculogram, and characteristic dark-adaptation time abnormalities. In general, dark-adaptation cone and rod thresholds are normal, but the time when each occurs, as well as the rod-cone break time, is slower than normal (Fig. 3-16 and Table 3-5). The b-wave of the electroretinogram, which is usually of normal amplitude, takes longer than normal to reach a maximum amplitude in the dark-adapted eye. Occasionally,

* No pathology has yet been obtained from an eye with fundus albipunctatus.

TABLE 3-5
Flecked Retina Group Dark-Adaptation Times *

	Cone Threshold		Rod-Cone Break		Rod Threshold	
	Mean	Standard Deviation	Mean	Standard Deviation	Mean	Standard Deviation
Normal Group †	3.1	1.0	9.1	1.5	30.5	2.6
Flecked Retina Group	7.5	5.5	17.0	5.6	41.5	11.4
Probability ‡	<.001		<.001		<.001	

* Time in minutes.
† Normal Group = 57 subjects.
‡ See *Arch. Ophthal.* 74:496, 1965, for statistical details.

the time of dark adaptation is so delayed that the patient will complain of "difficulty in adjusting to the dark," but most patients have no night visual complaints.

Fleck Retina of Kandori

This is a stationary, probably congenital, condition seen up to date only in Japan and characterized by large, discrete, irregularly shaped deposits in the midperipheral fundus.[32] There is a slower than normal dark-adaptation curve with normal final thresholds usually evident by 40 minutes after the start of testing.

In contrast to drusen, fundus albipunctatus, and fundus flavimaculatus, visual acuity is always normal in the fleck retina of Kandori. The scotopic b-wave of the ERG may take longer than normal to reach a normal maximum amplitude (See Chapter 16, Vol. 2).

STATIONARY ABNORMALITIES OF FINAL THRESHOLD

Congenital Stationary Night Blindness Without Fundal Changes

Congenital stationary night blindness with no fundal changes is characterized by the inability to see at night because of the complete absence of rod adaptation in affected individuals (Fig. 3-17). The condition may be inherited in an autosomal dominant, autosomal recessive, or X-linked recessive manner.

Vision is always normal in the dominant form but always abnormal

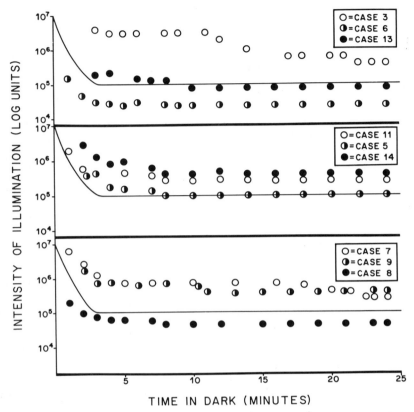

FIG. 3-17. *Dark-adaptation data from 9 patients with congenital night blindness. Solid curve in each section represents average normal cone curve. All patients' curves are monofunctional, showing only cone curves. All patients, except case 6, required a longer than normal time to reach a final cone threshold, and final cone thresholds were elevated in five patients (cases 3, 7, 9, 11, and 14). (From Krill, A. E., and Martin, D. Invest. Ophthal. 10:625, 1971.)*

in the X-linked recessive form. Vision may be normal or abnormal in the autosomal recessive type. Acuity may be as poor as 20/200 but is more likely, in patients with abnormal vision, to range between 20/40 to 20/100. Myopia is universal in the X-linked recessive type and frequent in the autosomal recessive form with abnormal vision.

Mild to moderate photopic abnormalities are common in all three hereditary types of congenital night blindness.[36, 61] In fact, the characteristic monophasic cone dark-adaptation curve is frequently slow and elevated as compared with normal controls (Fig. 3-17).

Congenital Stationary Night Blindness with Fundal Changes

Fundus Albipunctatus. An occasional patient with this diagnosis will show no secondary or rod adaptation. Most patients will show a delayed dark adaptation, as indicated in the previous discussion.

Oguchi's Disease. As indicated, patients with Type 2A Oguchi's disease show no secondary or rod dark adaptation.

Hereditary Vitreoretinal Degeneration and Night Blindness.[18] A pedigree was described in which a typical vitreoretinal degeneration of autosomal recessive inheritance was associated with a stationary form of congenital night blindness. The dark-adaptation and electroretinographic findings (see Chapter 4) were typical of stationary night blindness.

PROGRESSIVE ABNORMALITIES OF DARK-ADAPTATION THRESHOLDS

Diffuse chorioretinal degenerations—including retinitis pigmentosa; the choroidal atrophies, such as gyrate atrophy, and choroideremia; and the autosomal recessive form of vitreoretinal degeneration—are all characterized by early and diffuse involvement of the receptors. Therefore, afflicted patients complain of night blindness as an early symptom. Abnormal dark-adaptation curves are characteristic even in early stages of the disease. Frequently the rods are involved earlier and to a greater extent than the cones, so that there is a greater

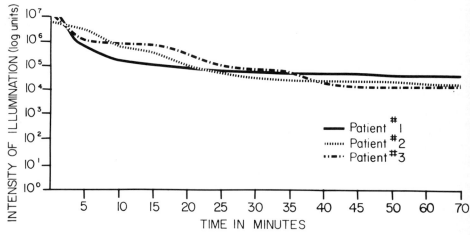

FIG. 3-18. *Dark-adaptation curves from three patients with retinitis pigmentosa. Note that both rod and cone segments are elevated.*

elevation of the rod portion of the dark-adaptation curve. Eventually, though, cone thresholds are usually also considerably elevated (Fig. 3-18).

An interesting finding that has been demonstrated in retinitis pigmentosa, which depicts the greater involvement of the rods as compared with the cones, is the so-called inverted profile (Fig. 3-19).[57, 58, 69] In the normal subject the thresholds are usually slightly higher (less sensitive) at 5 degrees than at 10 or 25 degrees retinal eccentricity. However, in the patient with retinitis pigmentosa the threshold at 5 degrees is almost always lower (more sensitive) than at the more peripheral areas, reflecting the greater involvement of rods, which are more concentrated in the peripheral areas tested.

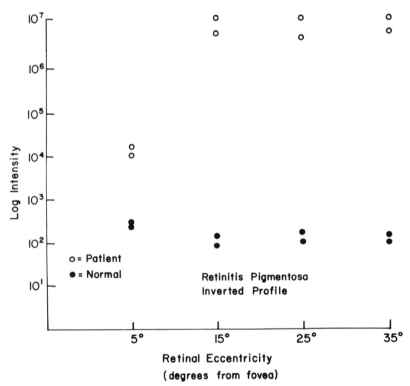

FIG. 3-19. Dark-adaptation data from two patients with retinitis pigmentosa and two normals at 5, 15, 25, and 35 degrees retinal eccentricities. Note that in the normal subjects thresholds are slightly higher at five degrees, whereas in patients with retinitis pigmentosa thresholds are lowest at this point. This characteristic greater involvement of areas away from the macula is related to a more pronounced effect of the disease on rods than on cones and is known as the inverted profile.

There is sometimes a problem as to whether eyeground changes represent scarring from a previous inflammatory process or a progressive retinal degeneration. An electroretinogram is markedly abnormal, frequently extinguished, in the latter, but only mildly abnormal or normal after chorioretinitis; but this test is not always available. Several dark-adaptation findings may aid in distinguishing the two conditions. The finding of an inverted retinal profile, as just described, favors a retinal degeneration. Severe elevation of both rod and cone thresholds is more characteristic of retinitis pigmentosa (Fig. 3-18). Finally, successive dark-adaptation determinations over a period of time (Fig. 3-20) indicate a progressive disorder (sometimes where distinct changes are not evident on less sensitive visual field testing).

A-beta-lipoproteinemia is associated with a retinal degeneration and typical functional changes such as severe night blindness. It has recently been shown that the retinal changes may be reversible. Carr[9] reported restoration of dark adaptation in two affected patients following administration of doses of 200,000 units of vitamin A and a continued maintenance of the serum vitamin A levels. It appears that the ability to dark-adapt closely parallels the serum vitamin A level in this condition.

Mytonic dystrophy is characterized by abnormalities of retinal function, in spite of frequent normal-appearing eyegrounds.[8] Burian and Burns[8] have shown elevated final rod thresholds, particularly with blue targets in this condition. It is not certain as yet, though, whether this is a progressive abnormality or not. The absence or presence of retinal involvement is not always obvious from the appearance of the

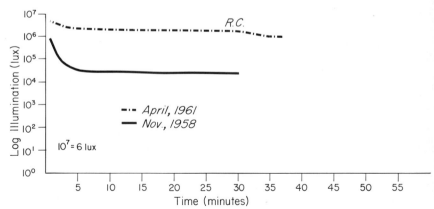

FIG. 3-20. *Progression of dark-adaptation abnormality in a patient with retinitis pigmentosa over a period of almost three years.*

eyegrounds. Dark-adaptation studies, as well as tests such as the elec-troretinogram and electrooculogram, may be helpful in evaluating the presence of and the type of retinal abnormality in various diseases.

CONVERSION REACTION AFFECTING VISION ("HYSTERICAL AMBLYOPIA")

Two dark-adaptation abnormalities may be found in patients with hysterical amblyopia.[22, 33] Elevated rod thresholds were found in 36 of 56 patients with this diagnosis that were tested. Thirty of the 36 showed another interesting phenomenon called the exhaustion phe-nonemon (Figs. 3-12 and 3-21).[33] Seven without elevated final thresh-olds also showed this finding. This exhaustion phenomenon com-prises a consistent upper shift in threshold of at least 0.5 log unit after prolonged testing. This finding is not seen in normals or in patients with organic disease (unless a superimposed conversion reac-tion is present). Repeated dark-adaptation studies in such patients may correlate with the psychological status of the individual (Fig. 3-21). Elevated absolute thresholds, not retinal in origin, have also been found in psychotics.[68]

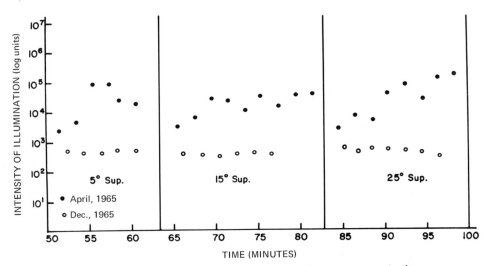

FIG. 3-21. *Initial and follow-up average threshold data after 50 minutes in the dark for a patient with hysterical amblyopia. Note that thresholds on the first test are elevated and also tend to shift upward (exhaustion phenomenon). On the second test thresholds were within normal limits and no longer showed fluctua-tion; at this time the patient's psychological status was also thought to be im-proved. (From Krill, A. E. Amer. J. Ophthal. 63:230, 1967.)*

MALINGERING

It is possible for a patient to choose and maintain a given test-light level above his absolute visual threshold if he can depend on clues other than the test light. The clues used may be such factors as the time between test-light exposures, the sound of a test-light shutter, or inadvertent signals from the examiner. It is possible to exclude mechanical or procedural techniques that might be used by a patient to give invalid test results. A specific technique called the double staircase method is particularly good for detecting falsely abnormal results.[16]

TOXIC RETINOPATHY

In toxic retinopathies due to a number of agents there may be severe retinal involvement, as evidenced by all tests of retinal function, including dark adaptation. Two examples of such drugs include quinine [21] and thioridazine.[11] Transient toxic retinopathy of a mild degree may be found in acute or subacute intoxication with ethyl alcohol.[66] In fact, slow dark adaptation with some elevation of final thresholds may be one of the major functional abnormalities in this condition.

Chloroquine Retinopathy

On the other hand, a striking exception is found in chloroquine retinopathy. An unusual finding in this condition is the presence of normal or close to normal final or rod adaptation in all areas of the retina, even in advanced stages of the disease, with an extinguished electroretinogram (Fig. 3-22).[37] However, cone function, as measured by initial dark-adaptation or by red-light thresholds, is usually abnormal, even in early stages of chloroquine retinopathy.[10] In fact, elevated red-light absolute thresholds may be the most sensitive criterion of early chloroquine retinopathy in most patients.[10] However, some patients have macular sparing, and therefore red-light thresholds may be normal.[37]

Contrary to what is found on subjective dark adaptation, no such distinction between the cone and rod portions of the ERG is evident in advanced cases. Indeed, no responses are observed, regardless of the conditions of testing. The explanation for this discrepancy between what is found on the ERG and on subjective dark adaptation in advanced chloroquine retinopathy is not clear.[37]

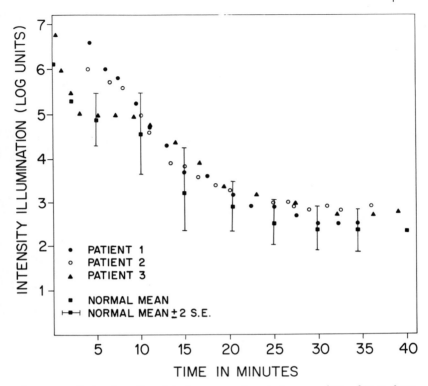

FIG. 3-22. *Dark-adaptation data from normal control group of 57 subjects showing mean (plus or minus two standard deviations from the mean for some values) together with data from the 3 patients with chloroquine retinopathy who had extinguished electroretinograms and eyeground changes similar to those seen in retinitis pigmentosa. Cases 1 and 2 did not see the test target for first four to five minutes, and both had elevated cone thresholds. All three patients had normal final rod thresholds. (From Krill, A. E., Potts, A. M., and Johanson, C. E. Amer. J. Ophthal. 71:530, 1971.)*

Since the eyegrounds of advanced chloroquine retinopathy may be similar to those seen in retinitis pigmentosa, it is important to know that dark-adaptation profiles easily distinguish the two conditions. As indicated previously, most patients with even early retinitis pigmentosa have markedly abnormal final thresholds. An occasional patient, particularly with an autosomal dominant or sector form of retinitis pigmentosa, will show close to normal thresholds in some retinal areas. However, in contrast to chloroquine retinopathy, when testing is done in several areas in the same quadrant (or in different quadrants with

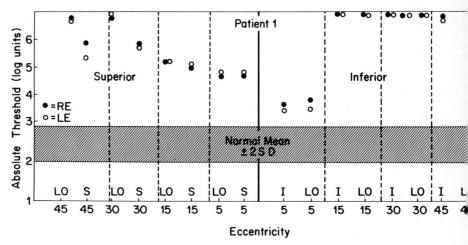

FIG. 3-23. *Absolute threshold values from normal-appearing superior retina and affected inferior retina from patient with sector retinitis pigmentosa plotted with data from normal control population (mean plus or minus two standard deviations). All thresholds were elevated. The greatest elevations were from the inferior retina. The symbols used to designate meridians are* L *for left,* O *for oblique,* I *for inferior, and* S *for superior. The position on a meridian (eccentricity) is shown along the X-axis in degrees. (From Krill, A. E., Archer, D., and Martin, D. Amer. J. Ophthal. 69:977, 1970.)*

sector retinitis pigmentosa), markedly elevated final thresholds are always seen in some areas (Fig. 3-23).

On the other hand, we have tested some patients with primary cone degenerations, who eventually had a severe abnormality of the scotopic ERG but retained a normal or only slightly abnormal dark adaptation in all areas tested.[34] These patients, though, usually have normal or close to normal peripheral visual fields, whereas patients with advanced chloroquine retinopathy always have abnormal peripheral visual fields.

REFERENCES

1. Adams, D. F., Johnstone, J. M., and Hunter, R. F. Vitamin A deficiency following total gastrectomy. *Lancet* 1:415, 1960.

2. Agacht, S., and Mandelbaum, J. The relation between vitamin A and dark adaptation. *J.A.M.A.* 112:910, 1939.

3. Arden, G. B., and Weale, R. A. Nervous mechanisms and dark adaptation. *J. Physiol.* 125:417, 1954.

4. Arroyave, G., Wilson, J., and Mendez, M. Alterations in serum concentrations of

vitamin A associated with hypoproteinemia of severe protein malnutrition. *J. Pediat.* 62:920, 1963.

5. Berry, W. *Review of War-time Studies of Dark Adaptation, Night Vision Tests, and Related Topics.* Ann Arbor, Mich., Armed Forces NRC Vision Committee, 1949.

6. Booker, L. E., Callison, E. C., and Hewston, E. M. An experimental determination of the minimum vitamin A requirements of normal adults. *J. Nutr.* 17:317, 1939.

7. Brenner, S., and Roberts, L. Effects of vitamin A deletion in young adults. *Arch. Int. Med.* 71:474, 1943.

8. Burian, H. M., and Burns, C. A. Electroretinography and dark adaptation in mytonic dystrophy. *Amer. J. Ophthal.* 61:1044, 1966.

8a. Campbell, C. J., and Rittler, M. C. "Clinical Adaptation Studies of the Human Retina," in Straatsma, B. R., Hall, M. O., Allen, R. A., and Crescitelli, F. (eds.). *The Retina. Morphology, Function, and Clinical Characteristics.* Berkeley, University of California Press, 1969, pp. 513–544.

9. Carr, R. E. Vitamin A therapy may reverse degenerative retinal syndrome. *Clinical Trends* 8:8, 1970.

10. Carr, R. E., Gouras, P., and Gunkel, R. D. Chloroquine retinopathy; early detection by retinal threshold test. *Arch. Ophthal.* 75:171, 1966.

11. Connell, M. M., Poley, B. J., and McFarlane, J. R. Chorioretinopathy associated with thioridazine therapy. *Arch. Ophthal.* 71:816, 1964.

12. Craik, K. J. W., and Vernon, M. D. The nature of dark adaptation. *Brit. J. Psychol.* 32: 62, 1941.

13. Dieterle, P., and Gordon, E. Standard curve in physiological limits of dark adaptation by means of the Goldmann-Weekers adaptometer. *Brit. J. Ophthal.* 40:652, 1956.

14. Dohrn, R. H. Effect of low level red or white light on dark adaptation. *Amer. J. Optom.* 44:103, 1969.

15. Dowling, J. E., and Wald, G. Nightblindness. *Proc. Nat. Acad. Sci.* 44:648, 1958.

16. Ernest, J. T. Night vision testing. *Milit. Med.* 136:381, 1971.

17. Ernest, J. T., and Krill, A. E. The effect of hypoxia on visual function. *Invest. Ophthal.* 10:323, 1971.

17a. Farkas, T. G., Krill, A. E., Sylvester, V. M., and Archer, D. Familial and secondary drusen: Histological and functional characteristics. *Trans. Amer. Acad. Ophthal. Otol.* 75:333, 1971.

18. Feiler-Ofry, V., Adam, A., Regenbogen, L., Godel, V., and Stein, R. Hereditary vitreoretinal degeneration and nightblindness. *Amer. J. Ophthal.* 67:553, 1969.

19. Fankhauser, F., and Schmidt, T. Studies of the functions of the dark-adapted eye with the Goldmann-Weekers adaptometer. *Ophthalmologica* 133:264, 1957.

20. Francois, J. La maladie d'Oguchie. *Bull. Soc. Belg. Ophtal.* 110:170, 1955.

21. Francois, J., Verriest, G., and DeRouck, A. Etude des fonctions visuelles dans deux cas d'intoxication par la quinine. *Ophthalmologica* 153:324, 1967.

22. Granger, G. W. Dark adaptation in anxiety states and hysterics. *Brit. J. Physiol. Opt.* 13:235, 1956.

23. Gunkel, R. D., and Gouras, P. Changes in scotopic visibility thresholds with age. *Arch. Ophthal.* 69:4, 1963.

24. Graham, C. H. *Vision and Visual Perception.* New York, John Wiley & Sons, 1965.

25. Hecht, S., and Mandelbaum, J. The relation between vitamin A and dark adaptation. *J.A.M.A.* 112:910, 1939.

26. Hecht, S., and Mandelbaum, J. Dark adaptation and experimental human vitamin A deficiency. *Amer. J. Physiol.* 130:651, 1940.

27. Hecht, S., Haig, C., and Wald, G. The dark adaptation of retinal fields of different size and location. *J. Gen. Physiol.* 19:321, 1935.

28. Hecht, S., and Hsia, Y. Dark adaptation following light adaptation to red and white lights. *J. Opt. Soc. Amer.* 35:261, 1945.

29. Hecht, S., Shlaer, S., and Pirenne, M. H. Energy, quanta and vision. *J. Gen. Physiol.* 25:819, 1942.

30. Heck, J. The flicker electroretinogram of the human eye. *Acta Physiol. Scand.* 39:158, 1957.

31. Jayle, G. E., Ourgaud, A. G., Baisinger, C. F., and Holmes, W. J. *Night Vision.* Springfield, Ill., Charles C Thomas, 1959.

32. Kandori, F., Tamai, A., Kurimoto, S., and Fukunaga, K. Studies on fleck retina. *Amer. J. Ophthal.* (In press).

32a. Klien, B. A., and Krill, A. E. Fundus flavim aculatus: Clinical, functional, and histopathologic observations. *Amer. J. Ophthal.* 64:3, 1967.

33. Krill, A. E. Retinal function studies in hysterical amblyopia: a unique abnormality of dark adaptation. *Amer. J. Ophthal.* 63:230, 1967.

34. Krill, A. E., and Deutman, A. F. Dominant macular degenerations. The cone dystrophies. *Amer. J. Opthal.* 72:352, 1972.

35. Krill, A. E., and Klien, B. A. Flecked retina syndrome. *Arch. Ophthal.* 74:496, 1965.

36. Krill, A. E., and Martin, D. Photopic abnormalities in congenital stationary nightblindness. *Invest. Ophthal.* 10:625, 1971.

37. Krill, A. E., Potts, A. M., and Johanson, C. E. Chloroquine retinopathy. Investigation of a discrepancy between dark adaptation and the electroretinogram in advanced stages. *Amer. J. Ophthal.* 71:530, 1971.

38. Krill, A. E., Smith, V. C., Blough, R., and Pass, A. An absolute threshold defect in the inferior retina. *Invest. Ophthal.* 7:701, 1968.

39. Lindstrom, E. E., Tredici, T. J., and Martin, B. G. Effects of topical ophthalmic 2% pilocarpine on visual performance of normal subjects. *Aerospace Med.* 39:1236, 1968.

40. McDonald, D. R., and Adler, F. Effects of anoxia on the dark adaptation of the normal and of the vitamin A deficient subject. *Arch. Ophthal.* 22:980, 1939.

41. McFarland, R. A. Psychophysiological studies at high altitudes. *J. Comp. Physiol. Psychol.* 21:1, 1937.

42. McFarland, R. A., and Evans, J. N. Alterations in dark adaptation under reduced oxygen tensions. *Amer. J. Physiol.* 127:37, 1939.

43. McFarland, R. A., and Fisher, M. B. Alteration in dark adaptation as a function of age. *J. Geront.* 10:424, 1956.

44. McFarland, R. A., and Forbes, W. H. Effects of variations in the concentration of oxygen and of glucose on dark adaptation. *J. Gen. Physiol.* 24:69, 1940.

45. McFarland, R. A., Halperin, M. H., and Niven, J. I. Visual thresholds as an index of physiological imbalance during anoxia. *Amer. J. Physiol.* 142:328, 1944.

46. McLaren, D. S. *Malnutrition and the Eye.* New York and London, Academic Press, 1963, pp. 166–207.
47. Moore, T. *Vitamin A.* London, Elsevier Publishing Co., 1957, pp. 357–364 and 418–441.
48. Mote, F. A. Variability of measurements of human dark adaptation. *J. Opt. Soc. Amer.* 45:7, 1955.
49. Norden, A., and Stigmar, G. Measurement of dark adaptation in vitamin A deficiency by a new quantitative technique. *Acta Ophthal.* 47:81, 1969.
50. Patek, A. J., and Haig, C. The occurrence of abnormal dark adaptation and its relation to vitamin A metabolism in patients with cirrhosis of the liver. *J. Clin. Invest.* 18:609, 1939.
51. Petersen, R. A., Petersen, V. S., and Robb, R. M. Vitamin A deficiency with xerophthalmia and nightblindness in cystic fibrosis. *Amer. J. Dis. Child.* 116:662, 1968.
52. Rodger, F. C., and Sinclair, H. M. *Metabolic and Nutritional Eye Diseases.* Springfield, Ill., Charles C Thomas, 1969.
53. Roels, O. A. Vitamin A physiology. *J.A.M.A.* 214:1097, 1970.
54. Rushton, W. A. H., and Cohen, R. D. Visual purple level and the course of dark adaptation. *Nature* 173:301, 1954.
55. Schmidt, I. Are meaningful night vision tests for drivers feasible? *Amer. J. Optom.* 38:295, 1961.
56. Sheard, C. Effect of anoxia. Oxygen and increased intrapulmonary pressure on dark adaptation. *Mayo Clin. Proc.* 20:230, 1945.
57. Sloan, L. L. Light sense in pigmentary degeneration of the retina. *Arch. Ophthal.* 28:613, 1942.
58. Sloan, L. L. Rate of dark adaptation and regional threshold gradient of the dark-adapted eye; physiologic and clinical studies. *Amer. J. Ophthal.* 30:705, 1947.
59. Sloan, L. L. The threshold gradients of the rods and cones in the dark-adapted and in the partially light-adapted eye. *Amer. J. Ophthal.* 33:1077, 1950.
60. Sloan, L. L. Perimetric procedures for detection of selective impairment of cone function. Presented at ARVO meeting in Sarasota, Florida, on April 26, 1971.
61. Sloan, L. L., and Brown, D. J. Area and luminance of test object as variables in projection perimetry. *Vision Res.* 2:527, 1962.
62. Someswara, R. K., De, N. K., and Subha, R. P. Relationship between anemia and nightblindness. *Indian J. Med. Res.* 41:349, 1953.
63. Steffins, L., Bair, H., and Sheard, C. Dark adaptation in dietary deficiency in vitamin A. *Amer. J. Ophthal.* 23:1325, 1940.
64. Stewart, W. C., Madill, H. D., and Dyer, A. M. Night vision in the miotic eye. *Canad. Med. Ass. J.* 99:1145, 1968.
65. Stiles, W. S., and Crawford, B. H. The luminous efficiency of rays entering the eye pupil at different points. *Proc. Roy. Soc. London (Biol.).* 112:428, 1933.
66. Verriest, G., and Laplasse, D. New data concerning the influence of ethyl alcohol on human visual thresholds. *Exp. Eye Res.* 4:95, 1965.
67. Wald, G., Jeghers, J., and Armino, J. An experiment in human dietary nightblindness. *Amer. J. Physiol.* 123:732, 1938.

68. Wolin, L. R., Meder, J., Dillman, A., and Solymos, M. Objective measurement of light thresholds of neuropsychiatric patients. *Int. J. Neuropsychiat.* *1*:504, 1965.

69. Zeavin, B. H., and Wald, G. Rod and cone vision in retinitis pigmentosa. *Amer. J. Ophthal.* *42*:253, 1956.

70. Zuege, P., and Drance, S. M. Studies of dark adaptation of discrete paracentral retinal areas in glaucomatous subjects. *Amer. J. Ophthal.* *64*:56, 1967.

4

Electroretinogram

The electroretinogram (ERG) is the record of an action potential produced in the retina by an adequate light stimulus. This response has been known to scientists since 1865, when Holmgren reported the first ERG. Dewar [17] in 1877 was the first to record this potential in humans. However, it was studied mainly in animals until 1941, when Riggs [76] constructed an electrode practical for human use. The stimulus and groundwork for clinical usage were provided by Karpe [44] in 1945, when he reported the results of a study of 64 normal and 87 abnormal eyes.

BASIC MATERIALS

The elements necessary for electroretinography are as follows: (1) A suitable device for stimulating the retina with light. (2) Electrodes for leading off the action current produced by the resulting retinal potential differences. These are an active corneal electrode (Fig. 4-1), an indifferent or inactive forehead or nasal electrode, and one or two ground electrodes usually placed on the ear. (3) An amplification system to enlarge (amplify) the small action current (Fig. 4-2). And (4) a device for registering or recording the amplified response.

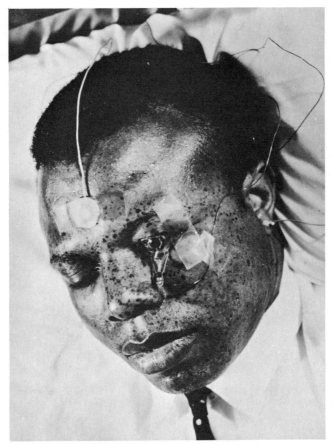

FIG. 4-1. *Patient with corneal contact lens (Burian-Allen type), which is an active electrode for electroretinography. A flat disc on the forehead is the inactive electrode. A ground electrode is attached to the ear.*

NORMAL ERG

COMPONENTS UNDER IDEAL CONDITIONS

Under the proper conditions the ERG consists of five components (Table 4-1). "Proper conditions" implies (1) a recording system that shows both fast and slow components (an oscilloscope is necessary rather than an electroencephalograph with an ink-writing apparatus which has inertia, and therefore cannot register either the very fast or very slow components); (2) an eye fixed in position (eye movements

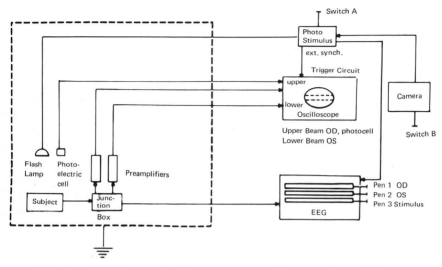

FIG. 4-2. Block diagram to illustrate two possible ways of amplifying and re-cording an ERG. One method involves amplification by the usual electroen-cephalograph machine and recording on paper of this machine via an ink-writer. The other method involves amplification with preamplifiers and an oscilloscope and photographing the record from the screen of the oscilloscope. Both can be used together as shown in this diagram where the leads go into a junction box and then separate into the two systems.

TABLE 4-1
Components of the ERG

Component	Principal Origin
Early receptor potential	Receptor outer segments
a-wave	Receptors
b-wave	Bipolar cell layer
1. Low-intensity d-c portion	?
2. High-intensity portion	Mueller cells
3. Oscillatory potentials	?
c-wave	Pigment epithelium
d-wave (off-response)	Interaction between a-wave and d-c portion of b-wave; possible additional source

will interfere with the slower components; therefore ideal conditions for seeing all components can be obtained, with rare exceptions, only in animals); (3) the proper state of adaptation (dark adaptation is neces-sary to visualize all the components); and (4) the proper light intensity (e.g., the early receptor potential requires a very bright light stimulus and the d-c potential of the b-wave requires a dim light stimulus).

Early Receptor Potential

A very rapid component seen immediately after the light stimulus is the early receptor potential (ERP). This component was first described by Brown and Murakami [13] in 1964, and is best seen after the use of a high-intensity stimulus, particularly in a dark-adapted eye. It consists of an initial positive and a subsequent negative peak (Fig. 4-3) and has a latent period of less than 60 microseconds. This response is thought to originate in the photoreceptor outer segments.[67] It is remarkably resistant to anoxia and most chemicals, as compared with the other components of the ERG. The ERP has proved to be useful in study-

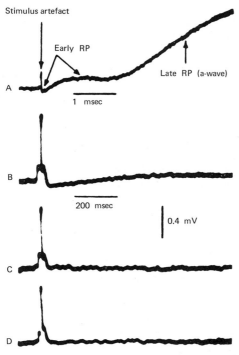

FIG. 4-3. Recordings of early receptor potential (ERP) and a-wave (late receptor potential). The ERP occurs almost instantly after the stimulus. Note that polarity is reversed so that the second, more prominent component of ERP and a-wave, normally displayed as negative waves, is shown as positive waves. (After Brown, K. T., and Murakami, M. Nature 204:739, 1964.)

Photopic Responses In Normals

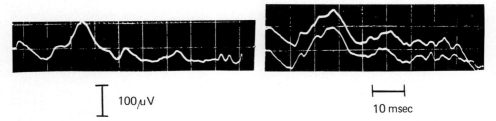

FIG. 4-4. *Single-flash photopic responses. The a-wave has only one component. There is a large b-wave which usually has one, rarely two, oscillations on its ascending limb. This is followed by two smaller positive components.*

ing the photochemistry of visual pigments, as its time course correlates with early steps of photopigment breakdown,[12] and its rate of recovery after a bleaching flash correlates with the regeneration of these photo-pigments.[15]

A-Wave (Late Receptor Potential)

This component is a negative deflection, following the ERP, which is monophasic in the light-adapted (photopic) eye (Fig. 4-4) and bi-phasic in the dark-adapted (scotopic) eye (Fig. 4-5). According to Brown,[12] the scotopic biphasic response consists of one component re-flecting cone activity and another component reflecting activity of the rods.* However, these two components appear to originate at slightly different levels of the retina,[80] and they manifest different sensitivities to certain poisons,[80] so that it is still an open question as to whether the two components both reflect activity from photoreceptors, or whether just one component does. The a-wave is more resistant to anoxia and to most drugs than the b- and c-waves.† Since the a-wave originates mainly or completely from retinal photoreceptors,[12,43] it is not affected by conditions that selectively affect only the bipolar and ganglion-cell layers, such as retinal vascular occlusions [14,26] or certain toxins (for example, sodium glutamate [75]).

* Brown [12] calls these two components the cone late receptor potential and the rod late receptor potential.

† Granit [37] divided the components of the ERG according to their sensitivity to ether anesthesia. The c-wave disappeared first and was called P_I. The b-wave was affected second and designated as P_{II}. Lastly, the a-wave was affected and thereby called P_{III}.

LOW INTENSITY SCOTOPIC

HIGH INTENSITY SCOTOPIC

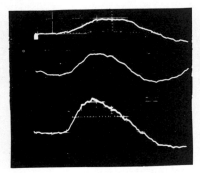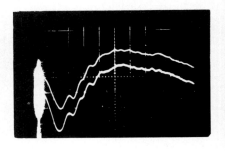

$$\text{I} \quad 100\ \mu\text{V}$$

$$\longmapsto \quad 10\ \text{msec}$$

FIG. 4-5. *Single-flash scotopic responses at low intensities (left) and high intensities (right). Low-intensity light stimulus produces a long-lasting slow-onset monophasic positive deflection, called the d-c potential. Note how the descending limb of the d-c potential swings below the base line before finally returning to it. A brighter light stimulus elicits a more rapid, larger positive deflection superimposed on the d-c potential; the latter becomes smaller as light intensity increases. Light of still higher intensity (right side of photo) produces two or three positive deflections superimposed on the ascending limb of the b-wave; these are known collectively as the oscillatory potential. At the higher intensities an a-wave with two components is also seen. It is noteworthy how the responses become faster as the stimulus intensity increases.*

B-Wave

The b-wave, a positive deflection following the a-wave, is quite complex. In the scotopic eye, it consists of three components that can be separated on the basis of intensity of light stimulus. Low-intensity light stimulus produces a long-lasting, monophasic, positive deflection called the d-c potential (Fig. 4-4). Brighter light stimulus elicits a much more rapid, larger, positive deflection superimposed on the d-c potential; the latter becomes smaller as light intensity increases (Fig. 4-5). Light of still higher intensity produces two or three positive deflections superimposed on the ascending limb of the b-wave; these are known collectively as the oscillatory potential (Fig. 4-6). In the photopic eye, the b-wave consists of four components (Fig. 4-4), which have not been separated. The second component is usually the most prominent one.

All components of the b-wave are very dependent on intactness of

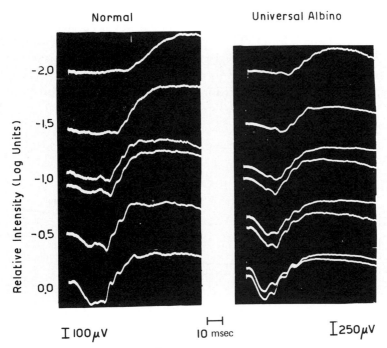

Normal   Universal Albino

Relative Intensity (Log Units)

-2.0

-1.5

-1.0

-0.5

0.0

$\mathrm{I}\,100\,\mu V$ 10 msec $\mathrm{I}\,250\,\mu V$

FIG. 4-6. *Scotopic responses of normal and universal albino subjects at five highest light intensities. Similar features described in Fig. 4-5 are shown. However, oscillatory responses are particularly prominent in the albino patient. (From Krill, A. E., and Lee, G. B. Arch. Ophthal. 69:32, 1963.)*

the bipolar cell layer and therefore on the retinal circulation. Recent evidence suggests that the fast portion of the b-wave probably originates from the Mueller cell secondary to increases in potassium ion concentration, which takes place in the extracellular space of the bipolar cell layer.[18] Neuronal activity in the bipolar cell layer may cause this potassium increase. The exact origin of the oscillatory potential and the d-c potential is unknown, although in the human these components undoubtedly depend on intactness of the bipolar cell layer.

Although originating in the bipolar cell layer, the b-wave and its components are not independent of events external to this layer. For example, destruction of the choroidal circulation eliminates the b-wave as well as the a-wave.[26] It appears that almost anything that affects the a-wave affects the b-wave as well; the histological and electrophysiological bases of this dependency are uncertain. However, as indicated, the opposite is not true: The a-wave may remain normal even with complete disappearance of the b-wave.

C-Wave

The c-wave is a monophasic positive deflection following the b-wave (Fig. 4-10). The c-wave originates from the pigment epithelium [87] and therefore is closely related to metabolism of this layer.[69] Like the a-wave, it is not altered by conditions that selectively affect the internal retina.[14, 26]

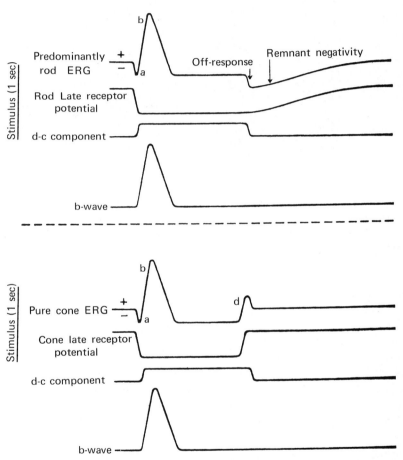

FIG. 4-7. *Brown's analysis of the d-wave (off-response), showing how this component may reflect interaction between two decaying earlier components, the a-wave (the late receptor potential) and d-c potential of the b-wave. Whether the d-wave will be negative or positive depends upon the duration of the a-wave and upon when it returns to the base line in relation to the c-wave. (After Brown, K. T. Vision Res. 8:633, 1968.)*

D-Wave ("Off-Response")

The d-wave, a positive or negative deflection, occurs approximately at the time the light stimulus is turned off. Therefore, it has been called an "off-response" in the past, implying that it is caused by turning off the light. In the analysis by Brown [12] this component reflects interaction between two decaying earlier components, the a-wave and d-c potential of the b-wave (Fig. 4-7). On the other hand, small wavelets may be superimposed upon the d-wave.[90] These wavelets are similar in appearance to oscillatory potentials and are affected in a like manner by diseases. They may therefore have a similar origin somewhere in the bipolar cell layer.

COMPONENTS IN CLINICAL ELECTRORETINOGRAPHY

COMMON COMPONENTS

Under the usual conditions of clinical recording, the ERG usually shows only two components, the a-wave and the b-wave, particularly because eye movements interfere with the recording of later occurring waves. Sometimes an ink-writer (on an electroencephalographic machine) is used for recording, and the a- and b-waves are greatly simplified, appearing as simple negative and positive deflections (Fig. 4-8). This contrasts greatly with the multiple components seen with the oscilloscope (Figs. 4-4 and 4-5).

RARE COMPONENTS

The early receptor potential has been recorded in the human by using a very bright light in a scotopic eye and a very fast sweep on the oscilloscope (because of the rapidity of this response).[7] Abnormalities of the ERP have been noted in patients with hereditary retinal diseases.[9] The c-wave has been recorded from well-dilated * eyes of patients under general anethesia.[27] The d-wave or "off-response" was recorded by one group from cooperative normals and a few patients with retinal degenerations.[90] Abnormalities of this component were noted in the patients with retinal degenerations. There is too little information from humans on any of these components as yet to be certain of their ultimate value in clinical electroretinography.

* Pearlman [73] showed that pupillary movement can produce a response identical in appearance with the c-wave. Therefore, a fixed pupil is essential before claims of a c-wave are acceptable.

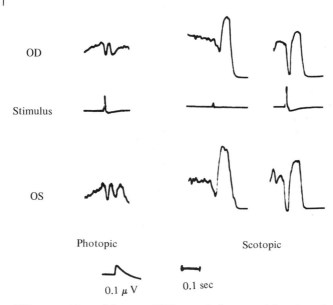

FIG. 4-8. *Normal human ERG recorded on an ink-writer showing simplified responses consisting usually of two single component responses called a- and b-waves. This photograph also demonstrates that a photopic response is quicker in onset and duration and smaller in amplitude than a scotopic response obtained with close to the same intensity.*

QUANTITATIVE EVALUATION OF THE CLINICAL ERG

Quantitatively the ERG is described by amplitude values and time relations (Fig. 4-9) and flicker fusion frequencies (see discussion under *Flicker Studies* in the next section). The a-wave amplitude is measured from the base line to the lowest point (trough) of this wave, the b-wave amplitude from the trough of the a-wave to the highest point on the b-wave (regardless of the number of components). If only a b-wave is present, the measurement is made from the base line to the highest point on the b-wave. In general, the b-wave varies between 75 and 600 microvolts, depending mainly on the intensity of light and the state of adaptation (see next section). The a-wave varies between 50 and 300 microvolts, depending mainly on the same factors. Time relations include the latent period (interval from the stimulus to the beginning of the wave), the implicit or peak time (interval from the stimulus to the highest point of the wave), and the duration of the wave (interval from the beginning to the end of the wave). The duration of the entire response is usually less than 250 msec.

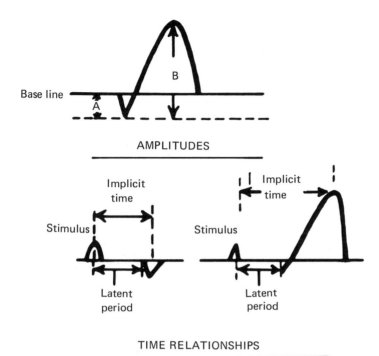

AMPLITUDES

TIME RELATIONSHIPS

FIG. 4-9. *Quantitative evaluation of the ERG showing measurement of amplitude and time relationships.* (*From Krill, A. E. "Clinical Electroretinography," in Hughes, W. F. Year Book of Ophthalmology,* Chicago, *Year Book Publishers, 1959, pp. 5–27.*)

In any quantitative assessment of the ERG the effect of the b-wave on the a-wave must be considered. The b-wave normally interferes with "full expression" of the a-wave because the falling phase of the a-wave is interrupted by the rising edge of the b-wave. This is best seen by studies that show the appearance of the a-wave before and after the development of the b-wave [70] or before and after the use of experimental methods that selectively eliminate the b-wave (for example, ligation of the central retinal artery [14]) (Fig. 4-10). Therefore, the a-wave implicit time is directly dependent on the b-wave latency. An increase in b-wave latency can occur with either an increase in the b-wave implicit time or a decrease in the b-wave amplitude.

MAJOR PARAMETERS AFFECTING THE CLINICAL ERG

The two major parameters affecting the clinical ERG (and the animal ERG as well) are the intensity of the light stimulus and the state of

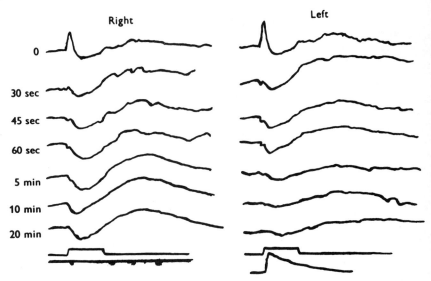

FIG. 4-10. *Comparison of the effect of occluding the retinal circulation (right eye) and choroidal circulation (left eye) in a monkey. Numbers at left represent times after the occlusion. Calibration 100 microvolts; time 1 sec. This photograph also is useful to demonstrate the c-wave, the positive deflection which follows the b-wave. Note how only the a- and c-waves remain in the right eye after occluding the retinal circulation. All components are eventually eliminated by occluding the choroidal circulation. (From Fujino, T., and Hamasaki, D. I. J. Physiol. 180: 837, 1965.)*

the eye's adaptation. However, other parameters to be considered have some importance as well.

STIMULUS INTENSITY

A dim light elicits only the b-wave (Fig. 4-5). A bright light, re-gardless of the state of adaptation, produces both a- and b-waves (Fig. 4-5). The elicitation of the a-wave, with usual clinical testing, requires about two more log units of light intensity than the b-wave. The a-wave amplitude and, within certain limits, the amplitude of the b-wave are proportional to the logarithm of the stimulus intensity (Figs. 4-16 and 4-17).* At higher intensities the large size of the a-wave prevents ac-curate interpretation of the b-wave amplitude; however, using ac-

* Because of this relationship, it is best to use a series of stimuli differing by partial or whole log steps so that when amplitude data are plotted against stimulus intensity a straight line will be obtained over most of the curve.

cepted means of measurement, this amplitude tends to decrease or remain about the same. The relationship of the various scotopic b-wave components to intensity has been discussed.

The latent and implicit times of the scotopic components shorten with an increase in intensity.[42] The flicker fusion frequency will be increased with an increase in intensity (see discussion under *Flicker Studies*, later).

ADAPTATION STATE

The photopic response is faster in origin, shorter in duration, and smaller in amplitude (Fig. 4-8) and reflects mainly cone activity. The larger and slower scotopic ERG is more complex and reflects both rod and cone activity, depending particularly on the light intensity used. As pointed out, the scotopic b-wave is monophasic at low intensities (the d-c potential), but has multiple components at higher intensities (Fig. 4-5).

PREADAPTATION

This factor is important mainly for the scotopic ERG. The intensity and duration of any preadapting light will affect the time of appearance of the maximum amplitude of the scotopic waves for a given light stimulus. Response to a particular spectral region will be reduced in size when the eye is subjected to preadaptation to the same or closely adjacent regions of the spectrum.[4]

WAVELENGTH

In general, blue light elicits the largest responses in the scotopic eye. Orange-red light in the scotopic eye produces a characteristic biphasic response (Fig. 4-11) utilized frequently in the evaluation of pure rod or cone disorders, such as congenital total color blindness and congenital night blindness. On the basis of changes noted in such diseases, the first portion of this response appears to relate to cone activity and the second portion to the rod activity.

INTERVAL BETWEEN SUCCESSIVE STIMULI

In light adaptation the ERG response to two successive stimuli is usually the same regardless of the interval; however, if intervals of less than about 50 msec are used, the two successive responses may partly

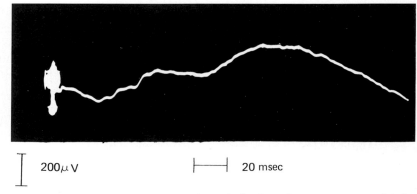

    200μ V   ⊢——⊣   20 msec

FIG. 4-11. *Normal response in a fully dark-adapted eye to orange-red light (about 600 nm). Note single component a-wave and slow double component b-wave.*

coincide on the record.[64] In dark adaptation it is important to keep successive stimuli far enough apart so that a minimum of light adaptation affects the succeeding response. If stimuli are repeated too soon, the components of the second complex will change in both amplitude and contour.

The value of an adequate interval will vary with the duration and intensity of the stimulation.

FLICKER STUDIES

Flicker studies analyze the response of the retina to repeated stimuli at increasing frequencies. The frequency at which each light flash is no longer accompanied by a corresponding response is defined as the fusion frequency (Fig. 4-12). Flicker studies permit separation of cone activity from rod activity. Fast flicker, in any state of adaptation — e.g., over 20 flashes per second — probably elicits only cone responses.[3, 29, 83] However, a flicker technique utilizing a patterned stimulus of alternating illuminated bars appears to elicit distinct cone responses even at low frequencies.[42a]

AGE OF THE SUBJECT

The ERG does not assume the adult appearance until toward the end of the first year of life.[99] In our experience, and that of others,[46] the b-wave amplitude is smaller in normals beyond the age of 50. It is therefore important to get normal controls from an older age group when evaluating retinal diseases from such patients.

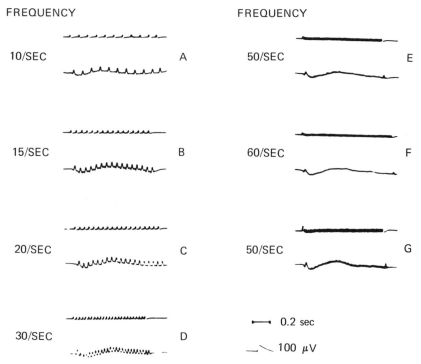

FIG. 4-12. *Photopic flicker ERG showing eventual canceling out of responses, other than the first and last of a series, until a fusion frequency is reached (60 in this record). (From Goodman, G., and Iser, G. Amer. J. Ophthal. 42:216, 1956.)*

REFRACTIVE ERROR

There appears to be a significant inverse relationship in normal eyes between b-wave amplitude and optic axis length.[72] Since refractive value and length of optic axis are also closely related, it is understandable why hyperopic eyes, on the average, have a larger b-wave amplitude than myopic eyes.[72] This explains why high myopes, with no evidence of retinal degeneration, may have at times a slightly subnormal ERG.

POSITION AND TYPE OF ELECTRODE

Recorded from the cornea, the amplitude of the potential is of maximum and practically constant value, decreasing rapidly, however, from the limbus posteriorly. With the active or recording electrode placed on the cornea, most investigators place the indifferent electrode on the bridge of the nose or the forehead. Eye movements decrease the amplitude of the components by shifting the electrode to the sclera and by changing the position of the base line. Flashes of short duration and fixation of the subject minimize eye movements; however, when movements do occur, it is important to wait for a return of the base line (monitored on the oscilloscope) to the original position. Eye blinks may alter the amplitude or shape of the positive waves. This effect is minimized by using a speculum type of electrode, such as that designed by Burian and Allen.[14a]

In our experience, the Burian-Allen speculum electrode is the easiest corneal electrode to keep in an eye over a long period of time. The lenses are made in three different sizes. We use methyl cellulose on the contact lens (no saline is necessary) to protect the cornea. Topical anesthesia may have to be repeated after 30 minutes of testing, but often this is not necessary.

In young or uncooperative patients or in patients with abnormalities preventing the placement of an electrode on the cornea, other types of electrodes have been tried.[41, 78] Cotton wick electrodes on the conjunctiva, hook electrodes on the eyelid, and electrodes on the skin have all been used.[41, 78] Responses are much smaller with these techniques, so that summation of a large number of responses on a computer may be necessary for assessment.

FIXATION

It is best to use some device (e.g., a red light) for fixation. The subject's fixation is easily monitored by reference to a base-line position on the oscilloscope. Therefore, it is not necessary to be in the same room with the subject being tested. In patients with nystagmus (e.g., albinos) it may help to have them look at a field containing two fixation lights on either side of the stimulus source. On the other hand, it is noteworthy that fixation nystagmus diminishes markedly (almost disappears at times) when the patient is dark-adapted and relaxed. Therefore, routine testing can usually be done without difficulty in the dark-adapted eye.

METHODOLOGY

Most workers in clinical electroretinography use a statistical approach in the evaluation of patients. A standard testing routine is followed, and the results are compared with those obtained under similar conditions from normal subjects.

It is important to obtain enough responses to permit quantitative comparisons with normal data. Whereas some diseases produce obvious qualitative ERG abnormalities, apparent after only a few responses under selected conditions, other diseases cause subtle abnormalities detectable only by quantitative comparisons. If insufficient responses are obtained, such differences may erroneously be dismissed as "normal variability." *

EQUIPMENT

Testing is done with the subject supine in a bed.† The active electrode is a Burian-Allen recording contact lens. Usually binocular recordings are obtained, and the data from each eye are evaluated independently. An indifferent electrode is centered on the forehead above the nose, and ground electrodes are placed on the ear. The light-adaptation source used before scotopic responses are obtained is a 61°-field provided by a 60-watt, 130-volt tungsten filament, illuminating a plastic diffuser in front of the bulb. This source produces a "white" light of 590 foot-lamberts luminance. Our test stimulus is a Grass model PS-2 photostimulator providing an estimated maximum illumination at the position of the subject's eye of 450,000 foot-candles, with the lamp centered about 18 inches away from the subject's eye. The brightest light stimulus we use is obtained with a maximum intensity setting on the instrument; and eight dimmer light stimuli, each differing by one-half log step, are obtained by interposing a series of 4-inch-square neutral density filters in front of the lamp. Control of eye position is attempted by having the subject fix on a 1.5 mm red fixation bulb placed below the center of the lamp.

The electrodes lead to a specially constructed junction box to allow the use of very short electrodes. The impulses lead to two RM 122 Textronix low-level preamplifiers from which all impulses are conducted into two parallel systems (Fig. 4-13). One set leads to a Nuclear-Chicago data retrieval computer, model 7100, which is used to study flicker responses. The other set leads to a dual beam type 512 Textronix

---

* Variability from time to time is minimal if curves of values are compared — not just single values, as has been done by some workers. Furthermore, it is important to know when one's light source is decreasing in intensity output.

† The equipment and test procedure described are those used by the author at the University of Chicago.

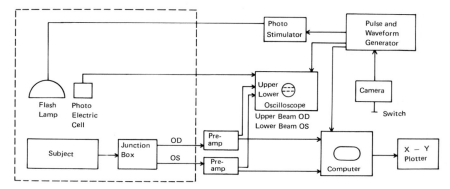

FIG. 4-13. *Schematic diagram of setup used at the University of Chicago. Pulse and wave-form generators are excited by camera shutter and trigger photostimulator, oscilloscope-sweep, and computer (if a flicker study is being done). Short electrodes from patient lead into a junction box that leads signal to two preamplifiers (one for each eye). Preamplifiers lead responses into oscilloscope and computer.*

oscilloscope. The oscilloscope is used to study single-flash responses, which are photographed with a Textronix C-13 oscilloscope camera. The responses on the computer are recorded on a type 700 4A Hewlett-Packard X-Y plotter.

TEST PROCEDURE

ERG testing is started with the room lights on. Two or three single-flash responses are recorded using the brightest light stimulus. The remainder of the examination is done in total darkness. The subject is initially light-adapted for 5 minutes; then responses to a constant single-light stimulus (obtained with a neutral filter of 2.0 log units) are recorded approximately every minute until a relatively constant b-wave amplitude is reached (usually 14 or 16 minutes). After 16 minutes, a series of responses is obtained using each of the nine intensities. Following this, additional responses to the initial constant test stimulus are again recorded at 1-minute intervals until at least 30 minutes of total dark adaptation have elapsed. After 30 minutes in the dark, two responses are obtained to an orange-red light (using no neutral density filter). A flicker study is then done with the room lights turned on again. The highest intensity setting is used, and responses to stimuli ranging from 1 to 70 flashes per second are obtained. Fifty responses are summated at each frequency with the computer.

ERG Test Routine

    Lighted Room

High-intensity single flash

    Dark Room

1. Five minutes light adaptation (590 ft-lamberts)
2. Constant stimulus until 14–16 minutes
3. Nine different intensities (0.5 log steps)
4. Constant stimulus until about 30 minutes
5. High-intensity orange-red stimulus

    Lighted Room

High-intensity flicker study summating 50 responses at each frequency

EVALUATION OF DATA

We calculate the following values for each patient: (1) photopic b-wave amplitudes, (2) b-wave amplitudes and implicit times at specific times in the dark (with the one intensity of stimulation used), (3) a- and b-wave amplitudes and implicit times from the fully dark-adapted eye at all intensities of testing used, (4) amplitudes and implicit times of the orange-red response components, and (5) the mean maximum amplitudes of the flicker responses calculated from the X-Y plotter at the various frequencies used with notation of the flicker fusion frequency.

The value of comparing a large number of responses under the same conditions is illustrated in Figures 4-14 through 4-20 in relation to albinos. Note the many differences, some of them subtle, between the albinos and the control group when quantitative comparison is made of the following parameters: (1) growth of the b-wave amplitude or the b-wave peak (implicit) time during dark adaptation (Figs. 4-14 and 4-15); (2) variation of the a-wave or b-wave amplitude with light intensity (Figs. 4-16 and 4-17); (3) relation of the a- or b-wave peak time to light intensity (Figs. 4-18 and 4-19); and (4) relation of the b-wave amplitude to flicker frequency (Fig. 4-20).

Quantitative Evaluation of ERG

1. Photopic b-wave amplitude
2. Scotopic b-wave
    a. Amplitude vs. time in dark (constant intensity)
    b. Amplitude vs. intensity in fully dark-adapted eye

    c. Implicit time vs. time in dark (constant intensity)
    d. Implicit time vs. intensity in fully dark-adapted eye
3. Scotopic a-wave
    a. Amplitude vs. intensity in fully dark-adapted eye
    b. Implicit time vs. intensity in fully dark-adapted eye
4. Orange-red response
    a. Amplitude of largest component
    b. Implicit times of both positive components
5. Summated photopic flicker
    a. Mean maximum amplitude at each frequency
    b. Fusion frequency

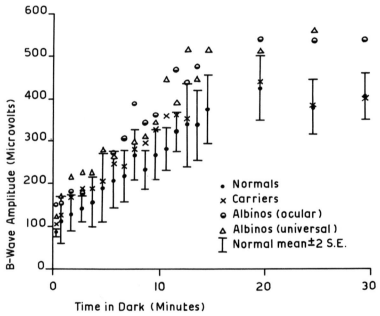

FIG. 4-14. *Growth of b-wave amplitude obtained with one intensity with time in the dark. Means of all b-wave amplitudes from a control group of eight normal subjects, from five universal albinos, from three ocular albinos, and from six carriers of ocular albinism are shown. The normal mean plus or minus twice its standard error is also shown. The means of the two albino groups are similar or slightly larger than the control group mean during the first ten minutes, but significantly larger after ten minutes. (From Krill, A. E., and Lee, G. B. Arch. Ophthal. 69:32, 1963.)*

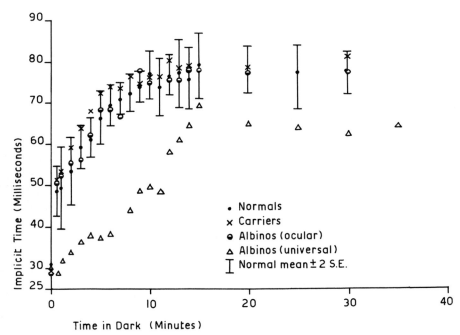

FIG. 4-15. *B-wave implicit time plotted in relation to time in the dark. Same groups as in Fig. 4-14. Note the consistently shorter implicit time in the universal albino. (From Krill, A. E., and Lee, G. B. Arch. Ophthal. 69:32, 1963.)*

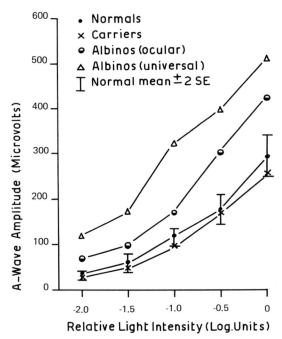

FIG. 4-16. *Means of all a-wave amplitudes for the same groups as in Fig. 4-14, plotted at five different light intensities. The normal mean plus or minus twice its standard error is also shown. The a-wave amplitude is larger in the two albino groups but largest in the universal albinos. (From Krill, A. E., and Lee, G. B. Arch. Ophthal. 69:32, 1963.)*

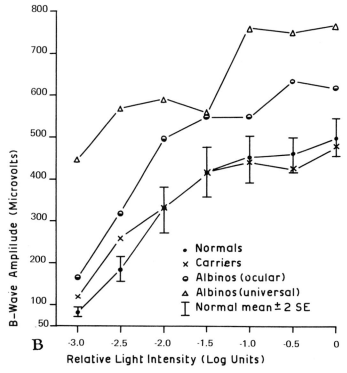

FIG. 4-17. *Means of all b-wave amplitudes for same groups in Fig. 4-14 are plotted at seven different light intensities. The normal mean plus or minus twice its standard error is also shown. Note the larger b-wave amplitudes for the two albino groups. (From Krill, A. E., and Lee, G. B.* Arch. Ophthal. 69:32, 1963.)

MODIFIED TESTING

Despite the statistical advantage of multiple responses, under certain test conditions only a few responses can be obtained, but these may be highly informative. For example, a few single-flash high-intensity responses under photopic conditions and a few single-flash responses under scotopic conditions usually suffice for diagnosis, as will be seen in the discussion of ERG patterns in specific diseases. Equally useful can be the precise determination of the flicker fusion frequency (a single value) under photopic or mixed conditions. The behavior of a young child or an uncooperative patient may permit only a few responses under any test condition, but even these can be informative if the disease is characterized by gross or unique ERG abnormalities.

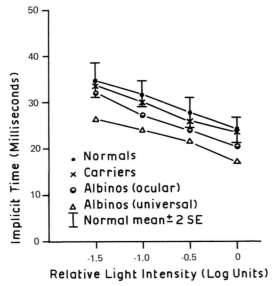

FIG. 4-18. *Means of all a-wave implicit times for each group in Fig. 4-14 for four different light intensities. Note the definitely shorter implicit time in the universal albino group for the a-wave at all intensities. These implicit times were second shortest in the ocular albino group. (From Krill, A. E., and Lee, G. B. Arch. Ophthal. 69:32, 1963.)*

GENERAL ANESTHESIA

For the infant or young child, anesthesia may be necessary,* and this in turn may affect the ERG. In our experience, anesthesia may cause up to a 50 percent reduction in the scotopic b-wave amplitude. However, the photopic responses, the scotopic a-wave, and the peak times of all responses are only minimally affected or not altered at all. Most diseases responsible for blindness in infants cause marked alteration of some or all of these usually unaffected components, as will be noted later. Some workers claim far less effect of anesthesia on the scotopic ERG,[79, 95] but unfortunately this has not been our experience. When anesthesia must be used, the infant or child to be tested is brought in at 8:00 A.M., without any food since the previous midnight or water after 4:00 A.M. The child has been previously evaluated by a pediatrician and has a normal hemoglobin value. Light anesthesia without

---

* Under a year of age it may be possible to do an ERG (like it is possible to fit contact lenses) with no or only a minimal amount of sedation simply by distracting the child (e.g., giving him a bottle of milk to suck on).

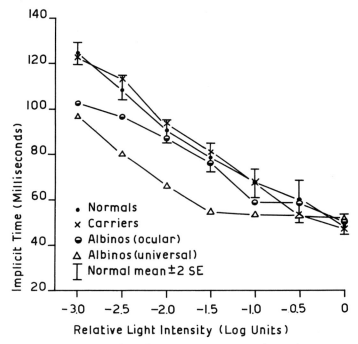

FIG. 4-19. *Means of all b-wave implicit times for each group in Fig. 4-14 at seven different light intensities. Note the definitely shorter implicit time in the universal albino group at the five lower intensities. The b-wave implicit times at the two lowest intensities were second shortest in the ocular albino group. (From Krill, A. E., and Lee, G. B. Arch. Ophthal. 69:32, 1963.)*

intubation (e.g., ketamine) is used, and the infant can usually be taken home by two hours after he wakes up. We are at present evaluating the effects of other anesthetics, such as rectal barbiturates, on the scotopic b-wave.

SPECIAL METHODS OF TESTING

The clinical ERG in the human is usually a mass response to stimulation of the entire external layer of the retina. It is a combination response to direct focal stimulation of a fairly large area, to light reflected from the retina, and to light scattered by the different media. However, with modifications and with specific instrumentation, small- and large-area electroretinograms are now being obtained.

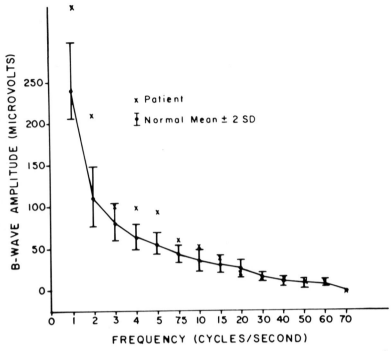

FIG. 4-20. *The b-wave amplitude from a universal albino are compared with normal data. Note the supernormal b-waves of the albino at the slower flicker frequencies (up to 10 cycles per second). (From Krill, A. E. Invest. Ophthal. 9: 600, 1970.)*

The Focal ERG

The ERG has been recorded from small areas of the retina with the assistance of a computer of average transients.[1, 6, 10, 39] Several hundred small responses obtained with small, dim stimuli, which are not discernible individually from background noise, are added up with the computer to a much larger size response which can be evaluated.* The most efficient methods are those that use a red stimulus and a blue background light to bleach the surrounding retina and prevent its participation in the ERG response.[1, 6] The large number of responses necessary to obtain useful information necessitates prolonged steady fixation, and therefore the technique is not yet feasible as a clinical procedure for most patients. Hopefully, though, this will be a useful tool for evaluating macular function in the future.

* See discussion under Theory of Summation, Chapter 6.

Total Area ("Ganzfeld") Direct Stimulation

With the standard ERG technique, a certain portion of the retina is stimulated indirectly by scattered light. With light stimulation presented as a ganzfeld[21,35] there is presumably direct homogeneous stimulation of most of the retina. This technique enhances the response, the a-wave, which is produced mainly by direct stimulation in comparison with the b-wave response, which is associated with a great amount of neural convergence[12] and thereby produced by both direct and indirect stimulation.* With the ganzfeld technique the advantage of convergent pathways is bypassed, so that the a-wave can be elicited at a lower light intensity than the b-wave. There probably should be a more precise correlation between psychophysical data and this method of stimulation.

THE ABNORMAL ERG

NOMENCLATURE

The various responses are illustrated in Figure 4-21.

Subnormal

Subnormal responses have amplitudes that are less than the normal (i.e., less than the normal mean minus two standard deviations). If the response consists of both a- and b-waves, both are smaller than normal (Fig. 4-21).

Negative

Negative responses are characterized by a selective reduction of the b-wave, so that the a-wave is the prominent portion of the response. These responses are commonly seen in retinal vascular abnormalities.

Supernormal

Supernormal responses are larger than normal (more than the normal mean plus two standard deviations). Only the b-wave or both the a- and b-waves may be supernormal.

---

* Indirect stimulation plays an important role in the usual ERG technique in elicitation of the b-wave due to light spread from directly stimulated areas over horizontal networks which are abundant in the bipolar cell layer.

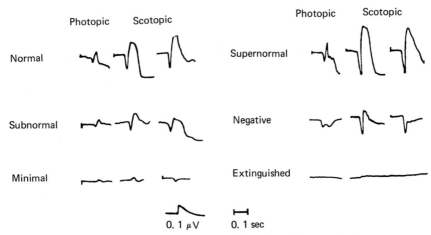

FIG. 4-21. *Pathological ERG patterns. One photopic and two scotopic responses are shown for each pattern. (From Krill, A. E. "Clinical Electroretinography," in Hughes, W. F. Year Book of Ophthalmology. Chicago, Year Book Publishers, 1959, pp. 5–27.)*

Minimal

A scotopic response less than 100 microvolts or a photopic response less than 50 microvolts is classified as minimal.

Extinguished

A record with no responses distinguishable from the base line is classified as extinguished.

CLINICAL INTERPRETATION OF THE ERG

The ERG is a record of all the electrical processes occurring in the external layer of the retina; thus, the proportion of healthy to diseased retina determines the response. If a large area of the retina is damaged or diseased, a subnormal ERG results. If almost the entire retina is damaged, an extinguished ERG is recorded. However, if only a small area is diseased (e.g., focal disease of the macula), a normal ERG is obtained (unless a technique for obtaining a focal ERG is used). Diseases affecting only the inner layer of the retina (e.g., glaucoma) are not reflected on the ERG. Any disease causing a generalized disturbance of retinal circulation or nutrition may produce a markedly abnormal ERG.

ERG PATTERNS IN SPECIFIC DISEASES

The following discussion does not tabulate ERG findings in all of the many diseases that have been studied; rather, it concerns only those conditions in which electroretinography aids in diagnosis, contributes to the understanding of a disease, or assists in following the course of a disease. Other specific uses for the ERG will also be discussed.

DIAGNOSIS OF UNEXPLAINED VISUAL LOSS IN INFANCY AND EARLY CHILDHOOD

The ERG may be a useful procedure in an infant or young child with poor vision whose ocular findings are insufficient to explain the visual deficit (Table 4-2). No or only minimal eyeground changes of questionable significance are noted. Subjective testing may be impossible or unreliable, so that objective testing is often the only method of evaluating the retina. Such a child has often been examined by many ophthalmologists; if cerebral blindness has been considered, because of the absence of retinal changes, the child may have even had an extensive neurological work-up, sometimes including pneumoencephalography. One of the most difficult concepts for the neurologist, pediatrician, or occasionally the ophthalmologist to accept is that severe retinal disease may exist *without* ophthalmoscopic changes.

Often a definite diagnosis can be made after ERG examination, and it may be then possible to predict the probable future course of the disease process, the type of schooling that will probably be needed, and the genetics of the condition. Obviously, an exact diagnosis is of epidemiological significance.

Four disorders of the retina that may cause a significant degree of blindness in an infant without producing obvious eyeground changes are (1) congenital retinal dystrophy (amaurosis congenita of Leber),

---

TABLE 4-2
Value of ERG in the Infant and Young Child

1. Diagnosis of unexplained visual loss
2. Evaluation of specific eyeground changes
   a. Pigmentary retinopathy
   b. Optic nerve atrophy
   c. Attenuated retinal vessels
3. Evaluation of early retinal degeneration

(2) total color blindness, (3) congenital stationary night blindness, and (4) albinism (the ocular and incomplete universal types).

Congenital Retinal Dystrophy (Amaurosis Congenita of Leber)

Congenital retinal dystrophy, first described as retinitis pigmentosa with congenital amaurosis by Leber[63] in 1869, was described by later workers under several headings including (1) hereditary retinal aplasia,[84] (2) dysgenesis neuroepithelialis,[91] and (3) heredoretinopathia congenitalis monohybrida recessiva autosomalis.[2] Fundal changes may be absent or minimal. Eyeground changes most commonly consist of diffuse pigmentary stippling and/or pale optic nerves,[52] but these changes may be absent. Associated ocular findings may include nystagmus, esotropia, cataracts, and high myopia. The ERG is diagnostic. The record is extinguished or only minimal responses are obtained under any test condition.

Congenital retinal dystrophy is usually a progressive disease that causes severe deterioration of visual acuity, visual fields, and night vision. Although the eyegrounds initially are normal or show only minimal abnormalities eventually, by the age of eight or later, extensive changes may be noted similar to those seen in retinitis pigmentosa. The condition is inherited as an autosomal recessive trait.

Total Color Blindness

In the complete form of total color blindness photophobia, nystagmus, and visual acuity of about 20/200 are usual findings. This is a stationary condition in which peripheral visual fields and night vision remain unaffected. The inheritance is autosomal recessive. Histological studies [20, 28, 62] have shown both a marked deficiency of cones and the presence of abnormal cones as well.

The two most common ERG abnormalities are a minimal or absent single-flash photopic response (Fig. 4-22) and a very low flicker fusion frequency (Fig. 4-23).[53] The fusion frequency hacomes lower as the stimulus intensity increases, and with very bright flickering lights sometimes no responses are noted. These abnormalities in the presence of a normal or only mildly abnormal scotopic record (particularly at high intensities) are diagnostic for total color blindness. A less frequently reported but also diagnostic finding in this condition is the loss or marked decrease of the entire first portion of the response to orange-red light in the fully dark-adapted eye (Fig. 4-24).

Single Flash Photopic Responses

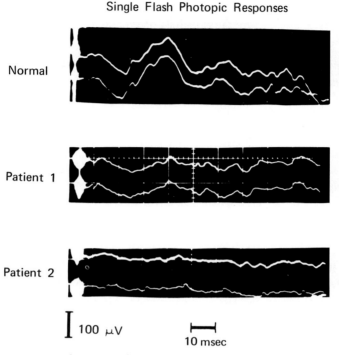

FIG. 4-22. *Shown are photopic responses from a normal subject, patient 1 with a cone degeneration and patient 2 with total congenital color blindness. Note that photopic responses are absent in patient 2 and minimal in patient 1. (From Krill, A. E. Trans. Amer. Acad. Ophthal. Otolaryng. 70:1063, 1966.)*

The findings in the incomplete form of total color blindness are the same as in the complete form, but less severe in degree. Photophobia and nystagmus may be absent and visual acuity less impaired. Sloan and Newhall [82] even reported one patient with acuity of 20/40. The chromatic defect is usually incomplete for certain colors. The ERG shows the same changes as in the complete form, but frequently to a lesser extent.

A unique group of patients are those in whom blue cones are minimally or not at all involved. If these cones constitute only a small portion of all retinal cones,[93] the ERG in such patients should be similar to that recorded from patients with complete achromatopsia, and indeed this is true.[25, 85] The female carrier of this condition may show minimal ERG abnormalities,[86, 49] such as a lower-than-normal flicker fusion frequency.

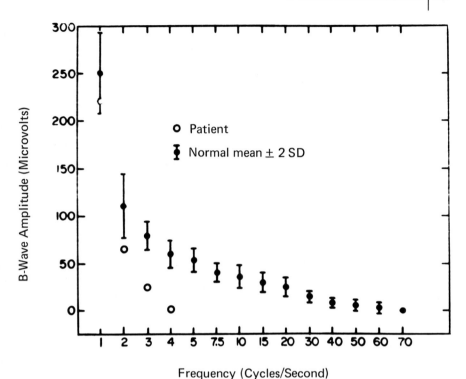

FIG. 4-23. *A comparison of flicker b-wave amplitudes from a patient with total congenital color blindness and a normal control group of 25 subjects (mean plus or minus two standard deviations). The patient has a fusion frequency of four cycles per second, and the normal control group about 70 cycles per second. (From Krill, A. E. Trans. Amer. Acad. Ophthal. Otolaryng. 70:1063, 1966.)*

Congenital Stationary Night Blindness

Congenital stationary night blindness may be inherited as an autosomal dominant, autosomal recessive, or X-linked recessive disorder. All males with the X-linked type have abnormal acuity, varying from 20/40 to 20/200, and myopia, usually of at least 4 diopters. Nystagmus may be noted with more severe reduction of acuity. Some patients with the autosomal recessive type have abnormal acuity. All patients with congenital night blindness have normal peripheral visual fields.

A unique ERG abnormality characteristic of all forms of congenital night blindness is the almost identical peak times of scotopic and photopic b-waves (Fig. 4-25) and sometimes a-waves. Normally the peak time of the scotopic b-wave is at least twice as long as that of

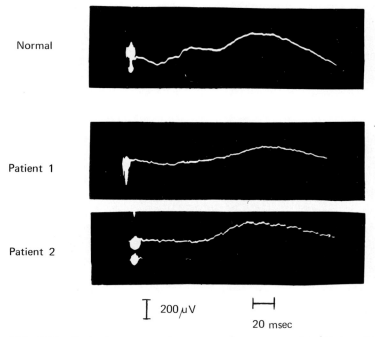

FIG. 4-24. *Scotopic orange-red responses from a normal subject, patient with total congenital color blindness (patient 1) and a patient with a cone degeneration (patient 2). Note that the first portion of the response is absent from the patient with the cone degeneration and only minimal from the subject with total color blindness. (From Krill, A. E. Trans. Amer. Acad. Ophthal. Otolaryng. 70:1063, 1966.)*

the photopic b-wave. Other less specific abnormalities may also be noted. A markedly subnormal scotopic b-wave is characteristic (Fig. 4-25), and in some patients the scotopic a-wave is also subnormal. Minimal photopic ERG abnormalities, such as subnormal photopic responses and low flicker fusion frequencies, are frequent.[59]

Albinism

Universal albinism is easily diagnosed. Incomplete universal albinism may be difficult to recognize, particularly in dark Caucasians or in Negroes, whose only visible abnormalities may be lighter skin and hair than unaffected members of their families. This type of albinism is usually inherited as an autosomal dominant but occasionally as an autosomal recessive trait.

Ocular albinism affects only the eyes and may be difficult to recog-

PHOTOPIC HIGH INTENSITY SCOTOPIC

NORMAL

PATIENT 1

PATIENT 2

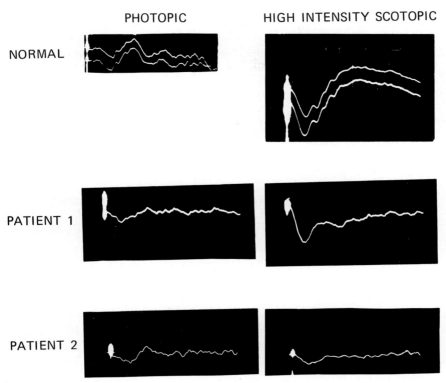

FIG. 4-25. Electroretinogram showing normal photopic and scotopic responses and responses elicited under same conditions from two patients with congenital night blindness. In the normal subject the peak (implicit) time of the scotopic a- and b-waves is considerably slower than that of the photopic a- and b-waves. Note how these times are almost identical in the two subjects with congenital night blindness. In both patients there is a marked reduction of the scotopic b-wave amplitude. However, in one patient there is reduction of the scotopic a-wave amplitude as well (bottom row). (From Krill, A. E. Invest. Ophthal. 9:600, 1970.)

nize. Both the iris and retina or only the retina may be deficient in melanin. This form of albinism is inherited as a sex-linked recessive trait and therefore affects males only. The female carrier may show typical minimal defects.[19]

The eyeground and iris changes characteristic of albinism are sometimes difficult to detect in the patient with incomplete universal or ocular albinism. The eyeground in particular often closely resembles that of a normal light-colored person, and the difficulty is compounded if the patient is an infant, since a normal blond baby's eyegrounds are almost albinotic during the first six months of life.

The scotopic ERG is supernormal in all forms of albinism, particularly during the first two decades of life[58] (Figs. 4-14 through 4-20). For some reason, normal or smaller-than-normal responses are seen in the older albino. This may reflect retinal damage secondary to chronic excessive exposure to light.

EVALUATION OF SPECIFIC EYEGROUND CHANGES IN INFANCY AND EARLY CHILDHOOD

PIGMENTARY RETINOPATHY

Pigmentary retinopathy in an infant or young child may have a number of different causes. Prenatal first trimester infection with rubella, and possibly other viruses, and irradiation may produce a prominent diffuse pigmentary retinopathy in the newborn.[24, 51] This type of retinopathy is of no visual consequence, and the ERG is normal. In congenital amaurosis of Leber, the eyegrounds show diffuse pigmentary stippling, and the ERG is severely abnormal. Syphilis also may produce diffuse pigmentary retinopathy and is associated usually with a normal, but sometimes with a subnormal, ERG pattern. Other diffuse inflammatory processes, such as diffuse chorioretinitis associated with virus inclusion disease, give a similar ERG pattern.

Pigmentary retinopathy that begins later in childhood is usually the result of infection or degeneration. Of infections, usually a virus is implicated; morbilli is by far the most common.[23] Other viral diseases responsible include variola, vaccinia, epidemic parotitis, encephalitis, and Bechet's disease (of questionable viral causation). Rubella contracted in childhood may produce a retinitis similar to that associated with congenital rubella.[22] Rarely, typhoid fever, diphtheria, scarlatina, and typhus cause pigmentary retinopathy.

With an infectious retinopathy, the child is normal at birth and abruptly loses vision in the course of convalescence from some childhood disease. The fundus at this stage may show a central retinal arterial occlusion or spasm. Although this is only transient, there is usually permanent impairment of retinal function. Acuity, visual fields, and dark adaptation are usually abnormal, and the ERG may show extinguished or minimal response. Eventually these children develop a pigmentary retinopathy.

Night blindness is usually the first complaint in early retinal degeneration. Gradual progression is characteristic. The ERG is markedly abnormal (minimal or extinguished) in most early retinal degenerations. However, in some children with either early autosomal dominant retinitis pigmentosa or early choroideremia, fairly large responses, classified as subnormal, may be noted. Studies of the families of such patients are usually quite informative.

OPTIC NERVE ATROPHY

Congenital or early-onset blindness with optic nerve atrophy as the only abnormal finding may have many causes, but in our experience amaurosis congenita of Leber, with a severely abnormal ERG, is the most common. Other causes include syphilis, diseases with ganglion-cell infiltration (infantile amaurotic idiocy, Niemann-Pick disease), discrete hereditary optic nerve atrophy without central nervous system involvement (either of autosomal recessive or of dominant inheritance), or optic nerve atrophy with central nervous system involvement (Behr's optic nerve atrophy [92]) or secondary to central nervous system involvement. The ERG may be abnormal, to a mild or moderate extent, in syphilis, but is normal in all the other causes of optic atrophy cited.

ATTENUATED RETINAL ARTERIOLES

This may be the sole finding in an infant with either congenital syphilis or amaurosis congenita of Leber. As indicated previously, the ERG easily distinguishes these two conditions.

DIAGNOSIS OF EARLY OR ATYPICAL RETINAL DEGENERATION AT ANY AGE

Early or even long-standing retinitis pigmentosa may show no or questionable eyeground changes. In such cases, the ERG examination may be diagnostic. An example is a 13-year-old girl who complained of poor vision and night blindness, but had normal eyegrounds. Several members of her family were known to have retinitis pigmentosa, with an autosomal dominant type of inheritance. A definitive diagnosis was made in this child after an extinguished ERG was noted. Another example is a 32-year-old male who had a long history of progressive night blindness, but only questionable eyeground changes. Only one of three ophthalmologists who examined the patient thought the eyegrounds were abnormal. A diagnosis of retinitis pigmentosa was made after an extinguished ERG was noted.

One of the five characteristic findings in the Laurence-Moon-Biedl-

Bardet syndrome is supposedly retinitis pigmentosa. However, only about 15 percent of patients with this syndrome have the typical ophthalmoscopic appearance of retinitis pigmentosa, but almost all of the patients develop night blindness, which indicates a diffuse disturbance of retinal function.[56] Of 16 patients we have studied, 15 had extinguished or almost extinguished ERG records. Eight of these patients had either no eyeground changes or minimal peripheral changes. Obviously, the demonstration of a diffuse disturbance of retinal function is a more meaningful criterion in this disease than the presence of retinitis pigmentosa.

Old inactive chorioretinitis may resemble retinal degeneration, but the finding of a markedly abnormal or extinguished ERG points to a diagnosis of the latter disorder. As indicated previously, a subnormal ERG may be obtained in early retinitis pigmentosa of autosomal dominant inheritance [23, 34] or in choroideremia. The demonstration of a changing ERG on follow-up studies is, of course, characteristic of retinal degeneration.

EVALUATION OF UNEXPLAINED VISUAL SYMPTOMS OR EYEGROUND CHANGES IN ADULTHOOD

TOXIC AMBLYOPIA

Toxic amblyopia, particularly if it results from a nutritional deficiency, may be difficult to diagnose. A patient may not admit to a history of alcoholism and not eating. Initially no eyeground changes may be seen, although visual acuity and visual fields may be abnormal. The presence of bilateral optic disc pallor may suggest a central nervous system lesion. The ERG findings are diagnostic. The ERG is always abnormal in nutritional amblyopia in our experience; in optic nerve disease secondary to central nervous system disease, the ERG is normal.

The b-wave amplitude and visual fields of a 41-year-old male are shown in Figures 4-26 and 4-27, at the time of initial evaluation and after treatment with large doses of vitamins. This patient had no eyeground changes.

Genest [31, 32] studied nutritionally deficient natives in Thailand and Indonesia and showed a clear-cut relationship between blood levels of vitamin A and a- and b-wave amplitudes of the ERG.

Drugs toxic to the optic nerve (quinine, methyl alcohol) are toxic to the outer retina as well. In spite of the absence of ophthalmoscopic

1–5–60   7–26–60

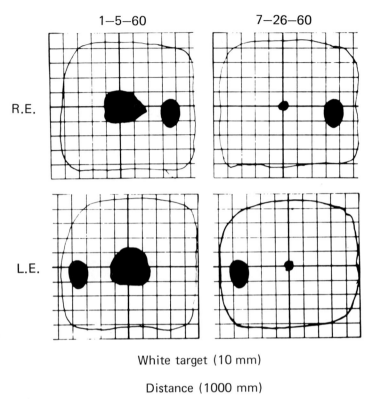

R.E.

L.E.

White target (10 mm)

Distance (1000 mm)

FIG. 4-26. *Visual fields of subject with nutritional amblyopia before and after treatment with large doses of vitamins.* (From Krill, A. E. Invest. Ophthal. 9:600, 1970.)

alterations, changes in the ERG may be noted even before changes in the optic disc are evident.[88] The ERG may be helpful in following such patients.

VASCULAR INSUFFICIENCY

The b-wave of the ERG reflects changes in retinal circulation. These changes may provide evidence of suspected previous central retinal artery spasm or transient occlusion. A marked loss of the b-wave with a normal a-wave is characteristic (Fig. 4-28). In contrast to congenital night blindness, which may elicit the same ERG pattern, the peak time of the scotopic b-wave in vascular disease is normal or slower than normal.

Changes in the b-wave on the side of diminished blood flow may aid

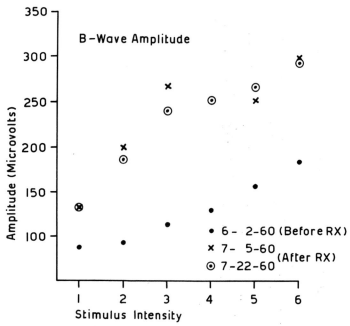

FIG. 4-27. *Plot of b-wave amplitudes from the same patient as in Fig. 4-26 before and after treatment with large doses of vitamins. Note the increase in the b-wave amplitudes after treatment recorded on two occasions. (From Krill, A. E. Invest. Ophthal. 9:600, 1970.)*

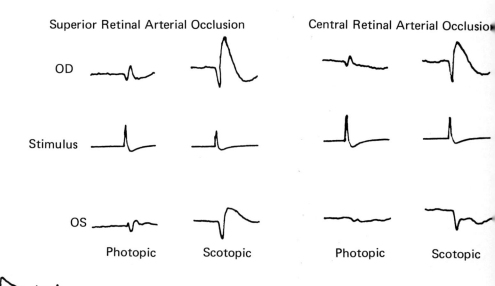

FIG. 4-28. *Electroretinograms from a patient with a left superior retinal arterial occlusion and from another with a left central retinal arterial occlusion. In each patient there is a smaller b-wave from the affected left eye. A much greater decrease is noted in the patient with the central retinal artery occlusion. (From Krill, A. E. Invest. Ophthal. 9:600, 1970.)*

in the diagnosis of carotid artery disease.[55] In some patients a consistently smaller b-wave, regardless of test conditions, may be noted from the eye with reduced blood flow (Fig. 4-29). In others, a significantly smaller b-wave can be demonstrated only under special conditions such as (1) during the early period of dark adaptation, (2) with the use of dim illumination (Fig. 4-30), or (3) with flicker studies. The flicker data from a patient with a right carotid insufficiency two days before and eight days after surgery are shown in Figure 4-31.

Wulfing [97] has used the ERG in conjunction with ophthaldynamometry and feels this is a more sensitive technique than either method alone for detecting carotid insufficiency.

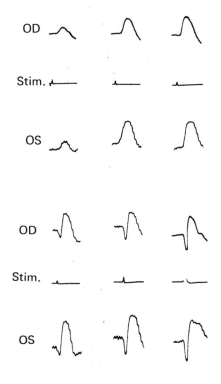

0.1 sec I 0.1 μV

FIG. 4-29. B-wave amplitudes at six intensities from normal left eye and right eye on side with proven carotid insufficienty (by arteriography). Note the smaller responses from the affected right eye.

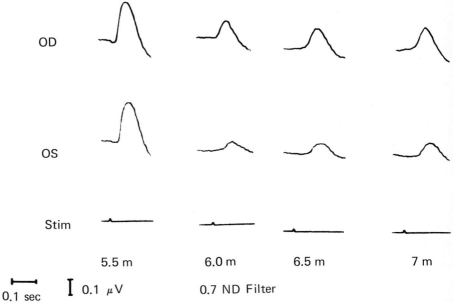

OD

OS

Stim

5.5 m   6.0 m   6.5 m   7 m

0.1 sec   I 0.1 μV   0.7 ND Filter

FIG. 4-30. *Responses from patient with aortic arch syndrome and proved left carotid insufficiency during early dark adaptation (5.5 to 7 minutes) to a constant stimulus intensity. Note that when light intensity is reduced with a neutral density (ND) filter of 0.7 log units (columns 2, 3, and 4) responses are much smaller from the involved left eye. At the higher intensity, responses are almost equal from the two eyes. (From Krill, A. E., and Diamond, M. Arch. Ophthal. 68:72, 1962.)*

CONE DEGENERATION

The onset of this condition is usually in the first two decades of life. The disease may be familial with autosomal dominant, or occasionally autosomal recessive inheritance.[8,54,89]

The characteristic findings are reduced visual acuity, severely defective color vision, and ERG changes often similar to those described for total color blindness[53] (Figs. 4-22, 4-23, and 4-24). In contrast to other types of macular degeneration, severe color blindness is usually an early complaint. Initially the changes in the macula may be quite

FIG. 4-31. *Preoperative (4-31A) and postoperative (4-31B) flicker responses from patient with partial right carotid obstruction. All b-waves from the right eye are smaller in amplitude before surgery; but after a right carotid endarterectomy, the b-waves are either equal from the two eyes, or small randomized differences at a few frequencies are seen.*

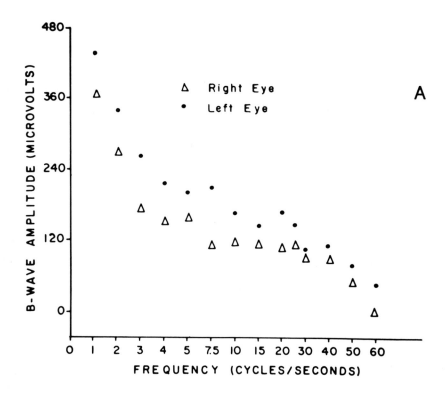

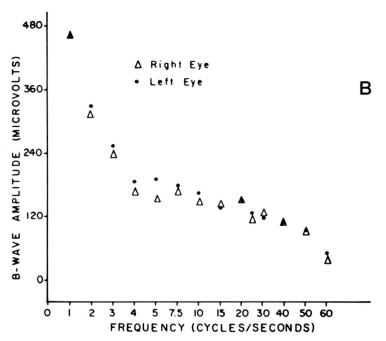

subtle and may even be overlooked. Temporal pallor, a frequent finding in this disease, may be the prominent feature in early stages, suggesting a central nervous system disorder. The characteristic ERG alterations, though, are diagnostic (Chapter 10, Vol. 2).

DETECTION OF TOXIC RETINOPATHY

Certain drugs (NP-207,[88] thioridazine,[94] LSD-25,[61] and chloroquine) exert a selective toxic effect on the retina. Such drug-induced changes may often be detected with the ERG before ophthalmoscopic or gross visual changes are evident.[30, 77] For this reason, the ERG is a useful screening procedure when drugs with proven or suspected retinal toxicity have to be used.

The ERG may be used to monitor the effects of certain physical agents that under certain circumstances may adversely affect retinal function. Low temperature,[65] hypoxia,[11] and continuous light[71] are examples of such physical agents.

The ERG should be one of the parameters used to determine whether a proposed vitreous substitute is safe enough to use in humans. Animal eyes in which vitreous substitutes are injected should be tested before injection and at definite intervals afterward.

EVALUATION OF RETINAL STATUS AFTER INTRAOCULAR FOREIGN BODIES

Changes in the ERG may enable prediction of the retinal status after a retained intraocular iron foreign body.[45, 47] Changes in the ERG appear before eyeground changes are seen and before visual field or dark-adaptation abnormalities can be detected. The time of initial occurrence of an abnormality, the severity of the abnormality, and its rate of progression depend on the nature of the metal, its alloy content, the degree of encapsulation, and the location. Iron and, to a lesser degree, copper affect the ERG rather rapidly. Aluminum only rarely produces a pathological ERG and then usually after a relatively long intraocular duration compared to iron.

Retinal damage after any metallic foreign body occurs only from particles in the vitreous, ciliary body, or retina. Recurrent vitreal hemorrhages from a foreign body may cause retinal changes similar to those produced by an iron foreign body and known as siderosis retinae.[47] Visualization of the eyegrounds may be impossible because of a vitreal hemorrhage, but retinal function can be assessed with the ERG.

EVALUATION OF RETINAL FUNCTION BEHIND CORNEA, LENS, OR VITREOUS OPACIFICATION

Focal disease of the macula and disease of the inner retina and optic nerve, as pointed out, cannot be detected with the ERG. However, most macular degenerations in the older patient are not really focal and are associated with a more widespread functional abnormality than predictable from ophthalmoscopic evaluation.[50, 66] Furthermore, most significant vascular abnormalities and a retinal detachment will cause pronounced ERG abnormalities. Therefore, the ERG may be of value in predicting visual results in the older patient with an opacity. In evaluating the ERG it should be noted that, because of the filter effect of an opacity, responses from a normal eye may be subnormal. In fact, the entire amplitude versus light intensity curve may be shifted. However, responses elicited with the brightest stimuli may be normal or even supernormal (in the absence of retinal disease) because of light scatter (occurring to a much greater extent with the brighter stimuli).

The ERG may aid in the evaluation of retinal status behind a vitreous hemorrhage of either spontaneous or traumatic origin, since a retinal detachment may be the cause of the bleeding. An abnormal ERG, depending on the size of the detached area, will be found in such cases.

EVALUATION OF COURSE OF DISEASE

In conditions characterized by abnormal ERG findings, the effectiveness of treatment can be evaluated by means of repeated ERG examinations. Disorders for which such ERG monitoring may be useful include toxic amblyopia, vascular deficiencies, such as carotid artery disease, vascular occlusion,[87] acute diffuse choroiditis (Fig. 4-32),[40, 48] retinal detachments, hyperthyroidism,[74] aldosteronism,[95] and, most recently, a reversible retinal degeneration associated with abetalipoproteinemia.[35] In this last condition, recovery to a normal ERG was seen after the use of large doses of vitamin A. Loss of the wavelets on the ascending limb of the scotopic b-wave, indicating early diabetic retinopathy, may be noted even before ophthalmoscopic changes are evident.[81, 98] The prognostic value of this finding is uncertain.

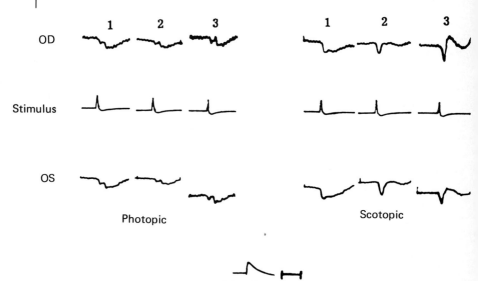

FIG. 4-32. *Electroretinogram of a patient with a diffuse choroiditis showing improvement of b-waves after treatment coincidental with subjective improvement. Column 1 shows responses before treatment, column 2, 15 weeks after treatment, and column 3, 8 months after treatment. (From Krill, A. E. "Clinical Electroretinography," in Hughes, W. F. Year Book of Ophthalmology. Chicago, Year Book Publishers, 1959, pp. 5–27.)*

One worker evaluated fluorescein angiography and the ERG in central retinal vein and artery occlusions within a week after onset and at successive intervals afterward.[68] He found correlations between the initial angiographic findings and ERG abnormalities and the extent of subsequent visual recovery.

ESTIMATION OF EXTENT AND NATURE OF INVOLVEMENT IN RETINAL DISEASES

Both the ERG and the electrooculogram (see Chapter 5) are helpful in this area. As pointed out previously, certain diseases (e.g., central choroidal sclerosis, cone degenerations) that appear to be confined to the macula on ophthalmoscopic evaluation show evidence of widespread functional involvement.[50, 66] Some diseases with frequent macular involvement, such as familial drusen, fundus flavimaculatus, and fundus albipunctatus,[57] show evidence of a significant diffuse abnormality of the pigment epithelium, since the electrooculogram (EOG) is usually abnormal, whereas the ERG (and subjective dark adaptation) is usually normal or close to normal. Vitelliruptive macular degeneration always shows an abnormal EOG with a normal or close to normal ERG.[60]

In myotonic dystrophy a diffuse abnormality of the retina is noted with the ERG; however, the pigment epithelium is spared, since the EOG is normal.[5] In juvenile retinoschisis, retinal splitting occurs in the internal retina as usually only the b-wave of the ERG is affected.[16,38] In senile retinoschisis extensive enough to affect the ERG, both the a- and b-waves are affected, so that retinal splitting must occur at a more external level than in the juvenile type.

AREAS OF FUTURE VALUE FOR ERG TESTING

As noted earlier in this chapter, small-area electroretinography is now possible. Theoretically, focal electroretinography could be used as an objective method of evaluating macular function or an objective method of perimetry. A basic problem, however, is that a very large number of responses must be obtained and summated to permit evaluation of differences among retinal areas.[1,6,10,39] This necessitates an impractically long period of steady fixation. A few groups, however, have now had limited success in some patients in showing alterations of the focal ERG in macular disease.[6,36,39] One group [9] used a ratio of macular and optic disc responses as a parameter, eliminating the necessity of "pure" focal responses at either area and thereby decreasing the total number of responses needed at either area. This latter technique may prove suitable for clinical use, but more data must be seen before its ultimate value can be assessed.

There is need for more stress tests designed specifically for individual diseases. The combination of ophthaldynamometry and electroretinography to detect carotid artery disease is one such test.[97] Perhaps the performance of exercises before an ERG in patients with suspected carotid artery disease would also be of value.

Eventual understanding of the significance of all the subcomponents of the ERG and of newly discovered major components, such as the early receptor potential, hopefully may broaden the clinical value of the ERG.

REFERENCES

1. Aiba, T. S., Alpern, M., and Masseidvag, F. The electroretinogram evoked by the excitation of human foveal cones. *J. Physiol. 189*:43, 1967.

2. Alstrom, C. H., and Olson, O. Heredoretinopathia congenitalis monohybrida recessiva autosomalis. *Hereditas 43*:178, 1957.

3. Armington, J. C., and Biersdorf, W. R. Flicker color adaptation in the human electroretinogram. *J. Opt. Soc. Amer. 46*:393, 1956.

4. Armington, J. C., and Thiede, F. C. Selective adaptation of components of the human electroretinogram. *J. Opt. Soc. Amer. 44*:779, 1954.

5. Anderson, R. A., and Burian, H. M. Ocular resting potential in myotonic dystrophy. *Amer. J. Ophthal. 68*:863, 1969.

6. Bankes, J. L. K. The foveal electroretinogram. *Trans. Ophthal. Soc. U.K. 87*:249, 1967.

7. Berson, E. L., and Goldstein, E. B. Recovery of the human early receptor potential during dark adaptation in hereditary retinal disease. *Vision Res. 10*:219, 1970.

8. Berson, E. L., Gouras, P., and Gunkel, R. D. Progressive cone degeneration, dominantly inherited. *Arch. Ophthal. 80*:77, 1968.

9. Biersdorf, W. R., and Diller, D. A. Local electroretinogram in macular degenerations. *Amer. J. Ophthal. 68*:296, 1969.

10. Brindley, G. S., and Westheimer, G. The spatial properties of the human electroretinogram. *J. Physiol. 179*:518, 1965.

11. Brown, J. L., Hill, J. H., and Burke, R. E. The effect of hypoxia on the human electroretinogram. *Amer. J. Ophthal. 44*:57, 1957.

12. Brown, K. T. The electroretinogram: its components and their origin. *Vision Res. 8*:633, 1968.

13. Brown, K. T., and Murakami, M. A new receptor potential of the monkey retina with no detectable latency. *Nature 201*:626, 1964.

14. Brown, K. T., and Watanabe, K. Isolation and identification of a receptor potential from the pure cone fovea of the monkey retina. *Nature 193*:958, 1962.

14a. Burian, H., and Allen, L. A speculum contact lens electrode for electroretinography. *Electroenceph. Clin. Neurophysiol. 6*:509, 1954.

15. Cone, R. A. Early receptor potential of the vertebrate retina. *Nature 204*:736, 1964.

16. Deutman, A. F. *The Hereditary Dystrophies of the Posterior Pole of the Eye.* Assen., Netherlands, Van Gorcum and Co., 1971.

17. Dewar, J. The physiological action of light. *Nature 15*:433, 1877.

18. Dowling, J. E. Organization of vertebrate retinas. *Invest. Ophthal. 9*:655, 1970.

19. Falls, H. F. Sex-linked ocular albinism displaying typical fundus changes in the female heterozygote. *Amer. J. Ophthal. 34*:41, 1951.

20. Falls, H. F., Wolter, J. R., and Alpern, M. Typical total monochromacy. *Arch. Ophthal. 74*:610, 1965.

21. Finkelstein, D., Gouras, P., and Hoff, M. Human electroretinogram near the absolute threshold of vision. *Invest. Ophthal. 7*:214, 1968.

22. Franceschetti, A., Dieterle, P., and Schwarz, A. Retinite pigmentaire a virus: Relation entre tableau clinique et electroretinogramme (ERG). *Ophthalmologica 135*:545, 1958.

23. Franceschetti, A., Francois, J., and Babel, J. Les heredodegenerescences (degeneres-cences tapeto-retiniennes). Paris, Masson et Cie, 1963, Vol. 1.

24. Francois, J. Embryopathie par radiations ionisantes. *Ophthalmologica* 143:163, 1962.

25. Francois, J., and Verriest, G. Trois nouvelles observations d'achromatopsie con-genitale atypique. *Ann. Oculist.* 193:123, 1960.

26. Fujino, T., and Hamasaki, D. I. The effect of occluding the retinal and choroidal circulations on the electroretinogram of monkeys. *J. Physiol.* 180:837, 1965.

27. Hanitzsch. R., Hammer, K., and Bornschein, H. Der nachweis lamgsamer potentials in Menschlichen ERG. *Vision Res.* 6:245, 1966.

28. Harrison, R., Hoefnagel, D., and Hayward, J. N. Congenital total color blindness: A clinical report. *Arch. Ophthal.* 64:685, 1960.

29. Heck, J. The flicker electroretinogram of the human eye. *Acta Physiol. Scand. 39:* 158, 1957.

30. Henkind, P., Carr, R., and Siegel, I. Early chloroquine retinopathy: clinical and functional findings. *Arch. Ophthal.* 71:157, 1964.

31. Genest, A. Vitamin A blood serum level and electroretinogram in five- to fourteen-year age group in Indonesia and Thailand. *Amer. J. Clin. Med.* 20:1275, 1967.

32. Genest, A. "Vitamin A and the Electroretinogram in Humans," in Francois, J. (ed.) *The Clinical Value of Electroretinography.* Basel, Karger, 1968, pp. 250–259.

33. Goldstein, E. B., and Berson, E. L. Rod and cone contributions to the human early receptor potential. *Vision Res.* 10:207, 1970.

34. Goodman, G., and Gunkel, R. Familial electroretinographic and adaptometric studies in retinitis pigmentosa. *Amer. J. Ophthal.* 46:142, 1958.

35. Gouras, P. Electroretinography. Some basic principles. *Invest. Ophthal.* 9:557, 1970.

36. Gouras, P., Gunkel, R. D., and Jones, J. Spatial differences in the human ERG. *Invest. Ophthal.* 1:333, 1962.

37. Granit, R. *Receptors and Sensory Perception.* New Haven, Yale University Press, 1955.

38. Guyot-Sionnest, M. A propos d'une famille atteinte de retinoschisis idiopathique recessive lie au sexe. *Ann. Oculist.* 202:573, 1969.

39. Jacobson, J. H., Kawasaki, K., and Hirose, T. The human electroretinogram and occipital potential in response to focal illumination of the retina. *Invest. Ophthal.* 7:472, 1968.

40. Jacobson, J. H., Popkin, A., and Hirose, T. The electroretinogram in Harada's disease. *Amer. J. Ophthal.* 64:1152, 1967.

41. Jayle, G. E., and Tassy, A. F. Prognostic value of ERG in severe recent trauma. *Brit. J. Ophthal.* 54:51, 1970.

42. Johnson, E. P. The character of the b-wave in the human electroretinogram. *Arch. Ophthal.* 60:565, 1958.

42a. Johnson, E. P., Riggs, L. A., and Schick, M. L. "Photopic Retinal Potential Evoked by Phase Alternation of a Barred Pattern," in Burian, H. M., and Jacobson, J. H. (eds.). *Clinical Electroretinography.* London, Pergamon Press, 1966.

43. Kaneka, A., and Hashimoto, H. Recording site of the single cone response deter-mined by an electrode marking technique. *Vision Res.* 7:847, 1967.

44. Karpe, G. Basis of clinical electroretinography. *Acta Ophtal.* (Suppl.) 24:1, 1945.

45. Karpe, G.   Indications for clinical electroretinography. *Trans. Ophthal. Soc. U.K.* 78:373, 1958.

46. Karpe, G., Rickenbach, K., and Thomasson, S.   The clinical electroretinogram: the normal electroretinogram above 50 years of age. *Acta Ophthal.* 28:301, 1950.

47. Knave, B.   Electroretinography in eyes with retained intraocular metallic foreign bodies. *Acta Ophthal. (Suppl.)* 100, 1969.

48. Krill, A. E.   "Clinical Electroretinography," in Hughes, W. F. (ed.). *Year Book of Ophthalmology.* Chicago, Year Book Publishers, 1959–1960.

49. Krill, A. E.   A technique for evaluating photopic and scotopic flicker function with one light intensity. *Docum. Ophthal.* 18:452, 1964.

50. Krill, A. E.   The electroretinographic and electrooculographic findings in patients with macular lesions. *Trans. Amer. Acad. Ophthal. Otolaryng.* 70:1063, 1966.

51. Krill, A. E.   Retinal disease of rubella. *Arch. Ophthal.* 77:445, 1967.

52. Krill, A. E.   "Congenital Retinal Degenerations," in *Trans. New Orleans Acad. Ophthal.*: Symposium on Surgical and Medical Management of Congenital Anomalies of the Eye. St. Louis, C. V. Mosby, 1968.

53. Krill, A. E.   "The ERG in Congenital Color Vision Defects," in Francois, J. (ed.). *The Clinical Value of Electroretinography.* Basel, Karger, 1968, pp. 205–214.

54. Krill, A. E., and Deutman, A. F.   The cone degenerations. *Amer. J. Ophthal.* (In press).

55. Krill, A. E., and Diamond, M.   The electroretinogram in carotid artery disease. *Arch. Ophthal.* 68:72, 1962.

56. Krill, A. E., Folk, E., and Rosenthal, I. M.   Electroretinography in the Laurence-Moon-Biedl syndrome. *Amer. J. Child.* 102:205, 1961.

57. Krill, A. E., and Klien, B. A.   Flecked retina syndrome. *Arch. Ophthal.* 74:496, 1965.

58. Krill, A. E., and Lee, G. B.   The electroretinogram in albinos and carriers of the ocular albino trait. *Arch. Ophthal.* 69:32, 1963.

59. Krill, A. E., and Martin, D.   Photopic abnormalities in congenital stationary night-blindness. *Invest. Ophthal.* 10:625, 1971.

60. Krill, A. E., Morse, P. A., Potts, A. M., and Klien, B. A.   Hereditary vitelliruptive macular degeneration. *Amer. J. Ophthal.* 61:1405, 1966.

61. Krill, A. E., Wieland, A., and Ostfeld, A.   The effect of two hallucinogenic agents on human retinal function. *Arch. Ophthal.* 64:724, 1960.

62. Larsen, H., and Lauber, H.   Demonstration mikroskopischer Praparate von einem Monochromatischen. *Klin. Mbl. Augenheilk.* 67:301, 1921.

63. Leber, T.   Ueber das Vorkommen von Anomalien des Farbensinnes bei Krankheiten des Auges. Nebst Bermerkungen uber einige Formen von Amblyopie. *Graefe Arch. Klin. Exp. Ophthal.* 15:26, 1869.

64. Mahneke, A.   Electroretinography with double flashes. *Acta Ophthal.* 35:131, 1957.

65. Massopust, L. C., Wolin, L. R., Albin, M. S., and Meder, J.   Evoked responses from the eye and visual pathways in the hypothermic cat. *Exp. Neurol.* 10:383, 1964.

66. Merin, S., and Auerbach, E.   The central and peripheral retina in macular degenerations. *Arch. Ophthal.* 84:710, 1970.

67. Murakami, M., and Pak, W. L.   Intracellularly recorded early receptor potential of the vertebrate photoreceptors. *Vision Res.* 10:965, 1970.

68. Nilsson, S. E. G. Human retinal vascular obstructions. A quantitative correlation of angiographic and electroretinographic findings. *Acta Ophthal.* 49:111, 1971.

69. Noell, W. K. The origin of the electroretinogram. *Amer. J. Ophthal.* 38:78, 1954.

70. Noell, W. K. Differentiation, metabolic organization and viability of the visual cell. *Arch. Ophthal.* 60:702, 1958.

71. Noell, W. K., Walker, V. S., Kang, B. S., and Berman, S. Retinal damage by light in rats. *Invest. Ophthal.* 5:450, 1966.

72. Pallin, O. The influence of the axial length of the eye on the size of the recorded b-potential in the clinical single-flash electroretinogram. *Acta Ophthal.* (Suppl.) 101, 1969.

73. Pearlman, J. T. The c-wave of the human ERG: its intensity dependence and pupil-lociliary origin. *Arch. Ophthal.* 68:823, 1962.

74. Pearlman, J. T., and Burian, H. M. The ERG in hyperthyroidism. *Amer. J. Ophthal.* 58:216, 1964.

75. Potts, A. M., Modrell, R. W., and Kingsbury, C. Permanent fractionation of the electroretinogram by sodium glutamate. *Amer. J. Ophthal.* 50:900, 1960.

76. Riggs, L. Continuous and reproducible records of the electrical activity of the human retina. *Proc. Soc. Exp. Biol. Med.* 48:204, 1941.

77. Schmidt, B., and Muller-Limroth, W. Electroretinographic examination following the application of chloroquine. *Acta Ophthal.* 70:245, 1962.

78. Schmidt, B., and Straub, W. Use of computers in clinical electroretinography. *Klin. Mbl. Augenheilk.* 156:808, 1970.

79. Schulze, H. "Scotopic Reaction of the ERG after Pentobarbital in the Frog," in Basar, D., and Bengisu, U. (eds.). *Symposium on Electroretinography.* Istanbul, University of Istanbul, 1971, pp. 299–306.

80. Sillman, A. J., Ito, H., and Tomita, T. Studies on the mass receptor potential of the isolated frog retina: I. General properties of the response. *Vision Res.* 9:1435, 1969.

81. Simonsen, J. E. Electroretinographic study of diabetes: preliminary report. *Acta Ophthal.* 43:841, 1965.

82. Sloan, L. L., and Newhall, S. M. Comparison of atypical and typical achromatopsia. *Amer. J. Ophthal.* 25:945, 1942.

83. Sokol. S., and Riggs, L. A. Electrical and psychophysical responses of the human visual system to periodic variation of luminance. *Invest. Ophthal.* 10:171, 1971.

84. Sorsby, A., and Williams, C. E. Retinal aplasia as a clinical entity. *Brit. Med. J.* 30:293, 1960.

85. Spivey, B. E. The X-linked recessive inheritance of atypical monochromatism. *Arch. Ophthal.* 74:327, 1965.

86. Spivey, B. E., Pearlman, J. T., and Burian, H. M. Electroretinography findings (including flicker) in carriers of congenital X-linked achromatopsia. *Docum. Ophthal.* 18:367, 1964.

87. Steinberg, R. H., Schmidt, R., Brown, K. T. Intracellular responses to light from cat pigment epithelium. Origin of the electroretinogram c-wave. *Nature* 227:728, 1970.

88. Straub, W. "ERG in Acute and Chronic Intoxications," in Francois, J. (ed.). *The Clinical Value of Electroretinography.* Basel, Karger, 1968, pp. 273–289.

89. Straub, W., and Schmidt, B. "Electrophysiological Investigations in a Family with

Central Retinopathy," in Basar, D., and Bengisu, U. (eds.). *Symposium on Electroretinography*. Istanbul, University of Istanbul, 1971, pp. 189–204.

90. Tsuchida, Y., Kawasaki, K., and Jacobson, J. H. Rhythmic wavelets of the positive off effect in the human electroretinogram. *Amer. J. Ophthal. 72*:60, 1971.

91. Waardenburg, P. J. Does agenesis or dysgenesis neuroepithelialis retinae, whether or not related to keratoglobus, exist? *Ophthalmologica 133*:454, 1957.

92. Waardenburg, P. J. *Genetics in Ophthalmology*. Springfield, Ill., Charles C Thomas, 1963, Vol. 2.

93. Wald, G., and Brown, P. K. Human color vision and color blindness. *Sympos. Quant. Biol. 30*:345, 1965.

94. Weekley, R. D., Potts, A. M., Reoton, J., and May, R. H. Pigmentary retinopathy in patients receiving high doses of a new phenothiazine. *Arch. Ophthal. 64*:65, 1960.

95. Wirth, A., and Tota, G. "Electroretinogram and Adrenal Cortical Function," in Schmoger, E. (ed.). *Advances in Electrophysiology and Pathology of the Visual System*. Leipzig, Thieme, 1968, pp. 347–350.

96. Wirth, A., Tota, G., and Vagelli, A. "The Effect of Fluothane Anesthesia on the Electroretinogram of the Rabbit," in Basar, D., and Bengisu, U. (eds.). *Symposium on Electroretinography*. Istanbul, University of Istanbul, 1971, pp. 289–292.

97. Wulfing, G. Clinical electroretinal-dynamometry. *Acta Ophthal. (Suppl.)* 73, 1953.

98. Yonemura, D., Aoki, T., and Tsuzuki, K. Electroretinogram in diabetic retinopathy. *Arch. Ophthal. 68*:19, 1962.

99. Zetterstrom, B. Clinical electroretinogram in children during first year of life. *Acta Ophthal. 29*:295, 1951.

5

Electrooculogram

THE NORMAL ELECTROOCULOGRAM

DEFINITION

A potential difference exists across a barrier somewhere in the retina, probably mostly across the pigment epithelium. This potential has been called the steady potential, static potential, standing potential, resting potential, dark potential, corneofundal potential, or corneo-retinal potential. However, when recording from the surface of the eye, this potential is seen as a difference between the cornea and the back of the eye, with the cornea being more positive. The potential is usually several millivolts. If two electrodes are placed below inner and outer corners of the eye and the eye is turned, then the electrode closest to the positive corneal pole will be positive in relation to the other electrode (Fig. 5-1). The recording of this potential difference, which is possible only when the eye is moved, is now known in ophthalmology as the electrooculogram (EOG), a term introduced by Marg [48] in 1951.

HISTORICAL BACKGROUND

This potential was discovered in 1849 by DuBois-Raymond and first recorded from a human eye by Dewar [14] in 1877. Its origin was

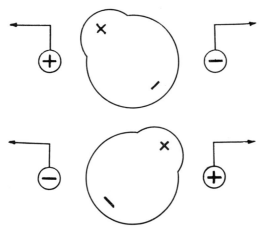

FIG. 5-1. *A potential difference exists between the front of the cornea and the back of the retina, with the cornea having a positive charge. If the eye is moved in either direction the electrode closest to the cornea becomes positive, and a deflection will be noted on a recording system. The direction of the deflection is opposite with the two electrodes.*

considered to be muscular until 1936, when Mowrer and co-workers [51] showed that the potential was unchanged after a cat was curarized but was eliminated after chemical destruction of the cat's retina. However, it was not until 1954 when Riggs [58] reported small values in a case of pigmentary degeneration of the retina and in 1956 that Francois and associates [20] reported abnormal data in several retinal diseases that the possible use of this technique as an objective test for retinal function was considered. Even then, there was the problem of large variation in amplitude due to electrode placement and sometimes to change in state of adaptation. Kris [47] in 1958 and Kolder [37] in 1959 demonstrated the remarkable oscillatory time course of the EOG and provided impetus for the classical work of Arden. Arden [2-4] in 1962 described how reproducible data could be obtained. He recommended studying the ratio of the maximum response obtained during light adaptation to the minimum response obtained during a period of dark adaptation (Fig. 5-2).

ORIGIN

Pigment Epithelium

When recorded from the cornea, this potential receives a slight contribution from the lens, cornea, and ciliary body, but its main

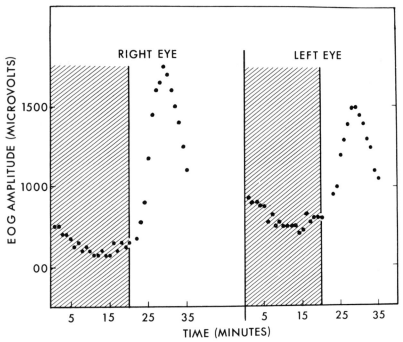

FIG. 5-2. In clinical electrooculography responses are recorded during a fixed period of dark adaptation and then during a fixed period of light adaptation, as shown for this patient. The record is evaluated by the ratio of the largest response obtained during light adaptation to the smallest during dark adaptation. Note how the amplitude decreases in size to reach a minimum during dark adaptation and increases in size to reach a maximum during light adaptation. In this patient the ratio is less for the left eye with a retinal detachment.

source is considered to be in the retina. On the basis of microelectrode studies,[9, 63] and a disappearance of this potential (and the c-wave of the ERG) after poisoning the pigment epithelium in rabbits,[53, 54] this potential is thought to originate mainly in the pigment epithelium. A clinical finding implicating the major role of the pigment epithelium in the genesis of this potential is the occurrence of a frequent markedly abnormal EOG in a disease such as fundus flavimaculatus, wherein there are histological changes only in the pigment epithelium.[36]

Internal Retina

Gouras and Carr [25] showed that a central retinal artery occlusion affects the EOG in monkeys, and some patients have shown an abnormal EOG following this type of occlusion.[5, 52, 21, 11] On the other hand, several patients with central retinal artery occlusions have been reported with a normal EOG.[11, 21, 26, 32] In one report,[11] two patients tested shortly after acute episodes showed pronounced abnormalities of the EOG, whereas a patient tested two years later showed a normal EOG. However, there is no doubt from some of the other reports that an abnormal EOG may be seen long after the acute episode. Therefore, it appears that although this response depends mainly on the integrity of the retinal pigment epithelium, it probably also depends to a much lesser degree on the integrity of the internal retina. This argument has been advanced particularly for the "light rise" portion of the response.

PARAMETERS AFFECTING AMPLITUDE

Position of Electrodes

In general, the response amplitude is markedly affected by the position of the electrodes. Usually, as indicated, these are placed at the medial and lateral canthi of each eye (Fig. 5-3).

Visual Angle

In our setup, the eye movements of the subject when looking from one fixation light to the other subtend a visual angle of 60 degrees.[39] Some laboratories use other visual angles (e.g., Francois and co-workers[21] have the subject look to the extreme right and extreme left; Arden and co-workers[2] use a 40-degree visual angle). With alternating-current amplification, it is probably better to use a smaller visual angle, since there may be more distortion of amplitudes with larger responses (see next section); however, this is not important with direct-current amplification. If a patient moves his head his eyes will not move throughout the standard angle chosen. Patients should be told, before the test, not to move their head, and the use of a fixed chin-rest will usually prevent this problem.

Amplification System

If possible, direct-current (dc) amplification is preferred, as this gives a slow, long-lasting response.[66] Also, there is a direct relationship to the angle of ocular rotation with dc amplification. With some direct-current amplifiers, base-line drift may occur, particularly if there is a potential difference between the electrodes. Frequent chlori-

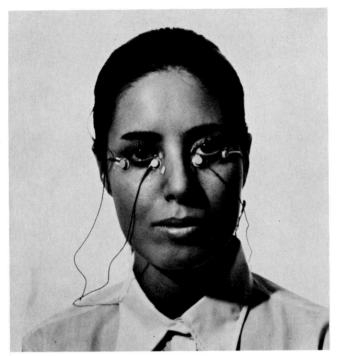

FIG. 5-3. Placement of electrodes at the outer and inner canthi of each eye for the recording of horizontal eye movements in electrooculography. Ground electrode is placed on one earlobe.

nation of electrodes may minimize or eliminate this problem — by eliminating the potential difference between the electrodes. In our experience, nonpolarizable electrodes prevent this occurrence. If alternating-current (ac) amplifiers are used, a very slow time constant is necessary (for example, one second), or else the full amplitude of a response will not have time to develop. For uninterrupted recording over several hours, an automatic method is probably preferable.[38]

Adaptation State

In general, the response remains at about the same amplitude unless there is a fairly rapid change in illumination. Slow changes are much less effective. The changes that occur with rapid onset of dark adaptation or light adaptation will be discussed under the headings *Dark-Adapted Responses* and *Light-Adapted Responses*. These changes are the basis of modern clinical electrooculography.

Light Intensity

The amplitude of light-adapted responses is directly related to the intensity of the adapting light.[4, 49]

Spectral Sensitivity

The spectral sensitivity of the responses is similar to the absorption curve of visual purple, suggesting a close relationship to rods; [4, 17] however, it has been shown that cones also contribute to this response.[15, 23]

Age

There appears to be a decrease in response amplitude with age,[55] although this has not been clearly worked out. It is probably best to obtain normals from several age groups for comparative purposes.

Time of Day

The amplitude varies slightly with the time of day in a diurnal rhythmic manner.[37, 47, 67] Therefore, if possible, patients should be reexamined during the same time of day.

TECHNIQUE

We routinely use four nonpolarizable Beckman skin electrodes placed in the positions described and a ground electrode on the left ear. These electrodes are coated inside with electrode paste and fastened to the skin (which is cleansed with acetone) with adhesive tape. The subject is seated one meter from a point midway between two fixation lights. Each patient is light-adapted for five minutes to a light source with a luminance of 590 foot-lamberts (Fig. 5-4). The room is then darkened and the patient is instructed to fix alternately four times on two red fixation lights subtending an angle of 60 degrees (Fig. 5-4). Test periods are repeated every minute for 20 minutes. The room illumination is then restored, and the test is continued as in the dark for 15 additional minutes.

Most workers use a somewhat similar technique, except for time differences. For example, some workers initially preadapt for a longer period of time (10 minutes with a weaker light), then test the patient in the dark for 10 minutes and in a lighted environment for an addi-

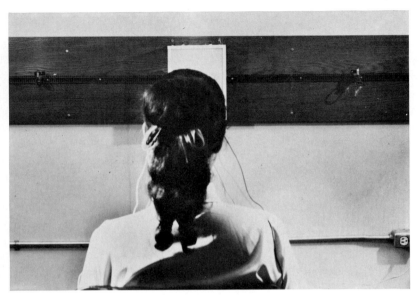

FIG. 5-4. *Subject being tested is seated one meter from preadapting light source, which is centered between two fixation lights that subtend a visual angle of 60 degrees.*

tional 10 minutes.[67] The important point is to note the sequence of three phases: Phase 1 (preadaptation); Phase 2 (dark-adaptation testing); and Phase 3 (light-adaptation testing).

Infants

Obviously, routine electrooculography cannot be done in infants and younger children. However, one group [27] has devised an ingenious device for use under anesthesia. A low-vacuum contact lens is employed which automatically moves the eye through a fixed visual angle at fixed time intervals.

DARK-ADAPTED RESPONSES

In general, the response remains at about the same amplitude unless there is a fairly rapid change in the degree of illumination. With the rapid onset of dark adaptation there is a fall in amplitude over the first 8 to 12 minutes to reach a minimum level and then a gradual rise to a steady-state level at almost 20 minutes (Fig. 5-2). The amplitude of the minimum response is about 30 percent of that of the steady-state response.

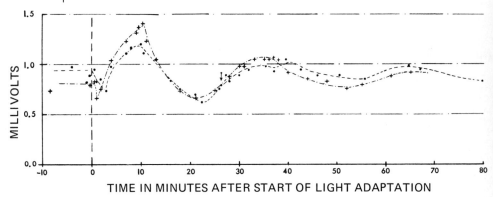

FIG. 5-5. *With a rapid change in light adaptation there is an initial large increase in the amplitude of the response and then one or two smaller secondary rises with gradual settling to a steady-state level.*

LIGHT-ADAPTED RESPONSES

With a rapid change to light adaptation there is an initial large increase in the amplitude of the response, depending on the intensity of light adaptation, then one or two smaller secondary rises with gradual settling to a steady-state level (Fig. 5-5). After the onset of light adaptation, the first peak occurs at about 8 to 12 minutes, the second peak at 21 to 29 minutes, and the third about 32 to 40 minutes.

EVALUATION OF RECORD

In evaluating the record, the average amplitude of each test period is measured and the ratio of the maximum light-adapted to the minimum dark-adapted response is calculated. (Some workers multiply this ratio by 100.) This ratio is compared with a similar value obtained from our control group. We consider ratios less than 2.00 (normal mean ±2 standard deviations) unusual in normals less than 50 years of age. In general we call a ratio of 1.80 abnormal in this group, with 1.90 being borderline (Table 5-1). In subjects over 50, ratios less than

TABLE 5-1
Evaluation of EOG Ratios

Age	Borderline	Definitely Abnormal
Under 50 years	1.90	1.80 or lower
Over 50 years	1.80	1.70 or lower

1.85 are considered to be unusual. In this age group we consider 1.70 definitely abnormal with 1.80 as borderline. Another group considers ratios of 1.65 to less than 1.90 as borderline, and 1.90 or over as normal, regardless of age.[67a] Obviously, it is necessary for each laboratory to study a control group of normals before evaluating patients.

REPRODUCIBILITY

Our experience in regard to reproducibility of ratios in patients has been rather good. It is unusual to find a difference greater than .20 in repeated testing of patients with presumed stationary disease. We consider a ratio difference of at least .30 a significant change if at least one of the values is abnormal. This value is in range with that reported by another group [67] who have never noted ratio variations of greater than .25 on repeated testing in patients.

On the other hand, variation within a normal range appears to be greater than that observed in patients with abnormal ratios. Two groups [34, 67a] report variations up to .50 in normal subjects, however, in spite of this degree of variation, the ratios remain in a normal or borderline range.

PATHOLOGY OF THE EOG

The EOG is a mass response, similar to the ERG, so that changes occur only with widespread disease of the pigment epithelium. It must also be emphasized that the EOG measures the *function* of the pigment epithelium. Certain diseases, such as rubella retinitis [40] and the retinopathy seen in the choroideremia carrier,[46] have marked structural abnormalities on ophthalmoscopic evaluation, particularly noticed in fluorescein angiography (Fig. 5-6). However, the EOG is usually normal in these conditions,[40, 46] indicating normal function in spite of structural alterations. On the other hand, conditions such as vitelliruptive macular degeneration and fundus flavimaculatus, with limited pigment epithelium structural involvement by ophthalmoscopic and fluorescein evaluation, may have a marked EOG abnormality.[36, 45]

The pigment epithelium may be functionally abnormal as the result of a severe disease of adjacent structures (receptors or Bruch's membrane). For example, an abnormal EOG may be found in some patients with angioid streaks [39] or in many patients with acquired cone degenerations (see later discussion on this subject). In other words, it is not certain that an abnormal EOG always means that the primary abnormality is in the pigment epithelium.

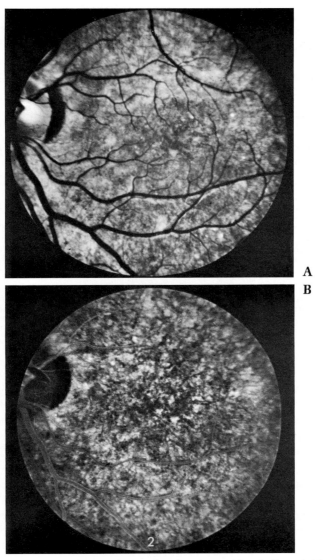

A

B

FIG. 5-6A and B. Left macula of patient with rubella retinitis showing white-light photograph (A) and same area during venous phase of fluorescein angiography (B). Diffuse fine pigment spots and small areas of atrophy are seen in white-light photograph (A). Pigment spots are accentuated in fluorescein photograph because of background contrast. Note multiple hyperfluorescent spots varying in size and configuration. The same changes are seen throughout most of the eyegrounds. In spite of widespread structural alteration of pigment epithelium, the EOG is normal. (From Krill, A. E., et al. Amer. J. Ophthal. 66:470, 1968.)

A possible relationship to severe diffuse disease of the internal retina must also be considered. However, other than in central retinal vascular occlusions, EOG abnormalities have not been reported in diseases of this portion of the retina (for example, a normal EOG is seen in glaucoma). Furthermore, cutting off the blood supply at a more proximal site (for example, at the carotid artery [5]) does not seem to affect the EOG. Therefore, with the possible exception of central retinal vascular occlusions (usually of the artery), an abnormality of the EOG probably reflects a functional abnormality of the pigment epithelium.

EOG IN SPECIFIC DISEASES

In general, the EOG is an adjunct to the ERG. The ERG is definitely more useful if one is limited to only one of these two tests. However, there are diseases, referred to in this section, where only the EOG is abnormal or where it may earlier show changes than the ERG. In addition, the use of both tests may provide more insight into the nature and extent of a disease process and at times provide a specific diagnosis.

AMAUROSIS CONGENITA OF LEBER

All infants with this disease have a severely abnormal ERG. However, according to Henkes and Verduin,[29] some infants have a markedly abnormal EOG, whereas others have a normal or close to normal EOG. They speculated that the first group has progressive disease (the more common type) and the latter group has stationary disease. Long-term data are needed to confirm or reject these speculations.

TOXIC RETINOPATHY

An abnormal EOG has been reported with several toxic retinopathies (e.g., phenothiazine [1,8]); however, the greatest amount of information published has been on chloroquine retinopathy. In spite of initial claims of great sensitivity of this test in detecting early chloroquine retinopathy, it now appears that either the EOG or the ERG or both may be abnormal in early chloroquine retinopathy.[30] Therefore, it is necessary to screen patients who are taking this drug with both tests.

SIDEROSIS RETINAE

The EOG may be abnormal before the ERG in this condition.[35] Therefore, this test is useful in detecting early retinal involvement.

DIABETIC RETINOPATHY

Henkes [28] found the EOG to be abnormal in some patients with early diabetic retinopathy, even at times before eyeground changes were seen. The long-term significance of these data are unknown. It has also been shown that the ratio increases after intravenous glucose infusion in normals, but not in diabetics.[6]

FLECKED-RETINA SYNDROME

Familial drusen, fundus flavimaculatus, and fundus albipunctatus are probably all a consequence of pigment epithelium disease. There are certain functional features that these three conditions have in common, which include minimal abnormalities demonstrated in subjective dark adaptation or by the ERG, but frequent moderate to severe abnormalities shown by the EOG.[43] The designation "flecked-retina syndrome" was originated to describe the features that the three diseases have in common.[43]

ALBINISM

One group has shown supernormal values in albinism,[56] and this finding may be helpful in arriving at a diagnosis in the incomplete universal and ocular forms of albinism, since both of these conditions are difficult to recognize.

VITELLIRUPTIVE (VITELLINE) MACULAR DEGENERATION

Vitelliruptive macular degeneration deserves special mention because in this condition the ERG is usually normal but the EOG is always abnormal,[18, 19, 42, 45] usually to a marked extent, regardless of the age of the patient or the apparent severity of the disease (Fig. 5-7). In fact, the EOG is even abnormal in carriers of this condition, who show no ophthalmoscopic changes or visual acuity abnormality [13] (Fig. 5-7). Therefore, this test serves as a genetic marker to trace this autosomal dominant disease in families where a "skipped generation" is part of the picture. Recently a condition has been described, called

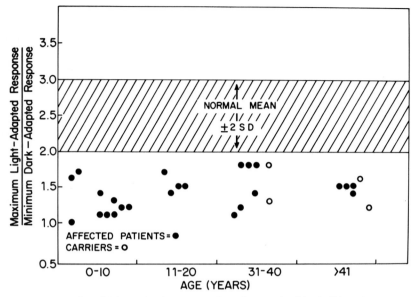

FIG. 5-7. *A plot of EOG ratios from 18 patients (25 eyes) with vitelliruptive macular degeneration and two carriers (4 eyes) of this condition. The normal group (the mean plus or minus two standard deviations is shown) is not broken up according to age. The affected individuals and carriers are divided according to age. It can be seen that the ratios are abnormal in all subjects and bear no relationship to age, and therefore to duration of the disease. (From Krill, A. E. Invest. Ophthal. 9:600, 1970.)*

butterfly-shaped dystrophy of the fovea, which also has an abnormal EOG with a normal ERG (Chapt. 15, Vol. 2).

DIFFUSE RECEPTOR DISTURBANCES

Diffuse Cone Abnormalities

The EOG is usually normal in congenital total color blindness.[11, 16, 21, 25b] We have found an abnormal EOG in only one of seven patients we tested with this condition. On the other hand, we have noted the EOG to be abnormal in 16 of 25 patients with diffuse cone degenerations. The abnormality was noted even in patients with normal rod function, as evidenced by a normal scotopic ERG and final threshold on dark adaptation. Patients with cone degenerations may eventually have abnormal rod function. Such patients (cone-rod degenerations) usually have an abnormal EOG (Chapt. 10, Vol. 2).

Congenital Stationary Night Blindness

It has been claimed, on the basis of the few patients studied, that the EOG is abnormal in the autosomal dominant form of congenital night blindness but normal in patients with the autosomal recessive form of the disorder.[10] However, a normal EOG has been reported in a patient with dominant stationary night blindness,[22] and an abnormal EOG has been found in patients with an autosomal recessive abnormality.[16,44] We have found an abnormal EOG in two patients with an X-linked recessive form,[44] and another group [25b] has found a normal EOG in this type. Therefore, either a normal or an abnormal EOG may appear in any of the three hereditary types of congenital stationary night blindness.

Diffuse Rod-Cone Degenerations

Diseases such as retinitis pigmentosa, diffuse choroidal sclerosis and choroideremia have pronounced abnormalities of the EOG, even in relatively early stages. However, in our experience and that of others,[24,52] the electroretinogram is a more sensitive and probably more reliable index of early disease.

SUMMARY

The specific diseases in which the EOG may be decidedly abnormal in relation to an ERG that is either normal or only mildly abnormal are early chloroquine retinopathy, early siderosis retinae, early diabetic retinopathy, drusen, fundus albipunctatus, fundus flavimaculatus, and vitelliruptive macular degeneration.

ELECTRONYSTAGMOGRAPHY (STUDY OF EYE MOVEMENTS)

The methodology for electrooculography can be used to evaluate eye movements in various oculomotor disorders or in cognitive processes such as reading.[12,31,59,60,64] Customarily the electrodes are placed at the outer and inner canthi to study horizontal eye movements; however, vertical eye movements can also be studied by placement of electrodes above the center of the upper eyelid and below the center of the lower eyelid. The EOG may also be of value in defining the amplitude, frequency, and variability of nystagmus in various

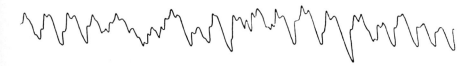

20 Feet

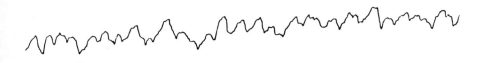

14 Inches

FIG. 5-8. *Recording of nystagmus from universal albino at 20 feet and at 14 inches (same calibration). Note lesser amplitude of movements at 14 inches. (From Krill, A. E. "Hereditary Macular Degenerations," in Symposium on Surgical and Medical Management of Congenital Anomalies of the Eye. St. Louis, C. V. Mosby Co., 1968.)*

neurological or neuromuscular abnormalities, in vestibular disorders, and in primary ocular abnormalities.[50, 61, 62, 64, 68] For example, in this last area it has been shown, by recordings on the EOG (Fig. 5-8), that in albinism, near vision is usually better than distance vision because of less nystagmus (Fig. 5-8) in the near position.[41]

There are several methods of recording eye movements.[7, 57, 61, 69] Probably, though, photoelectric techniques [57, 65] are best for the most sensitive and accurate study of eye movements. With photoelectric techniques, evaluation of normal oculomotor behavior and measurements of eye movements during reading are among some of the studies undertaken that cannot be done with sufficient accuracy with other techniques of recording eye movements.

REFERENCES

1. Alkemade, P. P. Phenothiazine-retinopathy. *Ophthalmologica* 155:70, 1968.
2. Arden, G. B., Barrada, A., and Kelsey, J. H. New clinical test of retinal function based upon the standing potential of the eye. *Brit. J. Ophthal.* 46:449, 1962.

3. Arden, G. B., and Fojas, M. R. Electrophysiological abnormalities in pigmentary degenerations of the retina. *Arch. Ophthal. 68:*369, 1962.

4. Arden, G. B., and Kelsey, J. H. Changes produced by light in the standing potential of the human eye. *J. Physiol. 161:*189, 1962.

5. Ashworth, B. The electrooculogram in disorders of the retinal circulation. *Amer. J. Ophthal. 61:*505, 1966.

6. Balik, J., and Van Lith, G. H. M. The influence of glucose loading on the electrooculographic ratio (EOG) in normal subjects and diabetics. *Acta Ophthal. 48:*1097, 1970.

7. Bengi, H., and Thomas, J. G. Three electronic methods for recording ocular tremor. *Med. Biol. Engin. 6:*171, 1968.

8. Boet, P. J. Toxic effects of phenothiazines on the eye. *Docum. Ophthal. 28:*1, 1970.

9. Brown, K. T., and Wiesel, T. Intraretinal recording in the unopened cat eye. *Amer. J. Ophthal. 46:*91, 1958.

10. Carr, R. E., Ripps, H., Siegel, I. M., and Weale, R. A. Rhodopsin and the electrical activity of the retina in congenital nightblindness. *Invest. Ophthal. 5:*497, 1966.

11. Carr, R. E., and Siegel, I. M. Electrophysiological aspects of several retinal diseases. *Amer. J. Ophthal. 58:*95, 1964.

12. Cohen, N. L. Clinical applications of electronystagmography. *New York J. Med. 67:*407, 1967.

13. Deutman, A. F. Electrooculography in families with dystrophy of the fovea. *Arch. Ophthal. 81:*305, 1969.

14. Dewar, J. The physiological action of light. *Nature 15:*443, 1877.

15. Elenius, V., and Karo, T. Cone activity in the light-induced response of the human electrooculogram. *Pflueger Arch. Ges. Physiol. 291:*241, 1966.

16. Elenius, V., and Karo, T. "Observations on the ERG, EOG and the Perimetric Areal Summation in a Case of Stationary Congenital Nightblindness," in *Clinical Electroretinography,* ed. by Burian, H. M., and Jacobson, J. H. *Vision Res. (Suppl.).* London, Pergamon Press, 1966.

17. Elenius, V., and Lehtonen, J. Spectral sensitivity of the standing potential of the human eye. *Acta Ophthal. 40:*559, 1962.

18. Francois, J. Vitelliform degeneration of the macula. *Bull. N.Y. Acad. Med. 44:*18, 1968.

19. Francois, J., DeRouck, A., and Fernandez-Sasso, D. Electrooculography in vitelliform degeneration of the macula. *Arch. Ophthal. 77:*726, 1967.

20. Francois, J., Verriest, G., and DeRouck, A. Electrooculography as a functional test in pathological conditions of the fundus. I. First results. *Brit. J. Ophthal. 40:*108, 1956.

21. Francois, J., Verriest, G., and DeRouck, A. L'ectrooculographie en tant qu'examen fonctionnel de la retine. *Progr. Ophtal. (Basel) 7:*1, 1957.

22. Francois, J., Verriest, G., and DeRouck, A. A new pedigree of idiopathic congenital nightblindness: transmitted as a dominant hereditary trait. *Amer. J. Ophthal. 59:*621, 1965.

23. Gouras, P. Cone activity in the light induced D-C response of monkey retina. *Invest. Ophthal. 4:*318, 1965.

24. Gouras, P., and Carr, R. E. Electrophysiological studies in early retinitis pigmentosa. *Arch. Ophthal.* 72:104, 1964.

25. Gouras, P., and Carr, R. E. Light induced D-C responses of monkey retina before and after central retinal artery interruption. *Invest. Ophthal.* 4:310, 1965.

25b. Gouras, P., and Gunkel, R. D. The EOG in chloroquine and other retinopathies. *Arch. Ophthal.* 70:629, 1963.

26. Hecht, J., and Papst, W. Ueber den Ursprung des corneoretinalen Ruhepotentials. Elektroretinographie, Hamburger Symposium 1956. *Bibl. Ophthal.* 48:96, 1957.

27. Henkes, H. E., Denier Van der Gon, J. J., Van Marle, G. W., and Schreinemachers, H. P. Electrooculography: a semi-automatic recording procedure. *Brit. J. Ophthal.* 52:122, 1968.

28. Henkes, H. E., and Houtsmuller, A. J. Fundus diabeticus. *Amer. J. Ophthal.* 60:662, 1965.

29. Henkes, H. E., and Verduin, T. E. Dysgenesis or abiotrophy? A differentiation with the help of the electroretinogram (ERG) and electrooculogram (EOG) in Leber's congenital amaurosis. *Ophthalmologica* 145:144, 1963.

30. Henkind, P., Carr, R. E., and Siegel, I. M. Early chloroquine retinopathy, clinical and functional findings. *Arch. Ophthal.* 71:157, 1964.

31. Hood, J. D. Electronystagmography. *J. Laryng.* 82:167, 1968.

32. Imaizumi, K. "The Clinical Application of Electrooculography," in *Clinical Electroretinography*, ed. by Burian, H. M., and Jacobson, J. H. London, Pergamon Press, 1966, pp. 311–326.

33. Jayle, G. E., Boyer, R. L., and Sarracco, J. B. *L'Electroretinographie.* Paris, Masson et Cie., 1965, Vol. 2, pp. 1085–1122.

34. Kelsey, J. Variations in the normal electrooculogram. *Brit. J. Ophthal.* 51:44, 1967.

35. Kelsey, J. H. The combined use of the EOG and ERG as a routine clinical procedure, in *Advances in Electrophysiology and Pathology of the Visual System*, ed. by Schmoger, E. Leipzig, Veb. Georg Thieme, 1968, pp. 19–28.

36. Klien, B. A., and Krill, A. E. Fundus flavimaculatus: clinical, functional and histopathologic observations. *Amer. J. Ophthal.* 64:3, 1967.

37. Kolder, H. Spontane and experimentelle Änderungen des Bestandpotentials des menschlichen Auges. *Pflueger Arch.* 268:258, 1959.

38. Kolder, H. Automatic recording and evaluating oscillations of indirectly measured corneoretinal potential in man. *Med. Res. Engin.* 6:26, 1967.

39. Krill, A. E. The electroretinographic and electrooculographic findings in patients with macular lesions. *Trans. Amer. Acad. Ophthal. Otolaryng.* 70:1063, 1966.

40. Krill, A. E. Retinal disease of rubella. *Arch. Ophthal.* 77:445, 1967.

41. Krill, A. E. "Hereditary macular degenerations," in *Trans. New Orleans Acad. Ophthal.: Symposium on Surgical and Medical Management of Congenital Anomalies of the Eye.* St. Louis, C. V. Mosby, 1968, p. 444.

42. Krill, A. E. The electroretinogram and electrooculogram: clinical applications. *Invest. Ophthal.* 9:600, 1970.

43. Krill, A. E., and Klien, B. A. Flecked retina syndrome. *Arch. Ophthal.* 74:496, 1965.

44. Krill, A. E., and Martin, D. Photopic abnormalities in congenital stationary nightblindness. *Invest. Ophthal.* 10:625, 1971.

45. Krill, A. E., Morse, P. A., Potts, A. M., and Klien, B. A. Hereditary vitelliruptive macular degeneration. *Amer. J. Ophthal. 61*:1405, 1966.

46. Krill, A. E., Newell, F. W., and Chishti, M. I. Fluorescein studies in diseases affecting the retinal pigment epithelium. *Amer. J. Ophthal. 3*:470, 1968.

47. Kris, C. Corneo-fundal potential variations during light and dark adaptation. *Nature 182*:1027, 1958.

48. Marg, E. Development of electrooculography. *Arch. Ophthal. 45*:169, 1951.

49. Miles, W. Modification of the human eye potential by dark and light adaptation. *Science 91*:456, 1940.

50. Milojevic, B. Electronystagmographical study of vertigo. *Trans. Amer. Acad. Ophthal. Otolaryng. 70*:931, 1966.

51. Mowrer, O., Ruck, T., and Miller, N. The corneo-retinal potential difference as the basis of the galvanometric method of recording eye movements. *Amer. J. Physiol. 114*:423, 1936.

52. Nagaya, T. The standing potential of the eye in vascular and degenerative disease of the retina. *Bull. Yamaguchi Med. Sch. 11*:187, 1964.

53. Noell, W. K. Experimentally induced toxic effects on structure and function of visual cells and pigment epithelium. *Amer. J. Ophthal. 36*:103, 1953.

54. Noell, W. K. The origin of the electroretinogram. *Amer. J. Ophthal. 38*:77, 1954.

55. Perdriel, G. Electrophysiologie clinique de la retine et du cortex visuel. *Arch. Ophtal. (Paris) 31*:287, 1971.

56. Reeser, F. W., Weinstein, G. W., Feiock, K. B., and Oser, R. S. Electrooculography as a test of retinal function. *Amer. J. Ophthal. 70*:505, 1970.

57. Richter, H. R. Comparison of different electronystagmographic, photoelectronystagmographic, and oculographic methods using contact lenses. *Rev. Neurol. (Paris) 117*:301, 1967.

58. Riggs, L. A. Electroretinography in cases of nightblindness. *Amer. J. Ophthal. 38*:70, 1954.

59. Robinson, D. A. The oculomotor control system: a review. *Proc. Inst. Elect. Engin. 56*:1032, 1968.

60. Rosen, S., and Czech, D. The use of electrooculography for identifying phases of cognitive process. *Psychophysiology 3*:203, 1966.

61. Rubin, W. Nystagmography: terminology, technique and instrumentation. *Arch. Otolaryng. 87*:266, 1968.

62. Toglia, J. U., and Cole, W., Jr. Electronystagmography in clinical neurology. *Dis. Nerv. Syst. 26*:630, 1965.

63. Tomita, T., Murakami, M., and Hashimoto, Y. On the R membrane of the frog's eye; its localization and relation in the retinal action potential. *J. Gen. Physiol. 43* (Suppl. 2):81, 1959–60.

64. Torok, N. Nystagmography. *Arch. Otolaryng. 84*:630, 1966.

65. Torok, N. Analysis of the nystagmogram utilization of the photoelectric principle. *Arch. Otolaryng. 84*:641, 1966.

66. Tursky, B., and O'Connell, D. N. A comparison of A-C and D-C eye movement recording. *Psychophysiology 3*:157, 1966.

67. Van Lith, G. H. M., and Balik, J.   Variability of the electrooculogram (EOG). *Acta Ophthal.* 48:1091, 1970.

67a. Van Lith, G. H. M., and Balik, J.   The variability of the EOG in the same person. *Ophthalmologica* 163:63, 1971.

68. VonNoorden, G. K., and Preziosi, T. J.   Eye movement recordings in neurological disorders. *Arch. Ophthal.* 76:162, 1966.

69. Young, L. R.   Measuring eye movements. *Amer. J. Med. Electronics* 2:300, 1963.

6

Visually Evoked Responses

An electrical response from the visual cortex after a flash of light before the eye was described initially in 1933 for animals [12] and in 1937 for humans.[5] This response, because of its small size (5 microvolts) and the rather large size of electroencephalographic responses (50 to 200 microvolts) could not be adequately studied until summating techniques were utilized. Initially this was done by photography,[6] but eventually the computer was used for algebraic summation.[22] Copenhaver [3] in 1963 was the first to use this technique for clinical purposes.

TERMINOLOGY

The preferred term at present for this light-induced response is visually evoked response (VER); other terms, though, such as electrocortical potential, evoked visual response (EVR), visually evoked cortical potential (VECP), cortically evoked potential (CEP), photically evoked potential (PEP), etc., have been used.

COMPONENTS

The VER is a complex polyphasic wave of both positive and negative components. The number of positive and negative components are a function of the experimental conditions and the subject. The responses may be quite different in appearance for unpatterned and patterned light flashes.[15, 16, 26, 29] There are usually five to seven components, depending primarily on the amplitude and latency criteria that are used.[22] In general, the latency of the response is about 30 to 45 milliseconds. The portion of the response occurring during the first 240 milliseconds after the light stimulus is the most constant segment of this response. Some waves, though, are known to occur as late as 750 msec after the flash.

RECORDING CONDITIONS

The response is greatly variable, and even the attention of the subject can alter its amplitude. Therefore, it is absolutely necessary to record from a relaxed subject away from distraction. Usually repetitive light stimuli of one flash per second are used, but up to five flashes per second have been utilized.[22] Obviously, if one wants to visualize the entire response (which may be as long as 750 msec after a flash), one-second intervals should be used.

The electrode position depends on whether monopolar or bipolar recording is desired. With bipolar recording the electrodes are usually placed along the vertical midline about 5 to 8 cm apart, with the posterior electrode just anterior to the inion. With monopolar recording, the active electrode is usually placed over the right occipital lobe and the indifferent electrode on the right earlobe. However, it should be emphasized that there has been considerable variation in the placement of electrodes.

The usual setup includes preamplifiers with a gain of at least 10,000, in addition to a computer of average transients. The data can be photographed from the face of the computer; however, the summed readout signals from the computer are usually printed out on a X-Y plotter. Most workers summate at least 100 responses, although 50 may suffice.

THEORY OF SUMMATION

The basic premise underlying this technique is that the cortical activity in the evoked response is time-locked with respect to the stimulus. In general, the average amplitude of such a response increases in direct proportion to the number of samples, while the amplitude of recurrent activity randomly related to the stimulus (noise) increases in relation to the square root of the number of samples.[31] With complete independence of random background activity and the time-locked response, the ratio of response amplitude to that of noise will grow in the proportion $N/\sqrt{N}$.

As an example, assume that the amplitude of background noise was about 25 microvolts while the amplitude of a signal of interest might be 5 microvolts, the response thus exhibiting a 1:5 signal-to-noise ratio. The averaging of 50 responses would produce a signal-to-noise ratio of approximately $50/\sqrt{50} \times 1/5 = 10/7$, while the averaging of 100 responses would produce a signal-to-noise ratio of $100/\sqrt{100} \times 1/5 = 2/1$. Using this same formula, though, it becomes obvious that the "noise penetration" of an averaging system for a time coherent signal has diminishing returns. For example, adding 200 responses results in a signal-to-noise ratio of less than 3:1 and it is necessary to add 400 responses to get a signal-to-noise ratio of 4:1. Another factor to be considered when deciding how many responses to add is that the likelihood of condition-constancy in the brain diminishes rapidly with excessive repetition.

It is also important to remember that the computer will add up anything that is time-locked to the stimulus. A constantly occurring artifactual potential will be summated. Furthermore, distracting stimuli (e.g., noise) may be time-locked to the visual stimulus and may thus affect the amplitudes of the responses added (see *Parameters Affecting Responses*).

ORIGIN OF THE VER

Although the exact cellular basis of the VER is unknown, it is mainly a function of macular and particularly of foveal cones; therefore, very small stimuli which stimulate foveal cones will give large responses. This has been shown most vividly by Potts and Nagaya,[23] who use 0.06 degree red light as a stimulus. There is, though, under the proper conditions, definitely a peripheral contribution to this response.[1] In general, the amplitude of the response falls off rapidly with stimuli outside of the fovea. Under the usual conditions of stimulation, it is not surprising that the action spectrum of the response is well fitted by the photopic luminosity function curve.[2] The anatomical importance of the fovea in the striate cortex is evidenced by the fact that its projection

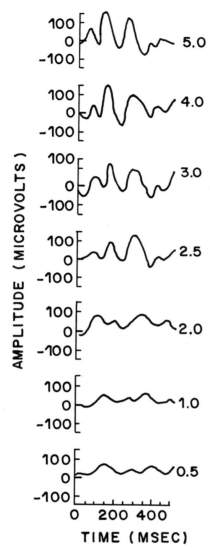

FIG. 6-1. *Effect of stimulus intensity upon the VER. Relative intensities are indicated on the figure in log units. Note larger responses with greater intensities. (From Shipley, T., Jones, R. W., and Fry, A. Intensity and the evoked occipitogram in man. Vision Res. 6:657, 1966.)*

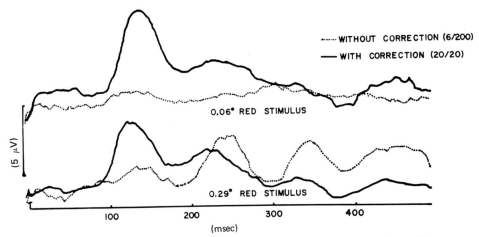

FIG. 6-2. *The effect of refractive error (myopia, 6 diopters) on VER. (From Potts,*
A. M., and Nagaya, T. Invest. Ophthal. 4:303, 1965.)

here occupies about 7.5 percent of this area, whereas foveal cones are
less than 0.2 percent of all retinal cones.

PARAMETERS AFFECTING RESPONSE

The amplitude of the response is proportional to the stimulus intensity [31] (Fig. 6-1). However, other factors can markedly affect amplitude. For example, the type of target [21, 24] (geometric forms, printed
words, etc.) can vary the response. A blurred target,[14, 20, 23, 27] because of
an uncorrected refractive error (Fig. 6-2), may reduce the amplitude of
response. The attention of the subject is important [23] (Fig. 6-3). The

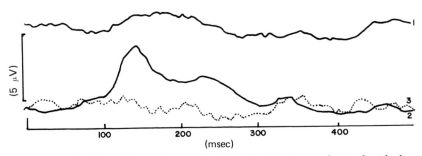

FIG. 6-3. *The effect of attention on the VER. Tracing 1 was obtained with the*
subject somnolent; tracing 2 was obtained with the subject alert; and tracing 3
was a control obtained with noise but no light. (From Potts, A. M., and Nagaya, T.
Invest. Ophthal. 4:303, 1965.)

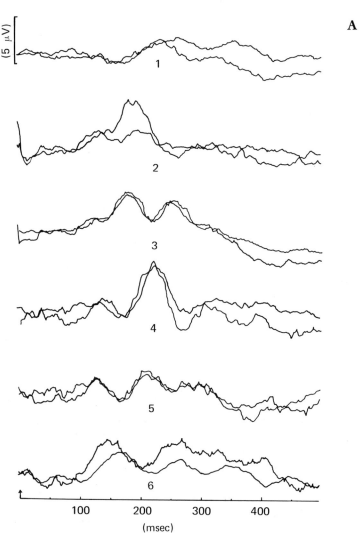

FIG. 6-4. *VER of 12 normal subjects (6-4A and 6-4B) to 0.06 degree red stimulus.*
(From Potts, A. M., and Nagaya, T. Invest. Ophthal. 4:303, 1965.)

level of subject excitability influences the response. The response can
be altered by having the subject perform mental tasks [13,24] or by background noise.[23,28] In fact, after about 10 minutes of exposure to a flash-
ing light stimulus, the VER has been found to diminish progressively.
The basis for this "habituation" is not entirely clear.[22] The latency of
the VER decreases with increasing stimulus intensity and also as the
stimulus area increases.[31]

(continued)

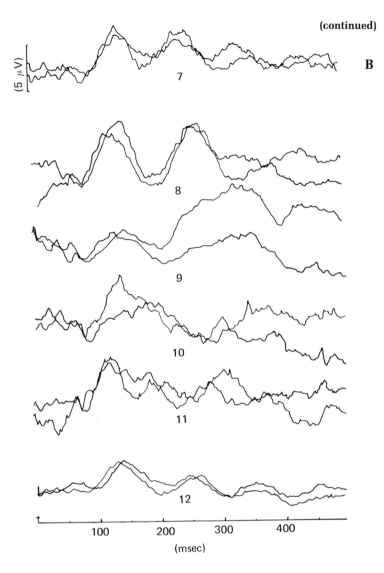

B

RELATION TO RETINAL AREA

As indicated, the largest responses are obtained from the macula; however, responses (depending on the size target used [23]) may be obtained outside of the area. The VER may be smaller in the nasal than in the temporal retina,[8] but smallest in the inferior retina.[9] The VER may be used to reveal the blind-spot scotoma.[4]

PROBLEM OF VARIABILITY

There is great variability among different subjects (Fig. 6-4), and even in the same individual from time to time. However, to some extent, the responses from a given individual are unique and identifiable over a period of time, particularly in adults and with a specific kind of stimuli.[7, 24] There are data that suggest that responses in infants show more variable wave forms, greater variability in amplitude, larger latency, and more marked fatigability than the adult VER. Probably the most important consideration is that the two eyes vary together, so that responses should be similar from the two eyes.

CLINICAL APPLICATIONS

Therefore, in certain unilateral diseases the VER may be helpful. The responses are abnormal from eyes with amblyopia ex anopsia (Fig. 6-5), but normal from eyes with hysterical or refractive amblyopia.[11, 22, 25] Unilateral optic nerve [19] or macular disease (Fig. 6-6) [11, 24] may produce significant differences in responses from the eyes. There are no data that indicate the degree of macular or optic nerve abnormality necessary to produce significant alteration of the VER.

It is obvious then that this test is of limited, if any, value in bilateral ocular disease. Furthermore, it is of no value in assessing macular function behind a corneal or lens opacity [23] because a smaller response can result from the intensity reduction and image blur produced by the opacity.

USE OF PATTERNED STIMULI

Up until now, the stimulus for clinical testing has usually been a diffuse light. However, there are several features of patterned stimuli (e.g., a checkerboard stimulus) which favor using this type of stimulus more frequently in patients: (1) A patterned stimulus elicits considerably larger responses than does plain light of the same intensity level.[15, 16, 26] (2) The response appears to be simpler in appearance than that elicited by diffuse light. A characteristic biphasic wave dominates the pattern stimulus response.[15, 16, 29] The diffuse light response is not

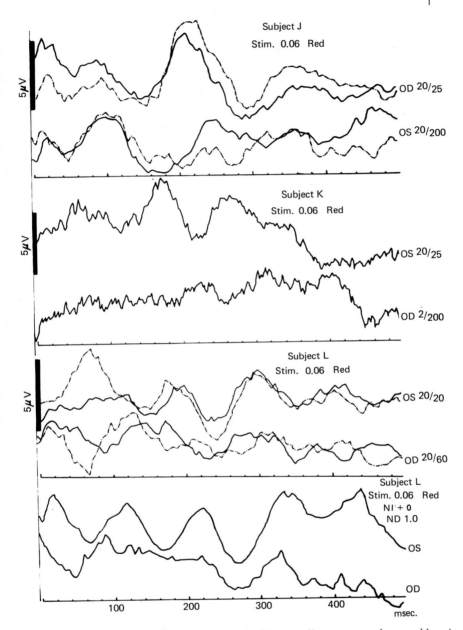

FIG. 6-5. VER in amblyopia ex anopsia. Note smaller responses from amblyopic eye. (From Potts, A. M., and Nagaya, T. Docum. Ophthal. 26:394, 1969.)

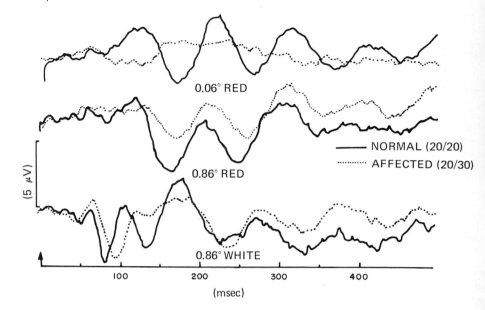

FIG. 6-6. VER from patient with unilateral macular disease. Note smaller responses, particularly with smallest target, from diseased eye. (From Potts, A. M., and Nagaya, T. Invest. Ophthal. 4:303, 1965.)

only more complex but more variable. (3) The responses are probably more consistent and predictable. In fact, the average amplitude of the characteristic biphasic wave increases almost in a linear manner with logarithmic increases in contour density within a certain range.[30] (4) Data from animal experiments (e.g., cat and monkey) indicate that most units of the visual cortex respond only to patterned illumination.[17, 18]

There appears to be a trend at present for using patterned, in place of diffuse, light stimuli. It remains to be seen whether the ultimate clinical value of the VER will be enhanced by this change.

REFERENCES

1. Adams, W. L., Arden, G. B., and Behrman, J. Responses of human visual cortex following excitation of peripheral retinal rods. Brit. J. Ophthal. 53:439, 1969.

2. Armington, J. C. "Spectral Sensitivity of Simultaneous Electroretinograms and Occipital Responses," in Clinical Electroretinography, Burian, H. M., and Jacobson, J. H. (eds.). New York, Pergamon Press, 1966, pp. 225–233.

3. Copenhaver, R. M., and Beinhocker, G. Evoked occipital potentials recorded from

scalp electrodes in response to focal visual illumination. *Invest. Ophthal.* 2:393, 1963.

4. Copenhaver, R. M., and Perry, N. W.   Factors affecting visually evoked cortical potentials, such as impaired vision of varying etiology. *Invest. Ophthal.* 3:665, 1964.

5. Cruikchank, R. M.   Human occipital brain potentials as affected by intensity duration variations of visual stimulation. *J. Exp. Psychol.* 21:625, 1937.

6. Dawson, G. D.   Central responses to electrical stimulation of peripheral nerve in man. *J. Neurol. Neurosurg. Psychiat.* 10:134, 1947.

7. Dustman, R. B., and Beck, E. C.   Long term stability of visually evoked potentials in man. *Science* 142:1480, 1963.

8. Eason, R. G., and White, C. T.   Averaged occipital responses to stimulation of sites in the nasal and temporal halves of the retina. *Psychonomic Science* 7:309, 1967.

9. Eason, R. G., White, C. T., and Oden, D.   Averaged occipital responses to stimulation of sites in the upper and lower halves of the retina. *Percept. Psychophysiol.* 2:423, 1967.

10. Ellingson, R. J.   Cortical electrical responses to visual stimulation in the human infant. *Electroenceph. Clin. Neurophysiol.* 12:663, 1960.

11. Fishman, R. S., and Copenhaver, R. M.   Macular disease and amblyopia: the visual evoked response. *Arch. Ophthal.* 77:718, 1967.

12. Gerard, R. W., Marshall, W. H., and Saul, L. J.   Cerebral action potentials. *Proc. Soc. Exp. Biol. Med.* 30:1123, 1933.

13. Glass, A.   Mental arithmetic and blocking of the occipital alpha rhythm. *Electroenceph. Clin. Neurophysiol.* 16:595, 1964.

14. Haider, M., Spong, P., and Lindsley, D. B.   Attention, vigilance, and cortical evoked potentials in humans. *Science* 145:180, 1964.

15. Harter, M. R., and White, C. T.   Effects of contour sharpness and check-size on visually evoked cortical potentials. *Vision Res.* 8:701, 1968.

16. Harter, M. R., and White, C. T.   Evoked cortical responses to checkerboard patterns: effect of check-size as a function of visual acuity. *Electroenceph. Clin. Neurophysiol.* 28:48, 1970.

17. Hubel, D. H., and Wiesel, T. N.   Receptive fields of single neurons in the cat's striate cortex. *J. Physiol.* 148:574, 1959.

18. Hubel, D. H., and Wiesel, T. N.   Receptive fields and functional architecture of monkey striate cortex. *J. Physiol.* 195:215, 1968.

19. Jacobson, J. H., Hirose, T., and Suzuki, T. A.   Simultaneous ERG and VER in lesions of the optic pathway. *Invest. Ophthal.* 6:279, 1968.

20. Jane, J. A., Smirnov, G. D., and Jasper, H. H.   Effects of distraction upon simultaneous auditory and visual evoked potentials. *Electroenceph. Clin. Neurophysiol.* 14:344, 1962.

21. Lifshitz, K.   The averaged evoked cortical response to complex visual stimuli. *Psychophysiology* 3:55, 1966.

22. Perry, N. W., and Childers, D. G.   *The Human Visual Evoked Response.* Springfield, Ill., Charles C Thomas, 1969.

23. Potts, A. M., and Nagaya, T.   Studies on the visual evoked response.   I. The use of the 0.06 degree red target for evaluation of foveal function. *Invest. Ophthal.* 4:303, 1965.

24. Potts, A. M., and Nagaya, T.   Studies on the visual evoked response.   II. The effect of special cortical activity. *Invest. Ophthal. 6:*657, 1967.

25. Potts, A. M., and Nagaya, T.   Studies on the visual evoked response.   III. The VER in strabismus amblyopia and hysterical amblyopia. *Docum. Ophthal. 26:*394, 1969.

26. Rietveld, W. J., Tordoir, W. E. M., Hagenouw, J. R. B., Lubbers, J. A., and Spoor, T. A. C.   Visual evoked responses to blank and to checkerboard patterned flashes. *Acta Physiol. Pharmacol. Neurol. 14:*259, 1967.

27. Ritter, W., and Vaughn, H. G.   Averaged evoked responses in vigilance and discrimination: a reassessment. *Science 164:*326, 1969.

28. Satterfield, J. H.   Evoked cortical response enhancement and attention in man: a study of responses to auditory and shock stimuli. *Science 19:*470, 1965.

29. Spehlmann, R.   The averaged electrical responses to diffuse and to patterned light in the human. *Electroenceph. Clin. Neurophysiol. 19:*560, 1965.

30. Venoyma, K.   Visual evoked response produced by patterned light stimulus. Presented at Western ARVO Meeting, September 11, 1970.

31. Vaughn, H. G.   The perceptual and physiologic significance of visual evoked responses recorded from the scalp in man, in *Clinical Electroretinography,* ed. by Burian, H. M., and Jacobson, J. H. New York, Pergamon Press, 1966, pp. 203–223.

7

Evaluation of Color Vision

Color is a subjective sensory experience, which is dependent on the "eyes of the beholder" and the presence of a specific kind of light stimulus. Some animals (e.g., horses and dogs) will always see things colorless regardless of the type of light stimulus. An object may appear red to a human with normal color vision but yellow to another human with abnormal color vision.

The human eye can perceive light that ranges in length from about 380 to 760 millionths of a millimeter (nanometers). Each visible wavelength produces a specific color sensation. Colored light is therefore produced by breaking up light into specific wavelengths (for example, by passing through prisms or thin films). Objects appear colored when they selectively absorb only certain wavelengths and transmit or reflect others (Table 7-1). The color of the object depends on the wavelengths of light reflected or transmitted.

An object reflecting most light striking its surface will appear white, whereas one absorbing most of this light will appear black (Table 7-1). An object that transmits most of the light hitting its surface will appear transparent. One that partially absorbs the same proportion of light at each wavelength will appear gray. An object will appear colored only when it absorbs *selective* wavelengths of visible light.

A colored light stimulus is best characterized by its three "attributes" —namely, its luminance, dominant wavelength, and purity. Each at-

TABLE 7-1

Light on Object	Appearance of Object
Reflected	White
Absorbed	Black
Similar partial absorption at each wavelength	Gray
Selective absorption of specific wavelengths	Colored
Transmitted	Transparent

tribute affects the individual's interpretation of the color in a specific manner (Table 7-2).

ATTRIBUTES OF COLOR

LUMINANCE; BRIGHTNESS

Luminance refers to the amount of light coming from the object being viewed. In daylight the luminance of an object will be much greater than at dusk. The individual's sensation of brightness (sometimes called lightness) is mostly dependent on the luminance of the object. An object interpreted as having very little brightness is said to be "dim," and a very bright object is said to be "dazzling."

Purkinje Phenomenon

As the luminances of colored stimuli are reduced, the brightnesses produced by long-wave stimuli decrease distinctly more rapidly than

TABLE 7-2
Primary Characteristics of Colored Light Stimulus

Physical Attribute	Corresponding Psychological Attribute
Luminance	Brightness
Dominant wavelength	Hue
Purity	Saturation

the brightnesses produced by short-wave stimuli. As a consequence, there is a remarkable difference in which colors appear the brightest at low and high luminances. With very dim lights, in a scotopic state, colors with a dominant wavelength close to 510 nm (blue-green) appear the brightest. With lights bright enough to produce a photopic state, colors with a dominant wavelength close to 555 nm (yellow) appear the brightest (Fig. 3-2). This change in brightness of colors with change in luminance is known as the Purkinje shift. It is dependent on a shift from rod vision at lower luminances to cone vision at higher luminances (see Chapter 3, *Evaluation of Night Vision: Dark Adaptation*).

DOMINANT WAVELENGTH; HUE

Dominant wavelength is simply the wavelength dominant in a light stimulus. Hue describes the color name the individual gives to the light stimulus (e.g., red, green, blue). Some of the more common hues and corresponding dominant wavelengths are shown in Table 7-3.

PURITY; SATURATION

Purity refers to the degree to which the dominant wavelength predominates in a light stimulus. This corresponds, in a sense, to the concentration of a solvent in a solution (e.g., salt in water). The greater the concentration of the solvent, the greater the purity. The individual's perception of purity is referred to as saturation. The greater the purity of a stimulus, the more saturated it appears.

Assume that a colored light stimulus with a dominant wavelength

TABLE 7-3
Hue Names Associated with
Various Wavelengths of Light

Approximate Wavelength Region (in nanometers)	Associated Hue
380–450	Violet
450–490	Blue
490–550	Green
550–590	Yellow
590–630	Orange
630–760	Red

producing a hue response of red is mixed with white light. (This would be the same as adding more water to a salt solution.) The change in the purity of the stimulus would be described by saying it is now more pink. Pink and red therefore refer to different saturations of the same hue. Eventually, if enough white light were added to the original red stimulus, it might be described by the individual as appearing almost the same as white light: "It has only a slight pinkish tinge." This stimulus has very little saturation. To continue the saltwater analogy, if enough water is added, one eventually barely tastes the salt, but it is still a saltwater solution.

INTERRELATIONSHIPS

It has been pointed out that luminance affects brightness, dominant wavelength affects hue, and purity affects saturation. However, there is not complete interindependence of these three perceptions. Some of these more important interrelationships will be considered.

Luminance

1. *Effect of Darkness*. All hue and saturation vanish except for the slightly bluish or greenish-blue cast often noticed in night vision.
2. *Bezold-Brucke Phenomenon*. This phenomenon occurs at higher luminances wholly within the photopic range. (The Purkinje phenomenon involves a shift from a photopic to a scotopic range.) As luminance is increased, all dominant wavelengths, with the exception of four near 474, 494, 506, and 571 nm, are described as appearing more blue or yellow and less red or green. The four exceptions are called the invariable hues. Another way of describing this phenomenon is to say that red-yellows and green-yellows become yellower, and red-blues and green-blues become bluer, as luminance is increased. Just the reverse occurs with decreasing luminance.
3. *Effect on Saturation*. The difference between the luminance when light is first perceived (absolute threshold) and the luminance when the hue of the light stimulus is first perceived is known as the photochromatic interval. This interval varies with wavelength. In fact, with wavelengths exceeding 650 nm, the hue of the light stimulus is identified when it is first seen so that there is no photochromatic interval.

Purity

Effect on Brightness. Purity exerts a considerable though somewhat confusing effect on brightness. There is a tendency for brightness to increase as purity increases, even when luminance, the principal correlate of brightness, is held constant. This relationship varies with the wavelength. There are also considerable individual differences, depending on the experience of the observer. A trained or experienced observer has much less of a tendency to confuse brightness and saturation. However, even with expert observers there is a definite brightness variation ascribable to purity. Brilliance is sometimes used to describe the sensation that depends on both brightness and saturation.

Chromaticity

This is a term used to describe both the purity and the dominant wavelength of a stimulus.

EVALUATION OF THREE BASIC ATTRIBUTES

RELATIVE LUMINOSITY CURVE

This refers to the apparent brightness of each wavelength to the human eye. Obviously, equal amounts of energy of different wavelengths do not produce visual sensations having equal brightness. Furthermore, as pointed out, the state of adaptation of the eye influences the apparent brightness of a given color. The measurement of the brightness produced by each color is usually done in an indirect manner. At each wavelength the light energy required to produce a constant value of brightness is determined. This requires the subject to match brightnesses, which is a relatively easy task. The data are usually plotted on a curve where the wavelength at which the least energy (in specified units of radiance) gives a match to a standard brightness is assigned a value of one and is the peak of the curve (Fig. 3-2). The other points of the curve are determined by taking the reciprocals of the radiances required for equal brightnesses, each expressed as a decimal fraction of the largest one used, and plotted against wavelength. The curve that results is called a relative luminosity curve, and it differs considerably from light-adapted (photopic relative luminosity curve) and dark-adapted (scotopic relative luminosity) eyes (Fig. 3-2).

HUE DISCRIMINATION

Sensitivity to dominant wavelength difference (hue discrimination) is usually measured with monochromatic stimuli of equal brightness in a bipartite field, by determining the just-noticeable difference in wavelength at different points in the spectrum. The resulting curve is known as a hue discrimination curve (Fig. 7-1). The normal observer is able to detect a difference in hue if two monochromatic stimuli differ by as little as 1 nm in wavelength in the regions of 490 (blue-green) and 585 (yellow). In other regions it is necessary to have a greater difference in wavelength, but only in the violet and red is a difference greater than 4 nm necessary.

SATURATION DISCRIMINATION

The study of sensitivity to differences in purity of a given color (saturation discrimination) requires the determination of the percentage of monochromatic light required in a mixture with white light to create a just-noticeable difference from the white light alone at equal brightnesses. This is done at wavelengths throughout the spectrum, and the reciprocal of this least-detectable change in purity for the first step away from white (or the logarithm of this reciprocal) is plotted against wavelength (Fig. 7-2). The ability to determine differences in saturation is greatest for blue, least for yellow, and intermediate for red. Note in the curve (Fig. 7-2) how the least-saturated part of the spectrum is in the yellow and saturation of color increases as the two ends of the spectrum are approached.

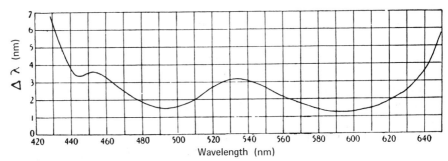

FIG. 7-1. *Mean hue discrimination curve of five normal subjects. Minimal difference in wavelength detected is plotted on Y-axis and dominant wavelength on X-axis. Note greatest ability to detect small difference in hues is in regions of 490 and 585 nm. Least sensitivity exists in the violet and red ends of the spectrum. (From Wright, W. D.* Researches on Normal and Defective Colour Vision. *London, H. Kimpton, 1946.)*

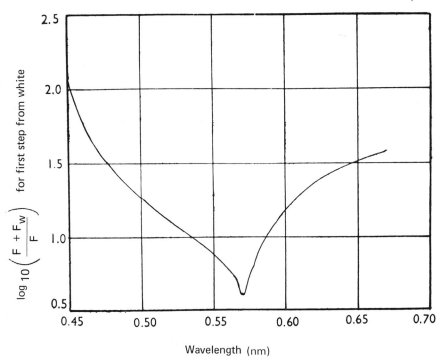

Wavelength (nm)

FIG. 7-2. *Mean saturation discrimination of curve of three normal observers. Logarithm of reciprocal of a just-noticeable difference of monochromatic light from white light (in a mixture) is plotted on Y-axis and dominant wavelength on X-axis. Higher number on Y-axis indicates more sensitive saturation discrimination. The most sensitive saturation discrimination is in the blue spectral region and the least sensitive is in the yellow area at 570 nm. Note how colors appear more saturated as the two ends of the spectrum are approached. (From* Wright, W. D. Researches on Normal and Defective Colour Vision. *London, H. Kimpton, 1946.)*

ANATOMY OF COLOR VISION

Color vision is well developed in birds, fish, reptiles, and certain insects (for example, bees) but is absent in most mammals. The human species is a notable exception, as we are able to perceive close to 200 hues. If there were receptors sensitive to every color perceived, there would have to be almost 200 kinds of cones, each responding to a different wavelength. But this is impossible, since visual acuity is almost as good in colored light (when presumably only 1 out of 200 cones would be stimulated) as it is in white light (when presumably all of the cones would be stimulated). This means that there must be only a very few kinds of cones. One of the greatest geniuses of all time, Thomas Young, saw this clearly in 1801. He presumed that there were only three color receptors—one sensitive to red, one to green, and one to violet light.

It was not until 1963 that two groups [31, 46] proved very definitely that Young was right. Three types of cone pigments were identified when measurements of the absorption characteristics of single cones in enucleated human eyes were made, using a recording microspectrophotometer. Additional data supporting the notion of three cone pigments are summarized elsewhere.[7] The three pigments identified consist of one most sensitive to blue light, one to green light, and a third to orange-red light. It is thought that the three pigments are each found in different cones, so that there are "red" cones, "green" cones, and "blue" cones. Cones containing the pigment most sensitive to blue light (blue cones) are thought to be by far in the minority.

The method of transmission of the colored message beyond the receptors is not completely understood as yet. There is evidence, though, based particularly on recordings of electrophysiological responses at different levels of the visual system in animals,[10] that the message is transmitted in a unique fashion. Some nerve fibers and cells probably send information only for red and green perception, since they produce electrical responses only when stimulated with red or green light. Other nerve fibers and cells, which produce electrical responses only when stimulated with blue and yellow light, probably transmit information only for blue and yellow perception. A specific feature of a nerve fiber or cell carrying information for two colors is that it responds in an opposite manner to each of the two colors. For example, certain ganglion cells respond by discharging when a red light is turned on ("on" or "excitatory" responses) or when a green light is turned off ("off" or "inhibitory" responses). Certain horizontal cells may show responses above the base line (depolarization or positive type) when stimulated with one color light, and responses below the base line (hyperpolarization or negative type) when stimulated with the other colored light.

This method of color information transmission fits in well with a theory originally developed by a German scientist, Hering, in the nineteenth century known as the "opponents' color theory." According to this theory, certain colors, known as complementary colors, are antagonistic to each other, so that when they are exhibited simultaneously their effects neutralize or oppose each other. Complementary colors are defined as two colors (red and green or blue and yellow) that give the sensation of white when added together in proper amounts.

These phenomena could be explained by this theory. It would also explain why each of two complementary colors placed side by side appears less saturated than if viewed separately (simultaneous contrast). Other psychological phenomena (e.g., colored afterimages, adaptation effects) could also be explained by this theory.

TRICHROMATIC COLOR VISION

It is understandable, then, that in tasks which reflect retinal response, such as performance on an instrument known as the colorimeter, a human is said to have trichromatic color vision. He can mix three specific colored lights (called primaries) in various proportions and produce all of the close to 200 hues he is capable of seeing. This can be visualized best by thinking of three movie projectors projecting superimposed lights—one a blue light, another a green light, and the third a red light (each of a specific wavelength and saturation). By changing the brightness of each light (placing neutral density filters in front of each projector as needed), all hues can be produced. This is known as additive mixing of colored lights. In contrast, in subtractive color mixing, done with pigments (or colored filters), the color that results after pigments are mixed depends on how much light is absorbed ("subtracted") by each pigment (or colored filter).

NOMENCLATURE OF ABNORMAL COLOR VISION

We prefer the terms "abnormal color vision" or "color defect" rather than "color blindness," because a complete absence of color vision is very rare. If "color blindness" is used, it should be qualified as partial or total.

Abnormal color vision is usually present at birth, is hereditary, and is characterized by specific inabilities in color vision as follows:

1. Incorrect identification of hues
2. Inability to discriminate certain closely related hues
3. Confusion of certain hues far apart in the light spectrum
4. Poor saturation discrimination
5. Certain hues appear gray
6. Certain hues appear very dim or even black

The individual with abnormal color vision fails to correctly identify many or most hues (for example, he calls green, yellow), has difficulty in distinguishing many closely related hues or closely related saturations of the same hue, sometimes finds certain hues gray and others very dim or even black, and confuses many hues that are often far apart in the light spectrum and therefore easily distinguished by individuals with normal color vision. There is a great variability in the severity of impairment among affected individuals.

PREFIX

The nomenclature of congenital color vision defects is derived from the classical concept that there are three fundamental colors — red, green, and blue — called respectively the first, second, and third primaries. By convention the Greek words for first, second, and third (*protos, deuteros,* and *tritos*) are substituted for red, green, and blue in naming partial color defects (e.g., any word for a red defect has the prefix *prot-*):

Trichromat
Normal
Protanomaly
Deuteranomaly
Tritanomaly
Dichromat
Protanopia
Deuteranopia
Tritanopia
Monochromat
Rod Monochromat
Cone Monochromat

SUFFIX

The suffix indicates whether there is a complete absence of the pigment (*-anopia*), whether the pigment is present but abnormal in some way (*-anomaly*), or whether the pigment is abnormal in some unspecified way (*-an*). This last category is less specific and lumps individuals with either an anopia or anomaly together.

COLORIMETRY PERFORMANCE

As indicated previously, a normal subject matches all spectral colors with mixtures of three properly chosen colors and is said to have trichromatic color vision. Subjects performing as if they had a deficiency of one cone pigment are called anomalous trichromats and require more than the normal amount of one color in a mixture.* A dichromat performs as if he had an absence of one cone pigment and can match all spectral colors with two properly chosen colors. A monochromat can match all spectral colors with different brightnesses of only one color. The monochromat has either a marked deficiency of normal cones (rod monochromat) or, more rarely, a transmission defect from the retina to the cerebral cortex (cone monochromat).

MINOR COLOR VISION DEFECTS

In addition, there are subjects with hypothesized minor color vision defects on the basis of slightly abnormal performance only on the anomaloscope.[33, 44] (See discussion of this instrument in next section.) In this group are subjects with only a wider than normal equation † or those who, after prolonged examinations, have wider than normal equations (color asthenopes), and those with a "shifted" equation just outside of the range of two standard deviations of the mean (color deviants). More data are necessary to define the color vision of individuals who have been included in these groups by some workers.

CLINICAL COLOR VISION TESTING

In defective color vision the three attributes of color sensation — brightness, hue, and saturation — are affected to a varying degree. Direct measurements of these three attributes by means of luminosity function, hue discrimination, and saturation discrimination are not usual clinical procedures. However, specific changes in these attributes enable a clearer understanding of each color defect, and therefore these will be discussed with the individual color defects.

The usual tests used clinically in evaluating color vision provide

---

* The actual defect may not be a deficiency of the pigment but rather something else (e.g., an abnormal type of pigment).

† The meaning of an "equation" on the anomaloscope is discussed with the instrument in the next section, *Clinical Color Vision Testing*.

data that may be dependent on more than one attribute. Sometimes the relative importance of each attribute in a test is not clear. Nevertheless, these tests are useful for the following purposes:

1. Screening
2. Type of color defect
3. Differentiation of acquired and congenital color defects
4. Severity of defect
5. Vocational suitability

The tests therefore answer the following questions in varying degrees: (1) Is the individual color-defective or not? (2) What is the precise nature of the defect? (3) Is the defect acquired or congenital? (4) How does the defect incapacitate the individual? (5) Can an individual, whether or not he has a color defect, qualify for a vocation involving certain color judgments? A summary of most of the clinical tests and their major value is shown in Table 7-4.

SORTING TESTS

The classical example of this type of test, the Holmgren wool test,[4] was developed in 1874 following a series of Swedish railroad accidents attributed to color blindness. The test involves the sorting of chromatic wool samples into three different groups, in relation to three larger standard wool samples. The three standard test skeins are a very pale green, a light purple or pink, and a full red. The examiner selects

TABLE 7-4
Specific Tests and Their Value

Test	Major Value
Holmgren wool test	Evaluation for fabric industry
Pseudoisochromatic plates	Screening
D-15 test	1. Type of defect
	2. Separation of severe and milder defects
100-hue test	1. Type of defect
	2. Quantitative evaluation of severity of defect
Inter-Society Color Council color aptitude test	Quantitative evaluation of severity of defect
Sloan achromatopsia test	Detection of total color blindness
Nagel anomaloscope	Precise diagnosis of deutan and protan defects
Lantern tests	Evaluation for transportation and communication industries

a standard test skein and the examinee sorts out eight or ten of the smaller skeins having nearly the same color. The procedure is repeated with the other two standard test skeins in turn.

The Holmgren wool test suffers from lack of standardization, detects only about half of the color-defectives examined, fails a number of "overanxious" normals, and permits easy improvement with practice. Its main use is in the selection of fabric inspectors. Its only other possible use would be to test infants. The Montessori educational movement has shown that the matching and grouping of dyed skeins of wool is an activity that develops quite spontaneously during the play of children.[31a]

PSEUDOISOCHROMATIC PLATES

The first series of pseudoisochromatic plates was published by Stilling [28] in 1878. Since then, there have been many modifications of this original series and many other types of plates that have been published from several countries. In general, pseudoisochromatic plates are most useful for screening color defectives from normals. Most of the data on incidence of color deficiency have been derived completely or in part from testing with plates.

Color-defectives confuse test symbols or numbers in pseudoisochromatic plates with the background. In most plates the colors of the test symbols and of the background are of such saturation, hue, and brightness that they are regularly confused by either the deutan or protan, or both. However, in one series, the American Optical Hardy-Rand-Rittler (H-R-R) plates, test symbol colors are close to the neutral points of deutans or protans and are thus confused to a varying degree with a gray background.

The most widely used set of pseudoisochromatic plates in the world at the present time is probably the Ishihara Series. In comparative studies these plates usually prove to be as good as, or better than, most other pseudoisochromatic series for screening purposes. These plates have been published in several editions since 1917. The most recent edition, published in 1962, consists of the 16 best plates from previous editions. In general, this test consists of some plates in which the normal sees one number and the color-deficient another (Fig. 7-3), some in which the numbers are read only by the normal subject, some in which the numbers are read only by the color-deficient subject, and some in which a path has to be traced. The larger editions contain plates of questionable value for distinguishing between protan and deutan defects. The background and test dots on each plate are of vary-

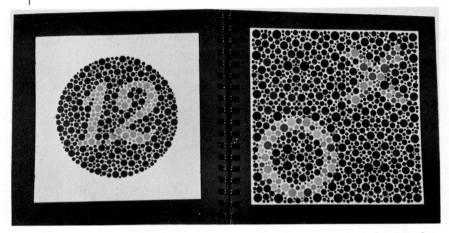

FIG. 7-3. *Photograph of Ishihara plate on left and American Optical H-R-R plate on the right. The Ishihara plate has a No. 12 which will not be seen by some color defectives because it is confused with the background color. The Hardy-Rand-Rittler plates have a cross in the upper right-hand corner and a circle in the lower left-hand corner, which are not seen by some individuals with a blue-yellow type of defect. The background, in this case gray, is close to the neutral point of individuals with a tritan type of defect. (Ishihara Plate, 1962 edition, reproduced with courtesy of Kanehara Shuppan Co., Ltd., Medical Book Publisher, Tokyo, and H-R-R plate reproduced with courtesy of American Optical Company, Buffalo, New York.)*

ing size and varying hue. The circular test dots form either arabic numerals or a multicurved continuous line. One criticism of the Ishihara plates is that some color-defectives may pass as normals if a cutoff of three errors is used.[40] A cutoff of two missed plates should detect most color-defectives, but it is likely that too many normals will be misclassified.[25] Our suggestion is to use more than one pseudoisochromatic series for screening (we also use the American Optical H-R-R plates).

Another popular test is in the second edition of the American Optical Company H-R-R plates published in 1957. It consists of 4 demonstration, 6 screening, and 14 diagnostic plates which test for both blue-yellow and red-green defects, and also attempt to grade the severity of either defect. All subjects, regardless of the severity of their color defect, should identify the symbols on the 4 demonstration plates. On each plate, there are circular dots of varying size. The background dots are neutral gray, and the test dots are colored to form a symbol (a circle, a triangle, or a cross) placed in one or two quadrants of each plate (Fig. 7-3). The dominant wavelengths of the test dots approximate the neutral points of deutans and protans.* Colors of low saturation are used as screening plates, and three higher saturations are used for the diagnostic plates. The screening series should be repeated twice, as some normals missing one or two plates on the first trial will score correctly on the second trial.

Major criticisms of the H-R-R test are the misclassification of some normals as color-defectives [9, 40, 45] and occasionally some color-defectives as normal.[12] However, there are several advantages that make this test quite useful in conjunction with another screening test such as the Ishihara: (1) it has blue-yellow plates which are not found in most of the other pseudoisochromatic series; (2) the symbols are easy to teach to young children, illiterates, or those trained in other languages with different-style numbers (e.g., Arabic or Chinese), and therefore the test can be used in most subjects; and (3) it is more accurate than most other pseudoisochromatic plates in classifying a defect as protan or deutan.[9, 17] The Rabkin plates are also good for this latter purpose.[17, 19] However, no pseudoisochromatic plates are completely reliable in classifying red-green defects. We have tested color-defectives in whom gross errors in classification were made with the H-R-R plates. Only the anomaloscope can be relied upon for the precise diagnosis of a red-green defect. Furthermore, no series of plates, including the H-R-R, should be used as the sole means of judging the severity of a defect.

Other pseudoisochromatic plates that have received acclaim as screening plates include the Dvorine series,[1, 8, 13, 17, 28] published since 1944, the Russian Rabkin series,[1, 17] published since 1939, and the Bostrom-Kugelberg series,[2] adopted as the official color test by the Royal Medical Board in Sweden. The Tokyo Medical College series attempts to classify and grade color defects just as the H-R-R series does, but a critical analysis has shown it to be useful only as a screening test.[39] It also has plates to detect blue-yellow defects.

FARNSWORTH'S HUE DISCRIMINATION TESTS

Farnsworth devised two tests from colored paper strips selected from the Munsell *Book of Color*, differing in hue but having approximately the same saturation and brightness for normal subjects.[14, 29, 32] In both tests the paper strips are mounted in black Bakelite caps, and a complete color circle of hues is formed with approximately equally discriminable hue steps between samples. The hue steps are much

---

* Colors appear gray at these neutral points.

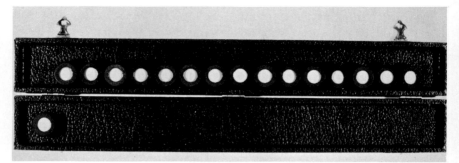

FIG. 7-4. *The Farnsworth D-15 test box consisting of one fixed blue violet cap and 15 removal caps with representative hues throughout the spectrum. The caps are to be arranged in sequential hue order. (Courtesy of Psychological Corp., New York City.)*

larger in the Farnsworth dichotomous (D-15) test with 16 paper strips than in the Farnsworth-Munsell 100-hue test with 85 paper strips.

The Farnsworth D-15 test was designed to distinguish more severe color-defectives from mild color-defectives and normals. Thus, there is a lower incidence of color blindness with this test than with pseudo-isochromatic plates (5 compared to 8 percent). The test consists of a blue violet cap fixed in position and 15 other caps presented in random array (Fig. 7-4). The subject attempts to arrange the caps in order starting with one having a color closest to the reference cap. Dichromats and sufficiently affected anomalous trichromats will make two or more errors. From the axis of confusion, easily determined from the cleverly designed score sheet (Fig. 7-5), the defect is classified as either protan, deutan, or tritan. According to some workers,[43] there are even characteristic axes for tetartanopia and total color blindness with this test.

The Farnsworth-Munsell 100-hue test was designed to separate persons with normal color vision into classes of superior, average, and low color discrimination and, second, to measure zones of color confusion in color-defective persons. The 85 paper strips of this test are mounted in 93 caps divided into four boxes. Each box samples about one fourth of the color circle and consists of 21 or 22 removable caps and two fixed pilot caps, one at each end of a case panel (Fig. 7-6). The second pilot cap of one box is the same as the first of another box. The boxes and caps within are presented in random order. The subject arranges the removable caps in hue sequence between the two fixed end caps of each box. Scoring evaluates both the total errors and the re-

FARNSWORTH DICHOTOMOUS TEST for Color Blindness—Panel D-15

Name..Age.............Date............................File No......................

Department..Tester..

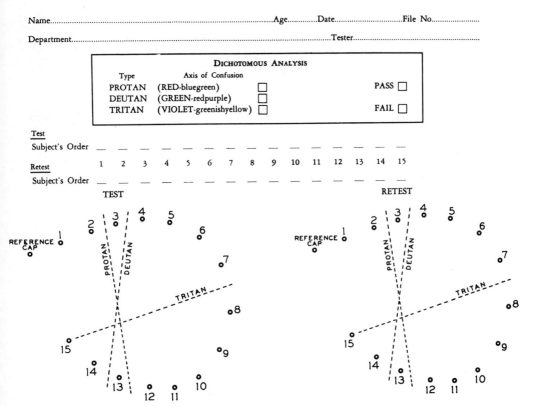

FIG. 7-5. Score sheet for the Farnsworth D-15 panel test. The dotted lines show characteristic confusion axes for the deutan, protan, and tritan defects. For example, an individual with a tritan type of defect would confuse caps Nos. 8 and 15 and therefore place cap No. 15 after cap No. 7. (Courtesy of Psychological Corp., New York City.)

gions of greatest error concentration. The data are plotted on a polar coordinate diagram with the circumference representing the 85 different caps and the radius representing the total number of errors for each removable cap (Fig. 7-7). Characteristic patterns (Fig. 7-8) readily identify the subject as deutan, protan, tritan, or as having poor color discrimination with no particular pattern. The age of the subject must also be considered, as normal older subjects (particularly beyond the age of 39) make more errors than younger subjects.[27, 41] A few mild color-defectives with good hue discrimination will be missed with this test; therefore, it is not recommended as a screening procedure.

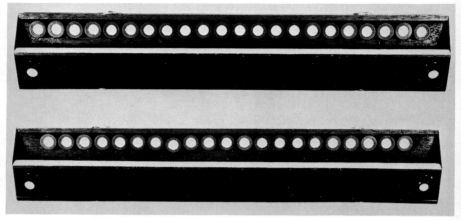

FIG. 7-6. *The Farnsworth-Munsell 100-hue test showing two of the four boxes in test. The four boxes contain hues from throughout the spectrum. In each box there are two fixed caps at each end of the case panel. The subject then takes the 21 or 22 removable caps and aligns them in sequential hue order from one fixed cap to the other fixed cap. (Courtesy of Munsell Color Co., Inc., Baltimore.)*

INTER-SOCIETY COLOR COUNCIL COLOR APTITUDE TEST

This test was developed to provide quantitative measures of color aptitude to be used in evaluating the suitability of workers for color-matching tasks and color-sorting operations.[5,9] An attempt is made to match 50 loose color samples to a panel of 50 fixed color samples. Color differences are small, so that the normal may make many errors. On the other hand, some color-defectives may perform adequately, for various reasons, so that this test cannot be used for screening or classification. Degree of color aptitude is indicated by the overall score on the test. The test can also be scored analytically with respect to per-

FIG. 7-7. *Score sheet for the Farnsworth-Munsell 100-hue test. A polar coordinate diagram is shown with the circumference representing the 85 different caps and the radius representing the total number of errors for each removable cap. The score for a particular cap is calculated by subtracting the difference between the number of this cap and that of each adjacent cap and adding up these two differences. If an individual makes no errors, then the score for each cap should be 2, and the score would be plotted on the closest circle to the center. For example, considering cap No. 2, if it were in proper sequence it would be preceded by cap No. 1 and be followed by cap No. 3. The difference between cap No. 2 and cap No. 1 is 1 and similarly 1 for the difference between cap No. 3 and 2. Each succeeding circle is an increase in error score of 1. (Courtesy of Munsell Color Co., Inc., Baltimore.)*

Name..Age.............   ....Date............/ ...../

85	1	2	3	4	5	6	7	8	9	10	11	12	13	14	15	16	17	18	19	20	21
22	23	24	25	26	27	28	29	30	31	32	33	34	35	36	37	38	39	40	41	42	
43	44	45	46	47	48	49	50	51	52	53	54	55	56	57	58	59	60	61	62	63	
64	65	66	67	68	69	70	71	72	73	74	75	76	77	78	79	80	81	82	83	84	

Lab................ Exp...............

Test.......................

Review......................

Retest...................

FARNSWORTH-MUNSELL 100-HUE TEST
For Color Vision

MUNSELL COLOR COMPANY, INC.
2441 North Calvert Street
Baltimore, Maryland 21218

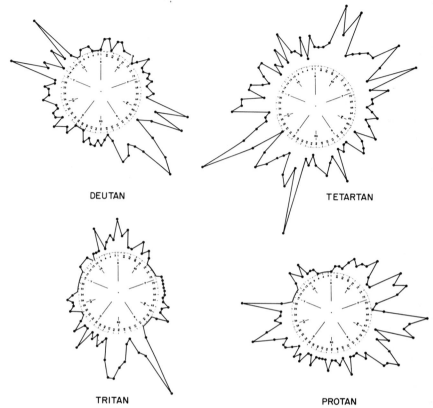

DEUTAN

TETARTAN

TRITAN

PROTAN

FIG. 7-8. *Characteristic distribution of errors on the F-M 100-hue test for deutan, tetartan, tritan, and protan individuals.*

formance in red, yellow, green, and blue areas. More control data are needed for this test.

SLOAN ACHROMATOPSIA TEST

This is a good screening test for total color blindness. This test uses six standard Munsell colors of high saturation covering the entire range of hues. Comparison of each color is made with a graduated series of 17 grays. Only the achromat makes a match with all or most of the six saturated Munsell colors shown. Data on matches from 19 patients with congenital total color blindness are used for comparison purposes.[38]

ILLUMINATION FOR TESTS

It should be emphasized that for all tests discussed so far, where pigments are used, the preferred illumination is that under which the test was standardized. In general, the light from a Macbeth easel lamp (Fig. 7-9), providing a white light of color temperature 6,740° Kelvin, is satisfactory. This light is equivalent to CIE (Commission Internationale de l'Eclairage) Illuminant C source, which is considered representative of average daylight.[6] It is our experience, and that of others,[18, 35] that results are most consistent when testing is done under

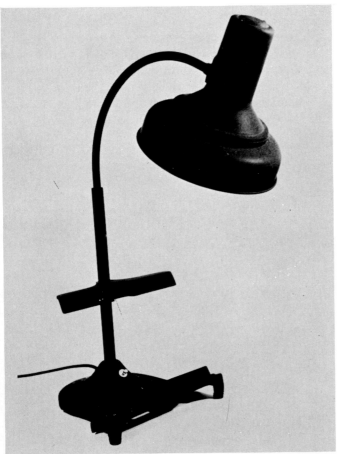

FIG. 7-9. *Macbeth easel lamp manufactured by Munsell Color Company in Baltimore.*

the Macbeth easel lamp. Results obtained in fluorescent or incandescent backgrounds are not considered reliable in our experience, although one worker [23] claims he gets consistent results on the Ishihara plates with a background of fluorescent lighting.

ANOMALOSCOPE

A normal subject can match yellow in both color and brightness with a proper mixture of red and green. This match is frequently called the Rayleigh equation after Lord Rayleigh,[34] who discovered its usefulness in differentiating red-green color-blind individuals from normals.

The anomaloscope is an instrument designed to measure the Rayleigh equation. It is the only instrument by which the exact diagnosis of red-green color vision defects can be made. Several anomaloscopes have been designed, but the Nagel anomaloscope (Fig. 7-10), named after the original designer, is most widely used. The instrument uses narrow-band spectral lights from a prism and is in essence a combination of a spectroscope and a comparison polarimeter. The subject

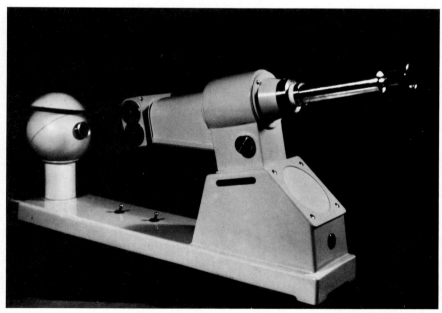

FIG. 7-10. *Nagel anomaloscope manufactured by Schmidt and Haensch Company in Berlin.*

views a bipartite circular field which is divided into a yellow half of variable luminance and a half with a variable red-green mixture of fixed luminance. Usually the examiner sets various red-green mixtures, and the subject attempts to make brightness and, when possible, color matches by varying the yellow half of the field (fixed matches). Initially the subject may be allowed to manipulate both halves of the circular field (free matches), but these are usually less accurate than fixed matches. The examiner selects red-green mixtures to determine the range of matches satisfying color and brightness equality (Rayleigh equation or Rayleigh match) and to obtain brightness values and color identification at points over the entire range of the instrument. Some of the problems encountered when testing with this instrument have been summarized.[36] The characteristic findings for the various color defects will be described in Vol. 2, Chapter 8.

LANTERN TESTS

These tests were designed primarily for occupations where the recognition of colored signals is the main or only discrimination involved. They are practical screening tests for these occupations but are useless for diagnosing type or degree of color defect. The examinee is required to name colored lights presented at different luminance levels and at different visual angles (simulating distance signal lights). The United States Air Force uses the Sloan color-threshold test,[37] and a popular lantern in the United States Navy is the Farnsworth New London Navy lantern.[6] The latter test presents paired, rather than single, colored signals. The brightness contrast between the paired test colors is chosen to eliminate cues from common brightness-hue relationships. Presumably, then, responses depend only on independent changes in brightness or hue and not on interrelationships between these two attributes.

SCREENING FOR VARIOUS OCCUPATIONS

Those interested in this area quickly learn that a color defect is not necessarily a contraindication to a job involving color judgments, as some color-defective individuals perform better than some normals. Therefore, a test that only distinguishes color-defectives from normals, such as the pseudoisochromatic plates, cannot be relied upon as a screening method for most occupations. This has been vividly demonstrated in a study comparing the colorimetric performance of 800 normals and 800 subjects classified as color-defectives by the Ishihara plates.[16] The performance of the color-blind group was close to normal, and most of the errors made were minor and described as "near-misses." However, it may be argued that screening with plates is adequate for certain individuals such as train drivers or aircraft pilots, where perfect color vision is essential. For example, a train driver passes a colored light only once, sees it for a relatively brief period, and if he has mistaken the color, there is no possibility of correcting his error. "Near-misses" cannot be accepted.

Screening color tests that simulate work conditions are useful, particularly when fairly close agreement between actual performance and test results has been demonstrated. Lantern tests are good for evaluating prospects for the transportation services or the armed forces. The Holmgren wool test may be good for fabric inspectors.

The Farnsworth D-15 test is of probable predictive value in many industries.[15, 29] In general, three out of eight color-defectives will pass the D-15 test. Therefore, some subjects failing the Farnsworth lantern test will pass even this test.[15] The number of errors made on the Farnsworth-Munsell 100-hue test is helpful in evaluating the performance of color-defectives. Those color-defectives with a precise narrow match on the Nagel anomaloscope, in our experience, make fewer errors on the Farnsworth-Munsell 100-hue test than those with wider equations. It was shown that the greater the number of errors congenital color-defectives make on a lantern test, the wider their equation on the Nagel anomaloscope.[3] Color-defectives classified as dichromatic or as having an extreme anomaly by the anomaloscope (see Vol. 2, Chapter 8) tend to perform poorly in most color vision tasks. However, protanomalous and deuteranomalous subjects have a great variation in performance, and therefore can be considered as possible candidates for several jobs involving color judgments.

In certain industries very critical color judgments are required (e.g., color coding in various electrical industries). Even some normal subjects may not have satisfactory color performance, and therefore screening with color aptitude tests may be helpful. The Farnsworth-Munsell 100-hue test is useful for dividing all subjects into three groups according to performance. An even more critical appraisal of color vision performance is given by the Inter-Society Council Color Aptitude test.

Color-defective individuals do just as well in traffic as normals.[47] In a study where the behavior of 169 color-defective drivers with normal vision and a control group were compared, no difference was found in accident and offense statistics.

ACQUIRED COLOR VISION DEFECTS

Acquired color vision defects are caused by diseases of the macula, optic nerve, or occipital cortex; or they may be due to cataracts. Certain findings aid in distinguishing acquired and congenital color vision defects (Table 7-5): (1) Congenital defects are likely to be bilateral and symmetrical. An acquired defect may be of greater degree in one eye than the other, may be unilateral, or may occasionally even be confined to various parts of the visual field of one eye. For example, a patient with a spotty macular lesion may give variable results on the anomaloscope by slight changes in direction of gaze. (2) Acquired defects frequently involve blue-yellow as well as red-green discrimination, whereas congenital defects usually involve only the latter. (3) Acquired color defects are usually associated with other evidence of abnormal retinal function (e.g., abnormal visual acuity, visual fields). Congenital color defects, except for total color blindness, are essentially associated with normal retinal function. (4) Congenital defects are less dependent on testing conditions. Size, brightness, and saturation of objects are more likely to affect color discrimination of an acquired defect. (5) A more rapid fatiguing develops for all colors on color vision testing with acquired color vision defects.[21] (6) Subjects with acquired defects name the color of objects as they see them, whereas patients with congenital defects or long-established acquired defects are markedly affected by psychological considerations as to what the color of an object should be.[22] Other differences have also been cited.[22, 44]

Kollner[24] originally proposed the often-quoted notion that retinal diseases are characterized by blue-yellow defects and optic nerve

TABLE 7-5
Differentiation of Acquired and Congenital Color Defects

Congenital	Acquired
1. Symmetrical	1. Asymmetrical
2. Usually R-G only	2. B-Y and R-G
3. Usually other visual functions normal	3. Other visual functions abnormal
4. More stable defect	4. More dependent on test conditions. Fatigues more rapidly
5. Names object color correctly	5. Names object color incorrectly

R-G = Red-Green
B-Y = Blue-Yellow

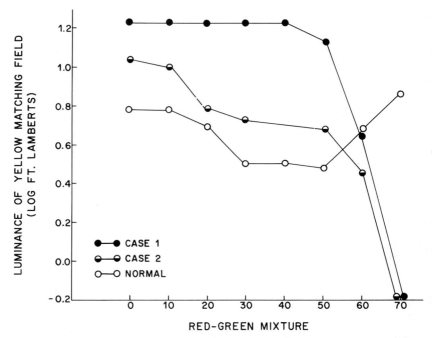

FIG. 7-11. *Yellow brightness values for various red-green mixtures over the range of the Nagel anomaloscope. On the X-axis pure red is No. 70 and pure green is 0. All possible red-green mixtures are represented by intervening numbers. Luminance of yellow light is indicated on Y-axis. Note that for the two patients with cone degenerations the yellow light is turned very bright at the green end of the instrument and very dim at the red end of the instrument.*

diseases by red-green defects. Several more recent studies,[20, 21, 30, 41, 42, 44] as well as our own data,[26] show notable exceptions to these classical notions. Two tests, the Nagel anomaloscope and the F-M 100-hue test, are particularly useful in characterizing acquired color vision defects.[26] These tests enable the division of acquired color vision defects into five distinct groups: *

1. Patients with cone degenerations often characterized initially by a deutan axis on the 100-hue test and a very wide Rayleigh equation on the anomaloscope.[26] Many of these patients find that pure green on the anomaloscope appears very bright and pure red very dim (Fig. 7-11). Their data may be similar to those of the patient with congenital total color blindness [26] (see Vol. 2, Chapter 8).

2. Patients with hereditary dominant optic atrophy initially charac-

* These distinctions tend to break down when vision is worse than 20/200.

terized by a tritan axis on the 100-hue test and usually a normal performance on the anomaloscope.

3. Patients with macular diseases, other than a cone degeneration, characterized usually by a wider than normal Rayleigh equation on the anomaloscope, requiring more red than normal in this equation, and having a tritan axis on the 100-hue test. The anomaloscope usually shows an abnormality before the 100-hue test.

4. Patients with optic nerve diseases, other than hereditary dominant optic atrophy and glaucoma, usually characterized initially by a deutan axis on the 100-hue test and a wider than normal Rayleigh equation on the anomaloscope. These patients also require more green than normal in their Rayleigh equation. Occasionally a patient in this category will show a tritan axis on the 100-hue test.

5. Patients with glaucoma, particularly with optic nerve damage, and those with cataracts may show findings similar to those with most macular diseases. However, an abnormality is seen with the 100-

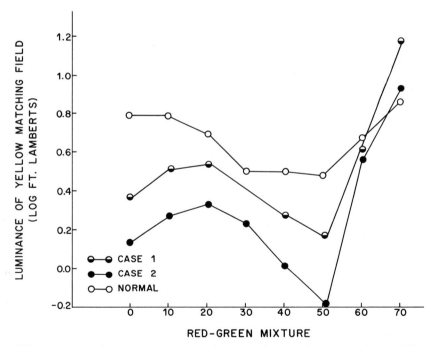

FIG. 7-12. A unique pattern seen on the anomaloscope in some patients with optic atrophy. The red-green mixtures, which are at the green end of the instrument (toward 0), appear dimmer than normal in relation to the red-green mixtures, which are at the red end of the instrument (toward 70).

March 1964

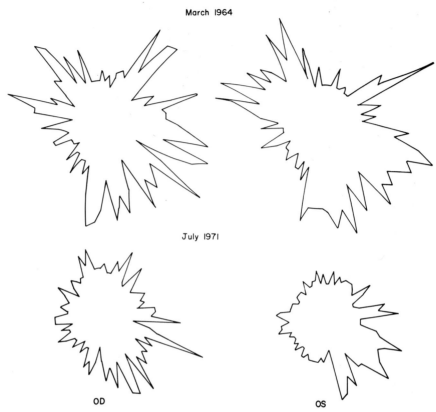

July 1971

OD   OS

FIG. 7-13.   *Patient initially seen in 1964 with history of alcoholism and diagnosis of nutritional amblyopia. Initial visions were 20/100. Initial scores on the F-M 100-hue test are shown in top half of photograph in which 652 errors were made with the right eye and 751 errors with the left eye. At that time, the patient was able to make a Rayleigh match over the entire anomaloscope. The patient stopped his drinking habit and started to eat normally. He was not seen until seven years later, at which time his vision had improved to 20/30 in the right eye and 20/20 in the left eye. Note the tremendous decrease in the number of errors made in both eyes (348 errors with the right and 276 with the left eye). Deutan axes with a slight tetartan component are evident on both occasions. At the last test time his Rayleigh matches on the anomaloscope were 7 with the right and 5 with the left eye and in a normal area.*

hue test before it is detected on the anomaloscope, in contrast to what is found in patients with macular disease.

In general, the brightness of pure red and green lights on the anomaloscope is normal in most patients with acquired retinal or optic nerve diseases. Notable exceptions are some patients with cone degeneration and a few with optic nerve disease who find predominately green lights to be brighter than normal and predominately red lights to be dimmer than normal (Fig. 7-11). A few patients with optic nerve disease find predominately red lights to be brighter than normal and predominately green lights to be dimmer than normal (Fig. 7-12).

As a rule, patients with amblyopia ex anopsia and congenital retinal abnormalities, such as albinism and congenital night blindness with abnormal vision, have only mild color vision abnormalities. On the other hand, patients with cone degenerations, chloroquine retinopathy, toxic amblyopia, and sometimes central serious choroidopathy are characterized by prominent color vision disturbances even with a minimal visual acuity abnormality.

Color vision testing may be another parameter to use in following patients with optic nerve and macular diseases (Fig. 7-13).

No specific color vision abnormalities characterize disease of the occipital cortex [27a] but not enough data are available.

REFERENCES

1. Babel, J. Diagnostic des dyschromatopsies congenitales et acquises. *Ophthalmologica 149*:277, 1965.
2. Bostrom, C. G., and Kugelberg, I. Official color sense control in Sweden. *Arch. Ophthal. 38*:378, 1947.
3. Cameron, G. R. Rational approach to color vision testing. *Aerospace Med. 38*:51, 1967.
4. Collins, M. *Color-Blindness*. New York, Harcourt, Brace & World, 1925.
5. Collins, W. E., Casola, A. S., and Zegers, R. T. The performance of color-blind subjects on the color aptitude test. *J. Gen. Psychol. 64*:245, 1961.
6. Committee on Colorimetry, Optical Society of America. *The Science of Color*. New York, Thomas Y. Crowell Co., 1953.
7. Cornsweet, T. N. *Visual Perception*. New York, Academic Press, 1970.
8. Crawford, A. The Dvorine pseudoisochromatic plates. *Brit. J. Psychol. 46*:139, 1955.
9. Crone, R. A. Quantitative diagnosis of defective color vision: a comparative evaluation of the Ishihara test, the Farnsworth dichotomous test, and the Hardy-Rand-Rittler polychromatic plates. *Amer. J. Ophthal. 51*:298, 1961.
10. DeValois, R. L., and Jacobs, G. H. Primate color vision. *Science 162*:533, 1968.
11. Dimmick, F. L. A color aptitude test, 1940 Experimental Edition. *J. Appl. Psychol. 30*:10, 1946.
12. Dreyer, V. Occupational possibilities of colour defectives. *Acta Ophthal. 4*:531, 1969.
13. Dvorine, I. Quantitative classification of the color blind. *J. Gen. Psychol. 68*:255, 1963.
14. Farnsworth, D. The Farnsworth-Munsell 100-hue and dichotomous tests for color vision. *J. Opt. Soc. Amer. 33*:568, 1943.

15. Farnsworth, D.   Testing for color deficiency in industry. *Arch. Indust. Health* 16:100, 1957.

16. Fetter, M. C.   Colorimetric tests read by color-blind people. *Amer. J. Med. Techn.* 29:349, 1963.

17. Frey, R. G.   Zur differentialdiagnore der angeborenen farbensinnstorungein mit pseudoisochromatischen Tafeln. *Ophthalmologica* 145:34, 1963.

18. Hardy, L. H.   Standard illuminants in relation to color testing procedures. *Arch. Ophthal.* 34:278, 1945.

19. Hardy, L. H., Rand, R., and Rittler, M. C.   Test for the detection and analysis of color blindness.   III. Rabkin test. *J. Opt. Soc. Amer.* 35:481, 1945.

20. Hong, S. M.   Types of acquired color-vision defects. *Arch. Ophthal.* 58:505, 1957.

21. Jaeger, W.   Defective colour vision caused by eye diseases. *Trans. Ophthal. Soc. U.K.* 76:477, 1956.

22. Jaeger, W., and Grutzner, P.   "Erworbene Farbensinnstorungen," in *Entwicklung und Fortschritt in der Augenheilkunde,* ed. by H. Sautter. Stuttgart, Enke, 1963, pp. 591–614.

23. Katavisto, M.   Pseudoisochromatic plates and artificial light. *Acta Ophthal.* 39:377, 1961.

24. Kollner, H.   *Die Storungen des Farbensinnes, ihre klinische Bedeutung und ihre Diagnose.* Berlin, Karger, 1912.

25. Krill, A. E., Bowman, J. E., and Schneiderman, A.   An investigation of so-called X-linked errors on the Ishihara plates. *Ann. Hum. Genet.* 29:253, 1966.

26. Krill, A. E., and Fishman, G. A.   Acquired color vision defects. *Trans. Amer. Acad. Ophthal. Otolaryng.* 75:1095, 1971.

27. Krill, A. E., and Schneiderman, A.   A hue discrimination defect in so-called normal carriers of color vision defects. *Invest. Ophthal.* 3:445, 1964.

27a. Lhermitte, F., Chain, F., Aron, D., Leblanc, M., and Souty, O.   Les troubles de la vision des couleurs dans les lesions posterieures du arveau. *Rev. Neurol. (Paris)* 121:5, 1969.

28. Linksz, A.   An Essay on Color Vision and Clinical Color-Vision Tests. New York and London, Grune & Stratton, 1964.

29. Linksz, A.   Farnsworth dichotomous test. *Amer. J. Ophthal.* 62:27, 1966.

30. Linksz, A.   Acquired color vision defects, in Strattsma, B. R., Hall, M. O., Allen, R. A., and Crescitelli, F. "The Retina: Morphology, Function, and Clinical Characteristics," *UCLA Forum Med. Sci.,* No. 8, Los Angeles, U. Calif. Press, 1969.

31. Marks, W. B., Dobelle, W. H., and MacNichol, E. F.   Visual pigments of single primate cones. *Science* 143:1181, 1964.

31a. Montessori, M.   *Dr. Montessori's Own Handbook.* Cambridge, Mass., Robert Bentley, Inc., 1964.

32. Perdriel, G.   Le test de Farnsworth 100-hue. *Ann. Oculist* 195:120, 1962.

33. Pickford, R. W.   The genetics of colour blindness. *Brit. J. Physiol. Opt.* 21:39, 1964.

34. Rayleigh, Lord.   Experiments on colour. *Nature* 25:64, 1881.

35. Schmidt, I.   Effect of illumination in testing color vision with pseudoisochromatic plates. *J. Opt. Soc. Amer.* 42:951, 1952.

36. Schmidt, I. Some problems related to testing color vision with the Nagel anomalo-scope. *J. Opt. Soc. Amer. 45*:514, 1955.

37. Sloan, L. L. A quantitative test for measuring degree of red-green color deficiency. *Amer. J. Ophthal. 27*:941, 1944.

38. Sloan, L. L. Congenital achromatopsia: a report of 19 cases. *J. Opt. Soc. Amer. 44*: 117, 1954.

39. Sloan, L. L. Evaluation of the Tokyo-Medical College color vision test. *Amer. J. Ophthal. 52*:650, 1961.

40. Sloan, L. L., and Habel, A. Tests for color deficiency based on the pseudoisochro-matic principle. A comparative study of several new tests. *Arch. Ophthal. 55*:229, 1956.

41. Verriest, G. Further studies on acquired deficiency of color discrimination. *J. Opt. Soc. Amer. 53*:185, 1963.

42. Verriest, G. Les deficiences acquises de la discrimination chromatique. *Bull. Mem. Acad. Roy. Med. Belg. 4*:37, 1964.

43. Verriest, G., Buyssens, A., and Vanderdonck, R. Etude quantitative de l'effet qu'exerce sur les resultats de quelques tests de la discrimination chromatique une diminution non selective du niveau d'un eclairage. *Rev. d'Opt. 42*:105, 1963.

44. Waardenburg, P. J., Franceschetti, A., and Klein, D. *Genetics in Ophthalmology.* Springfield, Ill., Charles C Thomas, 1963, Vol. 2.

45. Walls, G. How good is the H-R-R test for color blindness? *Amer. J. Optom. 36*:169, 1959.

46. Wald, G. The receptors of human color vision. *Science 145*:1007, 1964.

47. Zehnder, E. Die Bewahrung farbensinngestorter Motorfahrzeuglenker im Verkehr. *Schweiz. Med. Wschr. 101*:530, 1971.

Index

80–81—10–9–8–7–6–5–4